Current Clinical Strategies

---

Practice Parameters in Medicine, Primary Care, and Family Practice

1996 Edition

Paul D. Chan, M.D.

University of California, Irvine
College of Medicine
Clinical Practice Group

## Dedication

This book is dedicated to Camille, for her love, encouragement, and support.

Notice: The reader is advised to consult subspecialists, the drug package insert, and other references before treating any medical problem, and before using any therapeutic agent. Under no circumstances will this text supervene the experienced clinical judgement of the treating physician. No warranty exists, expressed or implied, for errors and omissions in this text.

Current Clinical Strategies Publishing
27071 Cabot Road, Suite 126
Laguna Hills, California 92653
Phone: 800-331-8227
Fax: 800-965-9420

Printed in USA                                                    ISBN 1-881528-33-2

# Contents

# *Cardiology*

---

## Myocardial Infarction

I. **Diagnosis of Acute Myocardial Infarction**
   A. MI can cause a constricting or squeezing sensation in the chest rather than pain per se; pain can radiate to the upper abdomen, back, either arm, either shoulder, neck, or jaw. Pain is of greater severity or longer duration (usually at least 30 minutes) than that seen with unstable angina.
   B. Assess cardiac risk factors and personal or family history of myocardial infarction.
   C. Diabetic patients may report unusual symptoms, such as a fluttering sensation, nausea, dyspnea, severe fatigue, or generalized malaise. Silent MI is more common among diabetics.
   D. Women tend to have more GI symptoms during acute MI than men.
   E. In younger patients without risk factors, cocaine-induced MI should be considered. Cocaine overdose is associated with pronounced anxiety, tachycardia, hyperpyrexia; consider a toxicology screen.
   F. Nicotine transdermal systems increase the risk of MI if the patient smokes while wearing a patch.
   G. Evaluate patient rapidly with history, physical exam, and electrocardiogram. Cardiac exam may reveal S3 or S4; an S4 may be more audible with the patient in a left lateral position

II. **Differential Diagnosis of Chest Pain**
   A. **Acute Pericarditis:** Pleuritic-type chest pain and diffuse ST segment elevation.
   B. **Aortic Dissection:** "Tearing" chest pain with uncontrolled hypertension and widened mediastinum on chest x-ray.
   C. **Esophageal Rupture:** Usually occurs after vomiting; x-ray may reveal air in mediastinum or a left side hydrothorax.
   D. **Acute Cholecystitis:** Characterized by right subcostal abdominal pain with anorexia, nausea, vomiting, and fever.
   E. **Acute Peptic Ulcer Disease:** Epigastric pain with melena or hematemesis and anemia.

III. **Electrocardiographic Findings in Acute Myocardial Infarction**
   A. ST elevations in two contiguous leads with ST depressions in reciprocal leads are strong predictors of MI and the need for thrombolysis. The earliest signs of transmural injury are hyperacute T waves. Q waves occur later.
   B. If the ECG is uninterpretable (left bundle-branch block), and the clinical signs strongly indicate an evolving infarct, reperfusion with thrombolytics or angioplasty should still be considered.
   C. When the 12-lead ECG suggests an inferior MI, consider obtaining ECG data from the right precordial leads. ST elevation in leads $V_{3R}$-$V_{5R}$ (especially $V_{4R}$) points to right ventricular involvement.
   D. About 2% of MI's occur without any ECG abnormalities. A negative result on the ECG does not completely exclude MI.

IV. **Diagnostic Testing**
   A. Blood for cardiac enzyme studies should be drawn after the ECG, and again every 6-12 hours; obtaining three samples is usually sufficient. CPK with isoenzymes and LDH should be measured. CPK levels may be normal early after acute myocardial infarction.
   B. **Creatine Kinase-MB Level** starts to rise within a few hours of infarction and peaks at 24 hours.
   C. **Echocardiography:**
      1. Useful when ECG is indeterminate in patients with chest pain. Normal left ventricular

wall motion confirms the absence of significant transmural ischemia.
2. A localized area of hypokinesia indicates possible coronary thrombosis. Echocardiogram may also reveal aortic dissection, mitral valve prolapse, or pericardial fluid.

## V. Emergent Therapy of Myocardial Infarction

A. **Initiation of Thrombolytic Therapy:** Time is a critical variable in MI management; therefore, it is often better to initiate treatment than to administer tests in the hope of achieving diagnostic certainty.

B. Thrombolytics are underutilized, and are the most efficient way to conserve heart muscle in MI, and are the most important element of acute-phase treatment.

C. Thrombolytics are no longer contraindicated by age older than 75 or by late initiation of treatment. They may be used up to 24 hours after MI.

D. **Indications for Thrombolytic Therapy in Myocardial Infarction:**
**Inclusion Criteria:**
1. Chest pain typical of acute myocardial infarction for longer than 30 min.
2. **Electrocardiography:** Changes consistent with acute myocardial infarction (ST-segment elevation $>1$ mV in two contiguous leads) or presence of left bundle-branch block pattern.
3. Presence of inferior infarction.
4. Age may exceed 75 years.
5. Initiation of treatment up to 24 hours after MI.

E. **Relative Contraindications:** Absence of ST-segment elevation, severe hypertension, cerebrovascular disease, relatively recent surgery ($>2$ wk), cardiopulmonary resuscitation.

F. **Absolute Contraindications:** Active internal bleeding, history of hemorrhagic stroke, head trauma, pregnancy, surgery within 2 weeks, recent non-compressible vascular puncture.

G. **Streptokinase (Streptase):**
1. Most commonly used and least expensive thrombolytic; offers about the same benefit as tPA for patients older than 75 and for those with small inferior infarctions; streptokinase confers greater benefit for patients presenting 6 hours or longer after pain onset. Can cause hypotension.
2. IV infusion of 1.5 million IU in 100 mL NS IV over 60 min. Diphenhydramine and steroids are often used to prevent allergic reactions.
3. The value of initiating IV heparin with streptokinase is controversial. Addition of intravenous heparin does not further reduce mortality when streptokinase is administered.

H. **Alteplase (tissue plasminogen activator, tPA, Activase):**
1. tPA is the quickest-acting of the available lytics; artery opening occurs 60 minutes faster than with other agents.
2. tPA should be used for patients who present early (within 4 hours) or who have an anterior MI (those in whom the best advantage for tPA has been demonstrated). Patients who present later, who have a relatively small predicted infarct size, or who are elderly ($>75$ yrs) and at increased risk for stroke should be given streptokinase. tPA should be use for patients at risk for allergy to streptokinase.
3. **Front-loaded Regimen:** IV bolus of 15 mg, then 0.75 mg/kg (up to 50 mg) over 30 min, followed by 0.5 mg/kg (up to 35 mg) infused over next 60 min, with total dose delivered over 1 ½ hours. Initiate IV heparin concurrently.
4. Intravenous heparin is strongly recommended to prevent infarct artery reocclusion with rTPA (because of the short half-life).

I. **Anistreplase (Anisoylated Plasminogen Streptokinase Activator Complex, APSAC, Eminase):**
1. Anistreplase is the agent of choice when ease of administration is important, as in prehospital therapy, because it is given as a single IV injection rather than a slow IV drip.
2. One IV bolus of 30 U, given over 2-5 min.

## VI. Percutaneous Transluminal Angioplasty

A. Direct PTCA offers advantages over thrombolytic therapy in patients with acute myocardial infarction.

B. **Indications for Immediate PTCA:**

1. Patients with a contraindication to thrombolytic therapy.
2. Sustained hypotension, severe pulmonary edema or cardiogenic shock related to a large acute MI. If delay is anticipated, lytic therapy with t-PA should be started in the interim.

C. If symptoms and ST-segment elevation do not resolve by the end of the thrombolytic infusion, consider referral of patients with anterior MI for emergency PTCA.

## VII. Drug Therapy for Acute Myocardial Infarction

A. **Aspirin:**

1. Patients with any sign of an acute coronary syndrome should immediately chew and swallow 160-325 mg of soluble aspirin. Follow with 80-325 mg enteric coated aspirin PO daily.
2. Aspirin is appropriate for either MI or unstable angina. In MI this drug can be lifesaving.
3. Contraindications to aspirin treatment under other circumstances do not outweigh the benefits of aspirin in an evolving MI.

B. **Beta Blockers:**

1. Patients with reflex tachycardia, systolic hypertension, continuing ischemic pain, or atrial fibrillation with fast ventricular response are excellent candidates for beta-blocker therapy.
2. **Contraindications to beta blockers:** Systolic pressure <100 mm Hg, pulse rate <50 beats per minute, second- or third-degree heart block, severe heart failure, bronchospastic lung disease.
3. **Atenolol (Tenormin),** 5 mg IV given over 5 minutes and repeated in 10 minutes if the pulse rate is more than 60 beats per minute.
4. **Metoprolol (Lopressor),** 5 mg every 5 minutes for three doses if tolerated; followed by oral maintenance therapy, 50-100 mg per day.
5. **Carvedilol (Coreg),** initiate at low dosage and increase dose slowly; 6.25-50 mg bid.

C. **Nitroglycerin:**

1. Intravenous nitroglycerin should be given to all patients with suspected MI as early as possible, unless hypotension is present.
2. Start infusion at a rate of 5 mcg/min and increase rate until the mean arterial blood pressure is reduced by 10%, but is not lower than 80 mm Hg. Continue for 48 hours; then, if free of chest pain for 24 hours, wean by gradually decreasing the rate of infusion. Oral nitrates may be substituted.

D. **Heparin:**

1. Initial 5000 units (100 U/kg) bolus, and an infusion of 1000 U/hr (15 U/kg).
2. Adjust heparin to prolong the activated partial thromboplastin time (PTT) to 2-2.5 times control. Continue heparin for 48-72 hours.
3. In patients not receiving intravenous heparin, prophylactic heparin is recommended (5,000 U SQ bid) to prevent venous thrombosis (or 12,500 U SQ bid in patients with anterior MI who are at risk for mural thrombus formation).
4. Warfarin following MI has a very high complication rate.

E. **Angiotensin Converting Inhibitors:**

1. ACE-inhibitors improve survival and decrease morbidity in patients with asymptomatic left ventricular dysfunction after myocardial infarction. ACE-inhibitor use for myocardial infarction patients is highly recommended for all patients.
2. An ACE-inhibitor should be started 3-16 days post-infarct.
3. Captopril, initial dose 6.25-12.5 mg PO, titrate to a target dose of 25 mg po tid; maximum of 50 mg PO tid as tolerated.

F. **Lidocaine:**

1. Lidocaine should not be routinely administered to patients with myocardial infarction.

2. Lidocaine should be administered only to patients who have more than six ventricular premature beats (VPBs) per minute, closely coupled VPBs (the R-on-T phenomenon), multiform VPBs, non-sustained, or sustained ventricular tachycardia or fibrillation.

G. **Calcium Channel Blockers** are useful for hypertension and stable angina pectoris, but they are not recommended for patients with MI.

H. **Magnesium** has not been shown to produce a significant benefit, and magnesium infusions should not be used routinely for MI.

## VIII. Myocardial Infarction Management After Thrombolytics

A. Monitor for a decrease in ST segment elevation either on 12 lead ECG (or monitor lead that shows the maximum ST elevation before treatment), every 5-10 minutes until evidence of reperfusion occurs.

B. If there are no signs of reperfusion (no significant relief of symptoms or no greater than 50% reduction in maximum ST elevation) within one hour of onset of therapy, consider urgent PTCA.

C. **Indications for Urgent PTCA:**
   1. Shock develops (before or after thrombolytic therapy).
   2. The patient develops signs and symptoms of reocclusion and recurrent ischemia after thrombolytics. In most patients with threatened reocclusion, another dose of thrombolytic therapy may abort reocclusion and buy time to perform angiography and angioplasty.

D. **Management after Thrombolytic Induced Reperfusion:**
   1. Continue patient on heparin plus aspirin until further decisions are made (usually heparin for 48-72 hrs and aspirin and beta-blockers, and nitroglycerine indefinitely).
   2. If patient remains clinically stable, then further management can proceed in one of the following routines: 1) stress testing around day 7-10 and if positive for ischemia, consider coronary angiography. 2) coronary angiography may be performed routinely around day 3-5 to decide need for angioplasty or surgery, or medical treatment only.

# Unstable Angina

## I. Initial Evaluation

A. The diagnosis of unstable angina depends on clinical history, physical examination, and 12-lead ECG.

B. Unstable angina typically presents with a prolonged episode of substernal chest pain, or as stable angina that has been increasing in frequency, severity, or duration.

C. Compared with patients with stable angina, those with unstable angina are more likely to have multivessel disease and progression of known atherosclerosis.

D. Pain may be accompanied by reversible, horizontal or down-sloping ST-segment depression or deep symmetric T-wave inversion.

E. **Factors that may Precipitate Unstable Angina:**
1. Lung disease (chronic obstructive pulmonary disease)
2. Anemia (occult gastrointestinal bleeding)
3. Fever or hyperthyroidism
4. Uncontrolled hypertension or arrhythmias

## II. Initial Medical Treatment of Unstable Angina

A. Begin individualized treatment in the emergency department. Institute antiischemic therapy as soon as the working diagnosis of unstable angina is made.

B. **Supplemental Oxygen:** Give oxygen at 2-4 L/min by nasal canula to patients with cyanosis, respiratory distress, or high-risk features.

C. Obtain a brief history, physical examination and, ECG (repeated every morning thereafter and whenever chest pain occurs).

D. **Initial Laboratory:** CBC count, random cholesterol and blood glucose levels; creatine kinase isoenzymes q8h over the next 24 hours; chest x-ray.

E. **Thrombolytic Therapy** is not indicated if there is no evidence of acute ST-segment elevation or left bundle branch block on 12-lead ECG. Thrombolytic agents do not have a beneficial effect in unstable angina.

F. **Invasive Therapy:** Angioplasty and coronary artery bypass surgery should not be considered as initial therapeutic approaches to unstable angina.

G. **Nitrates:**
1. Nitrates are indicated for ongoing anginal pain or ischemia.
2. Nitrates decrease oxygen demand by reducing preload, and they dilate coronary arteries. Reflex tachycardia increases oxygen demand; therefore, heart rate must be controlled.
3. **Contraindication:** Hypotension
4. Nitroglycerine 15 mcg IV bolus, then 5-10 mcg/min infusion (50 mg in 250-500 mL D5W, 100-200 mcg/mL). Titrate every 3-5 minutes to control symptoms in 5-10 mcg/min steps, up to 200-300 mcg/min. Avoid tachycardia and hypotension.
5. Nitroglycerine Sublingual, 1-3 tabs SL prn chest pain may also be used.

H. **Antiplatelet Agents:**
1. Aspirin should be given upon presentation, 160 mg chewed and swallowed immediately, then take 325 mg daily (range 160-325 mg daily).
2. **Contraindications:** Hypersensitivity, active bleeding. Peptic ulcer disease is not a contraindication in the setting of unstable angina.
3. **Ticlopidine (Ticlid)** has proved to be effective in unstable angina because it blocks fibrinogen binding to platelets. 250 mg bid is an alternative if aspirin is contraindicated or ineffective; may cause neutropenia, skin rash, diarrhea.

I. **Beta-Blockers:**
1. Beta-blockers reduce myocardial oxygen consumption and heart rate contractility. Monitor heart rate and blood pressure (target heart rate for beta-blockade is 50-60 beats per minute). Monitor for congestive heart failure and bronchospasm.
2. **Contraindications:** PR segment > 0.24 sec; 2 or 3 AV block; heart rate <60; systolic BP <90 mm Hg; CHF, severe reactive airway disease.
3. **Metoprolol (Lopressor)**, cardioselective beta1-blocker; 1-5 mg doses by slow IV

infusion over 1-2 min. q5min to 15 mg total; 100 mg PO bid; reduces the risk of recurrent ischemia or myocardial infarction within 48 hours.

4. **Atenolol (Tenormin)**, cardioselective beta1-blocker; 5 mg IV q5min to 10 mg total; 50-100 mg PO qd; water-soluble agent with less CNS side effects.

5. **Esmolol (Brevibloc):**
   a. Cardioselective beta1-blocker; has the advantage of a short half-life of 9.5 minutes; reduces the incidence of myocardial infarction.
   b. 2 mg/min IV infusion, increase up to 24 mg/min. The dose is increased at 5-minute intervals to achieve a 25% reduction in the heart rate-blood pressure product. May be immediate withdrawn if bradycardia, heart block, hypotension, bronchospasm, or heart failure.

J. **Heparin:**
1. Heparin in unstable angina reduces the risk of MI and recurrent unstable angina in high-risk patients if begun early. Patients with unstable angina and hypotension, pulmonary edema, significant prolonged rest pain, or other high-risk features, without contraindications, should receive aspirin and heparin, while those with lower-risk unstable angina would receive aspirin alone.
2. **Contraindications:** Active bleeding, severe bleeding risk, recent stroke.
3. 80 U/kg IV bolus, then IV infusion at 18 U/kg/h titrated to a activated partial thromboplastin time (aPTT) 1.5-2.5 times control.
4. Check the aPTT q6h until a therapeutic level has been achieved on two consecutive aPTT's. Obtain an aPPT every 24 hours thereafter.
5. Obtain hemoglobin/hematocrit and platelets daily for the first 3 days of heparin, or if bleeding, recurrent ischemia, or hypotension. Monitor for heparin-induced thrombocytopenia.

K. **Calcium Antagonists:**
1. Most trials with nifedipine have shown an increase in mortality, myocardial infarction rate, or myocardial ischemia; however, adding nifedipine to the regimen of patients with unstable angina who are already receiving beta blockers may be effective.

III. **Management of Stabilized Patients**

A. **Discontinuation of Intravenous Therapy:**
1. **Heparin:** Discontinue heparin after 2-5 days if used initially. Discontinue earlier in patients found to have a secondary cause for ischemia such as anemia.
2. **Aspirin:** Continue at 160-325 mg per day.
3. **Convert to oral beta blockers** after the initial intravenous beta blocker:
   -Metoprolol (Lopressor) 100 mg PO bid **OR**
   -Propranolol (Inderal) 20-40 mg PO q6-8h (160-240 mg/d) or Inderal-LA, 80-120 mg PO qd [60, 80, 120, 160 mg]
   **OR**
   -Atenolol (Tenormin) 50-100 mg PO qd.
4. Change to oral nitrate therapy when the patient has been pain-free for 24 hours. Tolerance to nitrates becomes significant after only 24 hours of continuous therapy.
   -Isosorbide dinitrate (Isordil Titradose) 10-40 mg PO bid-tid, with last dose no later than 7 pm [5,10,20, 30,40 mg].
   -Isosorbide Sustained Release (Isordil Tembids) 80-120 mg qd, or 40-80 mg bid, at 8 am and 2 pm.
   -Isosorbide Mononitrate (ISMO) 10-20 mg bid, with doses 7 hours apart **OR** Isosorbide Mononitrate Sustained Release (Imdur) 60-120 mg qd.
   -Nitroglycerine Sublingual, 1-3 tabs SL prn chest pain may also be used.

IV. **Indications for Cardiac Catheterization in Stabilized Patients**

A. **Early Conservative Strategy:** Unless contraindicated, cardiac catheterization is done if one or more of the following high-risk indicators are present: Prior revascularization; congestive heart failure or depressed left ventricular function (ejection fraction < 0.50); ventricular arrhythmia; persistent or recurrent pain/ischemia; functional study indicating high risk.

B. Patients with one or more recurrent, severe, prolonged (>20 minutes) ischemic episodes, should be considered for early cardiac catheterization.

## V. Progression to Nonintensive Medical Therapy

A. Most patients with unstable angina stabilize and become pain-free with appropriate intensive medical management.

B. **Requirements for Transfer from Intensive to Nonintensive Medical Management:**
1. Hemodynamically stable (no uncompensated heart failure) for 24 hours or longer.
2. Ischemia has been suppressed for 24 hours or longer.

C. Continue serial creatinine kinase and CK-MB q6-8 hours for the first 24 hours after admission. Lactate dehydrogenase levels may be useful in detecting myocardial damage in patients presenting 24-72 hours after symptom onset.

D. **12-lead ECG:** Repeat 24 hours after admission or whenever the patient has recurrent symptoms or a change in clinical status.

E. **Radionuclide Ventriculogram or a Two-Dimensional Echocardiogram:** Measure resting left ventricular function in patients who do not have early cardiac catheterization.

F. Encourage patient to gradually increase level of activity under supervision. Advise the patient regarding modification of cardiac risk factors.

G. Recurrent ischemic episodes should prompt an assessment and emergent ECG. Patients who have pain or ECG evidence of ischemia lasting 20 minutes or longer that is unresponsive to sublingual nitroglycerin, should be transferred back to the intensive medical management.

## VI. Noninvasive Testing

A. Noninvasive testing is used in recently stabilized patients to estimate prognosis, especially for the next 3-6 months, and to make adjustments in therapy.

B. Noninvasive testing may be considered within 72 hours of presentation in low-risk patients who are to be managed as outpatients. Noninvasive testing should be delayed until after the patient has stabilized, and has been free of angina and congestive heart failure for a minimum of 48 hours.

C. **Choice of Noninvasive Test**
1. Selection of stress testing method is based on an evaluation of the patient's resting ECG, ability to perform exercise, and the local technologies available.
2. **Exercise Treadmill Test:** Standard method of stress testing in male patients with a normal ECG who are not taking digoxin. In women, the stress echocardiogram is superior to exercise ECG for initial diagnostic testing for suspected coronary artery disease. Exclusions from exercise treadmill testing include S3 gallop, rales, hypertension, chest pain, unstable ECG.
3. **Imaging Modality Test:** Should be used for patients with an abnormal ECG, including widespread resting ST-segment depression, ST-segment changes secondary to digoxin, left ventricular hypertrophy, left bundle branch block or significant intraventricular conduction deficit. Imaging tests include technetium-99m sestamibi (Cardiolite) scan and stress echocardiogram.
4. **Pharmacologic Stress Testing with an Imaging Modality** are used if physical limitations prevent exercise. Pharmacologic studies include dipyridamole, adenosine, and dobutamine.
5. Ambulatory ECG can be used for testing if exercise treadmill testing and imaging are contraindicated.

# Congestive Heart Failure

## I. Clinical Evaluation of Heart Failure

A. All patients who complain of paroxysmal nocturnal dyspnea, orthopnea, or new-onset dyspnea on exertion should undergo evaluation for heart failure unless history and physical examination clearly indicate a noncardiac cause (such as pulmonary disease).

B. Chest pain may indicate that ischemia is the cause of heart failure; however, ischemia can also occur without chest pain, and can still cause depression of ventricular function.

C. Ascertain any history of edema, heart murmur, prior viral illness, hypertension, myocardial infarction, alcohol or drug use, thyroid disease, anemia, lung disease. Determine the degree of impairment.

## II. Physical Exam Findings

A. Elevated jugular venous pressure and a third heart sound are the most specific findings, and they are virtually diagnostic in patients with compatible symptoms.

B. Pulmonary rales or peripheral edema are relatively nonspecific findings.

C. Patients with symptoms highly suggestive of heart failure should undergo echocardiography or radionuclide ventriculography to measure left ventricular ejection fraction.

D. Abdominal jugular reflex is a better clinical indicator of heart failure than pulmonary rales. Have the patient breath normally, then press on the abdomen and observe jugular veins for distension.

## III. Conditions That Mimic or Provoke Heart Failure

Coronary artery disease and myocardial infarction

Hypertension

Aortic or mitral valve disease

Cardiomyopathies: Hypertrophic, idiopathic dilated, postpartum, genetic,

Pulmonary disease

Congenital abnormalities

High output states: Anemia, hyperthyroidism,

toxic, nutritional, metabolic

Myocarditis: Infectious, toxic, immune

Pericardial constriction

Tachyarrhythmias or bradyarrhythmias

Pulmonary embolism

A-V fistulas, Paget's disease, fibrous dysplasia, multiple myeloma

Renal failure, nephrotic syndrome

## IV. Laboratory Evaluation of Heart Failure

A. Echocardiogram, CXR, EKG

B. Electrolytes, BUN, creatinine, albumin, liver function tests

C. CBC, urinalysis

D. Thyroxine and thyroid stimulating hormone (if atrial fibrillation, evidence of thyroid disease, or age >65 yrs)

## V. Clinical Evaluation of Laboratory Studies

| Test | Finding | Possible Diagnosis |
|------|---------|--------------------|
| Electrocardiogram | Acute ST-T wave changes | Myocardial ischemia |
| | Atrial fibrillation, other tachyarrhythmia | Thyroid disease or heart failure due to rapid ventricular rate |
| | Bradyarrhythmias | Heart failure due to low heart rate |
| | Previous myocardial infarction (Q waves) | Heart failure due to reduced left ventricular performance. |
| | Low voltage | Pericardial effusion |
| | Left ventricular hypertrophy | Diastolic dysfunction |
| Complete blood count | Anemia | Heart failure due decreased oxygen carrying capacity |
| Urinalysis | Proteinuria | Nephrotic syndrome |
| Serum creatinine | Elevated | Volume overload due to renal failure |

| | | |
|---|---|---|
| Serum albumin | Decreased | Increased extravascular volume due to hypoalbuminemia |
| Free T4, thyroid-stimulating hormone | Abnormal | Heart failure due to hypothyroidism or hyperthyroidism |

A. **Common Laboratory Findings in Heart Failure:** Dilutional hyponatremia, hypo- or hyperkalemia, liver function abnormalities, hypoalbuminemia, hepatic hypoglycemia, elevated prothrombin time are common in heart failure.

B. **Chest Roentgenogram:** Cardiomegaly, pleural effusions, pulmonary vascular redistribution, Kerley's lines, perivascular cuffing, alveolar edema, and/or infiltrate may be seen.

C. **Electrocardiogram:** Often evidence of old myocardial infarction, hypertrophy, and/or conduction system delays.

D. **Echocardiography or Radiographic Ventriculography:**
   1. Left ventricular function should evaluated by measurement of left ventricular performance is a critical step in the evaluation and management of patients with suspected or apparent heart failure.
   2. Echocardiography or radiography ventriculography should be used to differentiate between dilated cardiomyopathy, left ventricular diastolic dysfunction, valvular heart disease, or a noncardiac etiology.
   3. **Left Ventricular Ejection Fraction:** Most patients with heart failure are found to have ejection fractions of less than 40%.

## VI. Management of Congestive Heart Failure

A. **Indications for Hospitalization:**
   1. Clinical or electrocardiographic evidence of acute myocardial ischemia
   2. Pulmonary edema or severe respiratory distress
   3. Oxygen saturation below 90 percent
   4. Severe complicating medical illness
   5. Anasarca
   6. Symptomatic hypotension or syncope
   7. Heart failure refractory to outpatient therapy

B. **Angiotensin Converting Enzyme Inhibitors:**
   1. ACE inhibitors should be prescribed for all patients with left ventricular systolic dysfunction unless contraindicated (serum potassium level greater than 5.5 mMol/L, or symptomatic hypotension).
   2. ACE inhibitors may be considered as sole therapy in patients with fatigue or mild dyspnea on exertion and no signs or symptoms of volume overload. Diuretics should be added if symptoms persist despite treatment with ACE inhibitors.
   3. ACE-inhibitors have an enhanced first-dose response that may occur in patients with hyponatremia or dehydration; very low initial doses should be prescribed. To avoid orthostasis, the dose of diuretic can be reduced or briefly discontinued as the dose of ACE inhibitor is increased.

C. **Diuretics:**
   1. Diuretics are extremely useful for reducing symptoms of volume overload, including orthopnea and paroxysmal nocturnal dyspnea. Diuretics should be started immediately when patients present with symptoms or signs of volume overload.
   2. Diuretics reduce intravascular volume and reduce preload, but have no beneficial effect on afterload.
   3. Adequate diuretic dosage is indicated by neck veins that are flat and by the absence of perforated edema. Physicians frequently prescribe inadequate doses of diuretics.
   4. Loop diuretics (furosemide [Lasix], bumetanide [Bumex]) are diuretics of first choice. Severe congestive symptoms require a twice daily regimen because of fluid accumulation during the day. The second daily dose should be given by mid-afternoon to avoid nocturnal diuresis.
   5. **Adverse Effects:** May cause orthostatic hypotension or abnormalities of fluid and electrolyte balance (hypokalemia, hypomagnesemia), which predispose to

arrhythmias. Elevated glucose and lipid levels, sexual dysfunction, fatigue, and muscle cramps can occur.

6. Serum magnesium and potassium levels should be monitored and supplemented when necessary.

D. **Digoxin:**

1. Digoxin increases the force of ventricular contraction in patients with left ventricular systolic dysfunction. Physical functioning and symptoms improved with digoxin.

2. Digoxin should be initiated along with ACE inhibitors and diuretics in patients with severe heart failure.

3. Patients with mild to moderate heart failure will often become asymptomatic with optimal doses of ACE inhibitors and diuretics, and these patients do not require digoxin. Digoxin should be added to the regimen if symptoms persist despite optimal doses of ACE inhibitors and diuretics.

4. For many patients the dose of digoxin is often too low, leading to sub-therapeutic levels. Digoxin level should be kept between 1.0 and 2.0 ng.

5. Digoxin is ineffective and contraindicated in patients without cardiomegaly who have preserved systolic function, reduced ventricular compliance, and diastolic disfunction.

| Drug | Initial Dose | Target Dose | Max Dose | Adverse Reactions |
|---|---|---|---|---|
| **Loop Diuretics** | | | | |
| Furosemide | 10 - 40 mg qd | As needed | 240 mg bid | Postural hypotension, hypokalemia, hyperglycemia, hyperuricemia, rash; rare severe reaction includes pancreatitis, bone marrow suppression and anaphylaxis. |
| **ACE Inhibitors** | | | | |
| Lisinopril (Prinivil, Zestril) | 5 mg qd | 20 mg qd | 40 mg qd | Same as enalapril |
| Quinapril (Accupril) | 5 mg bid | 20 mg bid | 20 mg bid | Same as enalapril |
| Enalapril (Vasotec) | 2.5 mg bid | 10 mg bid | 20 mg bid | Hypotension, hyperkalemia, renal insufficiency, cough, skin rash, angioedema, neutropenia |
| Captopril (Capoten) | 6.25 - 12.5 mg tid | 50 mg tid | 100 mg tid | Same as above |
| **Digoxin** | 0.125 mg qd | As needed | As needed | Cardiotoxicity, confusion, nausea, dizziness, tachycardia, lupus-like syndrome |

E. **Anticoagulation:** Routine anticoagulation for heart failure is not recommended. Patients with a history of systemic or pulmonary embolism or recent atrial fibrillation should receive warfarin to an International Normalization Ratio of 2.0-3.0.

**VII. Revascularization**

A. Coronary artery disease is the most common cause of heart failure, and some patients may benefit from revascularization. In particular, patients with viable myocardium, subserved by substantially stenotic vessels, may obtain benefits if stenosis is relieved.

B. In patients without a history of myocardial infarction or significant angina, physiologic tests for ischemia or coronary angiography should be completed. Patients should undergo scintigraphy (thallium scanning) with post-stress, redistribution and rest reinjection imaging.

C. Patients with heart failure who have exercise-limiting angina, angina at rest, or recurrent acute pulmonary edema should undergo coronary artery angiography.

VIII. **Management of Refractory Heart Failure**
   A. **Reasons for Resistance of Heart Failure to Therapy:**
   1. Inadequate diuretic dosage. Neck veins should be flat without any peripheral edema.
   2. Inadequate digoxin level; should be kept between 1.0 and 2.0 ng.
   3. Nonsteroidal anti-inflammatory drugs can cause Na retention in CHF or renal failure.
   4. Uncontrolled heart rate in atrial fibrillation can exacerbate or cause heart failure, heart rate should be aggressively controlled.
   5. Hypertension should be controlled with an ACE-inhibitor in maximum dosage if necessary.
   6. Dietary noncompliance, thyroid disease, or anemia.
   B. Patients with persistent dyspnea after optimal doses of diuretics, ACE inhibitors, and digoxin should be given a trial of hydralazine and/or nitrates.
   C. **Methods for Overcoming Diuretic Resistance:**
   1. Constant infusion of diuretic, 4-30 mg/hour furosemide
   2. Add distal convoluted tubule diuretic:
      Metolazone 2.5 to 10 mg/day
      HCTZ 25 to 100 mg/day **or** IV chlorothiazide 500-1000 mg/day
   3. High dose diuretic: Furosemide 160 mg IV bid or tid
   4. Long acting loop diuretic: Torsemide 100-200 mg IV.
   D. **Beta Blockers:**
   1. Low-dose beta blockers may produce long-term improvements in heart failure. In patients with catecholamine excess, beta blockers may be very beneficial. However, beta blockers may also cause acute deterioration.
   2. **Carvedilol (Coreg)** should be considered in virtually all heart failure patients if they are limited by symptoms or are deteriorating on conventional triple therapy of digoxin, diuretic, and an ACE-inhibitor. Initiate at low dosage and increase dose slowly; 6.25-50 mg bid.
   3. **Metoprolol (Lopressor)** may be given to patients with compensated CHF at 6.25 mg PO bid for 1 week followed by a doubling of the dose every week as tolerated until 50 mg bid or symptoms appear.

IX. **Non-Pharmacologic Measures**
   A. Patients should be informed about symptoms of worsening heart failure, and they should keep a record of their daily weights. If worsening of symptoms or a weight gain of 3-5 lb or more occurs within one week, the patient should advise physician and take an extra dose of diuretic.
   B. **Activity:** Regular exercise such as walking or cycling should be encouraged for all patients with stable heart failure.
   C. **Diet:**
   1. Dietary sodium should be restricted to 2 g per day.
   2. Total fluid intake of 1.5-2 L/day should be maintained, and excessive fluid intake should be avoided. Fluid restriction is not advisable unless hyponatremia.
   3. Alcohol should be discouraged, and patients should be advised to consume no more than one drink per day.

X. **Heart Transplantation**
   A. **Criteria for Cardiac Transplantation:** Age <60 years, end-stage heart disease refractory to medical treatment in whom revascularization is not likely to convey benefit, disabling symptoms, and estimated survival of less than 1 year.
   B. **Contraindications:** Pulmonary hypertension, hepatic or renal failure, other serious illness, active infection, recent pulmonary infarction, drug or alcohol abuse, and medical noncompliance.

# Cardiomyopathies

Some cases of cardiomyopathy have a specific etiology while many cases are classified as "idiopathic". The cardiomyopathies are divided into three categories: 1. Dilated, 2. Hypertrophic and 3. Restrictive. The broad functional abnormalities can also be referred to as defects in systolic and/or diastolic function. Echocardiography is essential in classifying cardiomyopathies.

I. **Dilated Cardiomyopathy**
    A. Characterized by a decrease in systolic function and a decrease in right and/or left ventricular ejection fraction.
    B. Characterized by decreased cardiac output and a clinical picture of "typical" congestive heart failure. Cardiomegaly is present secondary to dilatation of the chambers.
    C. **Etiologies of Dilated Cardiomyopathy:** 1. Ischemic, 2. Idiopathic (Peripartum), 3. Toxic (ethanol, heavy metals, doxorubicin), 4. Inflammatory (viral, bacterial, parasitic, collagen disease, vasculitis, sarcoidosis), 5. Metabolic (thiamine deficiency, myxedema, catecholamine excess).
    D. Diagnosis and Treatment, see section on "Heart Failure", page 12.

II. **Hypertrophic Cardiomyopathy**
    A. Hypertrophic cardiomyopathies may be either obstructive or non-obstructive. The non-obstructive type may be idiopathic or commonly secondary to systemic hypertension.
    B. Hypertensive cardiomyopathy is characterized by the presence of LVH and diastolic dysfunction. This may progress to eventual dilatation and systolic dysfunction. Clinical heart failure occurs in the presence of systemic hypertension and often coronary artery disease.
    C. **Complications:** Atrial fibrillation, mitral insufficiency, endocarditis, diastolic failure and sudden death.
    D. **Echocardiogram:** Often diagnostic, demonstrating asymmetric septal hypertrophy.
    E. **Treatment of Non-obstructive, Hypertrophic Cardiomyopathy:**
        1. Control of the hypertension, angiotensin converting enzyme inhibitors (ACEI), vasodilators, calcium channel antagonists, beta blockers and possibly diuretics.
        2. In patients with pure diastolic dysfunction inotropic agents such as digoxin may be ineffective and detrimental.
    F. **Treatment of Obstructive Hypertrophic Cardiomyopathy:**
        1. Beta blockers are the mainstay of treatment. Verapamil and disopyramide may be beneficial.
        2. Prophylactic treatment for infective endocarditis is indicated.
        3. Dual chamber pacemaker therapy; surgical myomectomy with mitral valve replacement may be indicated.
        4. The risk of sudden death increases with excessive physical exertion and should be avoided.

III. **Restrictive Cardiomyopathy**
    A. This group of cardiomyopathies is characterized by varying degrees of systolic and diastolic dysfunction secondary to myocardial and endocardial thickening. The myocardium may be infiltrated with cellular and/or abnormal substances such amyloid, iron deposits, connective tissue.
    B. **Etiologies:** 1. Amyloidosis, 2. Hemochromatosis, 3. Sarcoidosis, 4. Scleroderma, 5. Metastatic malignancy, 6. Glycogen storage disease.
    C. **Diagnosis:**
        1. May present with signs and symptoms of congestive heart failure secondary to systolic and/or diastolic dysfunction.
        2. Findings may mimic constrictive pericarditis, and myocardial biopsy may be helpful in obtaining a definitive diagnosis.

D. **Treatment:**
   1. Treatment of underlying etiology (e.g., hemochromatosis) is essential. Ace-inhibitors, diuretics, vasodilators may be beneficial.
   2. Inotropic agents are often ineffective and may be detrimental.

# Atrial Fibrillation

## I. Clinical Evaluation

A. Fatigue may occur because of impaired cardiac output; palpitations, shortness of breath, or chest pain may occur. Vague symptoms such as lack of energy or a change in the sense of well-being, or no symptoms may be noted. Syncope may infrequently accompany AF.

B. Paroxysmal AF may cause symptoms that abate and recur, especially with physical exertion or emotional stress.

C. The pulse has an irregular timing and amplitude. Rapid ventricular rate may cause hypotension, pulmonary congestion, or myocardial ischemia and angina.

D. The cause of the atrial fibrillation should be identified once the ventricular rate has been controlled.

E. Rule out precipitating causes such as hyperthyroidism, electrolyte abnormalities, drug toxicity (theophylline). Exclude stimulant abuse, excess tobacco, alcohol, caffeine, chocolate, over-the-counter cold remedies, and street drugs. AF may be associated with a recent acute illness such as pneumonia or a history of ischemic heart disease.

F. Examine for evidence of hypertension, rheumatic fever, valvular disease, pericarditis, coronary artery disease, hyperthyroidism, or chronic obstructive pulmonary disease.

G. Thoroughly evaluate cardiovascular system; murmurs or cardiac enlargement on chest x-ray should be investigated by echocardiogram. Peripheral bruits may be a marker for associated coronary artery disease.

## II. Diagnostic Evaluation

A. **12-lead Electrocardiogram:** Irregular R-R intervals with no P waves. Ventricular rate is irregularly irregular. No P-waves will be seen in AF. There is an irregular baseline with rapid fibrillary waves (more than 320 per minute). The usual ventricular response rate is 130-180 per minute.

B. Chest x-ray, electrolytes and screening labs, ECG, echocardiogram, free T4, TSH, drug levels (theophylline).

## III. Causes of Atrial Fibrillation

Hypoglycemia

Theophylline intoxication

Acute pulmonary disease (pneumonia, asthma, chronic obstructive pulmonary disease, pulmonary embolus)

Heavy alcohol intake or alcohol withdrawal

Hyperthyroidism

Severe acute systemic illness

Left or right ventricular failure

Mitral valve disease (stenosis or regurgitation)

Pericarditis

Hypertensive heart disease with left ventricular hypertrophy

Hypertrophic cardiomyopathy

Coronary artery disease

Atrial septal defect

Aortic stenosis

Infiltrative diseases (amyloidosis, cardiac tumors)

Acute myocardial infarction

Lone atrial fibrillation (No underlying disease state)

Electrolyte abnormalities

Stimulant abuse, excess tobacco, xanthine (tea), chocolate, over-the-counter cold remedies, street drugs.

## IV. Emergency Management of Unstable or Complicated Atrial Fibrillation

A. **Patients Who Develop Acute Hypotension, Angina or Heart Failure because of rapid heart rate should be treated as follows:**

1. Immediate direct-current cardioversion. Anesthesia or sedation and nasal oxygen are necessary in all but the most serious emergency situation.

2. After cardioversion, cardiac rhythm should be stabilized with intravenous procainamide (Pronestyl), followed by oral maintenance therapy (Procan).

3. These potentially unstable patients should also receive a maintenance, rate control drug such as digoxin (Lanoxin) or a beta-blocker.

## V. Initial Management of Uncomplicated Atrial Fibrillation

### A. Rate Control:

1. Control of the ventricular response is the first issue in patients who do not require immediate cardioversion. Ventricular rate should usually be brought below 100.

2. **Beta blockers:**

   a. Beta blockers should receive first consideration although digoxin has traditionally been used. One reason is that digoxin does not promote conversion to normal sinus rhythm. In contrast, beta blockers may have such an effect.

   b. Beta blockers have a more rapid onset of action than digoxin. Digoxin is relatively slow-acting, and slowing of the heart rate takes 6 hours. In contrast, the heart rate may decrease within minutes after a beta blocker.

   c. **Contraindications to Beta-Blockers:** Asthma, obstructive lung disease, heart failure.

   d. **Propranolol HCL (Inderal)** may be given IV in a dose of 1-4 mg at 1 mg/min. A second dose may be given after two minutes, if necessary. Thereafter, additional drug should not be given in less than 4 hours. Oral maintenance dosage is 10-30 mg tid or qid.

   e. **Esmolol HCL (Brevibloc)** loading dose infusion of 0.5 mg/kg IV over 1 minute, followed by a 4 minute maintenance infusion of 0.05 mg/kg/min. If an adequate therapeutic effect is not observed within five minutes, repeat the loading dose, and follow with a maintenance infusion increased to 0.1 mg/kg/min. Continue the titration procedure, repeating loading infusion and increasing maintenance infusion by increments of 0.05 mg/kg/min. As the target heart rate is approached, titrate the maintenance dosage up or down. Treatment is cumbersome because multiple bolus doses are required, but its rapid clearance from the circulation is an advantage if hypotension develops.

   f. **Atenolol (Tenormin)** 5-10 mg IV doses; 25-100 mg PO per day

   g. **Metoprolol (Lopressor)** 5-15 mg IV doses; 25-100 mg PO bid daily

3. **Calcium Channel Blockers:**

   a. The calcium channel blockers, verapamil (Calan, Isoptin) and diltiazem (Cardizem), are appropriate therapeutic options for patients with asthma or obstructive lung disease. Diltiazem has less intense negative inotropic effects than verapamil.

   b. Diltiazem HCL (Cardizem) is given in a 20-25-mg IV bolus over 2 min, followed by an infusion of 10-15 mg/h for up to 24 hours. Repeat bolus of 25 mg if the target rate is not achieved within 15 minutes.

   c. Verapamil HCL (Isoptin) is administered in an IV bolus of 5-10 mg over two minutes. If the target heart rate--less than 100 bpm or a 20% reduction from baseline--is not attained within 30 minutes, give another bolus dose of 10 mg.

   d. Calcium Channel Blockers are contraindicated in CHF

4. **Digoxin:**

   a. Useful in patients with left ventricular systolic dysfunction.

   b. Digoxin may be less effective when hypomagnesemia is present, and hypomagnesemia should be considered when the ventricular rate is refractory to digoxin.

   c. Digoxin is not useful, and may be harmful, in left ventricular diastolic dysfunction (hypertensive heart disease and hypertrophic cardiomyopathy). Beta blockers or calcium blockers are the preferred agents in diastolic dysfunction.

   d. Loading dose: IV 0.25 mg for 4 doses (total dose: 1.0 mg) maintenance: 0.125-0.25 mg/day. Oral Loading dose: 0.25 mg q6h for 5 doses (total: 1.25 mg); maintenance: 0.125- 0.375 mg per day.

## VI. Intermediate Management of Uncomplicated Atrial Fibrillation

### A. Consideration of Restoration of Sinus Rhythm:

1. After the ventricular rate has been controlled, cardioversion should be considered in all patients. Restoration of sinus rhythm improves cardiac output and exercise capacity, and reduces systemic embolization.

    2. Sinus rhythm can be restored by direct-current cardioversion or by antiarrhythmic drugs.

B. **Factors that Identify Patients who are Unlikely to Remain in Sinus Rhythm:**
1. The most important factor is duration of fibrillation. Uncorrected mitral valve disease, cardiomyopathy, advanced pulmonary disease, and ongoing binge alcohol drinking will also prevent sustained conversion to sinus rhythm.
2. Left atrial size by echocardiography is probably not as important.

C. **Anticoagulation:**
1. All patients should be anticoagulated before cardioversion. Hospitalized patients should receive heparin for at least 48 hours before cardioversion, and outpatients should receive warfarin (Coumadin) for two to three weeks before the procedure. The international normalized ratio (INR) should be maintained at 1.4 to 2.8.
2. After successful cardioversion, oral anticoagulants should be continued for three weeks, because atrial contraction does not immediately begin after conversion.

## VII. Antiarrhythmic Drug Therapy

A. After 48 hours of heparin therapy or two to three weeks of warfarin therapy, and after ventricular rate has been controlled, antiarrhythmic therapy should be initiated.

B. Type IA agents include quinidine, procainamide (Pronestyl), and disopyramide (Norpace) Patients taking type IA antiarrhythmics should be monitored closely by ECG. Marked prolongation of the QT interval may be an indication of impending Torsades de pointes.
1. **Quinidine:** Conversion success rate is 60%. Continue quinidine after sinus rhythm is restored to reduce the risk of recurrent atrial fibrillation. The dosage of quinidine gluconate is 324 mg PO bid or qid. Intravenous or IM quinidine is rarely used because of associated symptoms.
2. **Procainamide:**
    a. 43-58% convert to sinus rhythm with IV administration of procainamide.
    b. The loading dose is 500-1,000 mg IV over 30-60 minutes, followed by an infusion of 1-4 mg/min. Oral dosage of procainamide (Procan SR, Pronestyl-SR) is 500-1,000 mg tid or qid, using the sustained-release form. Long-term use commonly leads to increased antinuclear antibody levels and to a lupus erythematosus-like syndrome.
3. **Disopyramide** should be used only as a second-line agent, since it has an adverse side effect profile. 100-200 mg tid or qid for the immediate-release form and 100-300 mg bid.

C. Type IC antiarrhythmic drugs Flecainide (Tambocor) and Propafenone (Rythmol) can produce a negative inotropic effect and should not be used in patients with CHF.
1. The Class IC agents should be used with caution because of their association with serious proarrhythmic effects. Flecainide and propafenone are equally effective for AF and are more effective and better tolerated than the class IA agents.
2. Flecainide (Tambocor) initial dose, 50 mg q12h, and increase in increments of 50 mg bid every four days until desired effect; max dosage 300 mg/d.

D. **Class III antiarrhythmics:**
1. **Amiodarone (Cordarone)** has an advantage over other antiarrhythmic agents since it maintains sinus rhythm more frequently and has fewer proarrhythmic effects than other available. Loading dose of 600-800 mg/d po for 1-3 weeks; gradually reduce to a maintenance dosage of 200 mg/d (or less) after 6-8 weeks. Closely monitor for pulmonary toxicity, hepatic dysfunction, visual impairment, and thyroid abnormalities.
2. **Sotalol (Betapace)** has less toxicity than amiodarone and is well-tolerated; useful in patients unresponsive to other drugs. The initial dosage 80 mg PO bid, increase as needed to 240-320 mg/d divided into bid or tid doses.

## VIII. Elective Direct-Current Cardioversion

A. The ventricular rate should be controlled and the patient anticoagulated fully before undergoing elective cardioversion.

B. Patients undergoing elective DC cardioversion should receive a class IA antiarrhythmic agent (quinidine) for one or two days before cardioversion in order to increase the likelihood that a normal rhythm will be maintained.

C. Digoxin level should be checked before the procedure is performed because digitalis toxicity may predispose to ventricular fibrillation during electrical cardioversion.

D. Electrolyte imbalances, especially a low potassium level, should be excluded.

E. An anesthesiologist should administer a benzodiazepine and manage the airway.

F. Conversion usually can be accomplished with 50 to 100 joules (J), but up to 360 J may be required.

## IX. Long-Term Management of Chronic Atrial Fibrillation

A. **Stroke Prevention Therapy:**

1. Patients with risks factors for stroke should be treated with warfarin (Coumadin) unless contraindicated.

2. **Risk Factors for Stroke:** Increasing age (>75 years), previous stroke or transient ischemic attack, hypertension, diabetes, heart failure, myocardial ischemia or valvular disease.

3. In patients younger than 60 years of age and without a history of prior embolus, hypertension or diabetes, the annual stroke rate is very low (1.0 percent) and unchanged with warfarin therapy; such patients should not receive anticoagulant therapy. All others should.

4. For patients under 60 years old with lone or paroxysmal atrial fibrillation, 325 mg of aspirin a day again should be considered instead of heparin. Aspirin should be given to patients who are not given anticoagulants.

B. **Coumadin (Warfarin)** therapy for atrial fibrillation should be titrated to an international normalized ratio (INR) of 1.4 to 2.8.

# Hypertension

## I. Clinical Evaluation

A. The evaluation of hypertension should include an assessment of drug use, including missed doses of maintenance antihypertensive therapy, use of nonsteroidal anti-inflammatory drugs, cocaine, or amphetamines.

B. **Initial Physical Examination of the Hypertensive Patient:**
1. Blood pressure should be measured with the patient seated for at least 5 minutes, and the arm bared at heart level. Two or more measurements separated by a 2-minute interval should be averaged to determine the blood pressure.
2. Measure blood pressure in both arms.
3. Check for retinal hemorrhage, exudates, or arteriovenous crossing defects.
4. Evaluate for carotid bruits, left ventricular enlargement and hypertrophy, coarctation of the aorta, aortic aneurysm, and examine for absence of a peripheral pulse in an extremity.

C. **Initial Diagnostic Testing for Hypertension:**
1. **12 lead Electrocardiography:** Documents evidence of ischemic heart disease, rhythm and conduction disturbances; not sensitive for left ventricular hypertrophy.
2. **Urine Analysis:** Dipstick testing for glucose, protein, hemoglobin.
3. Complete blood cell count, blood glucose, cholesterol (total and high-density lipoprotein), triglyceride, potassium, calcium, creatinine, and uric acid.
4. Selected patients may require plasma renin activity, plasma catecholamines, 24 hour urine for metanephrines, renal function testing (glomerular filtration rate and blood flow). A sensitive thyroid stimulating hormone test identifies hypothyroidism.

## II. Classification of Blood Pressure

| Category | Systolic | Diastolic | Recommended Follow-up |
|---|---|---|---|
| Normal | <130 mm Hg | <85 mm Hg | Recheck in 2 years |
| High normal | 130-139 mm Hg | 85-89 mm Hg | Recheck in 1 year |
| Stage I hypertension | 140-159 mm Hg | 90-99 mm Hg | Reevaluate within 2 months |
| Stage II hypertension | 160-179 mm Hg | 100-109 mm Hg | Evaluate and treat within 1 month |
| Stage III hypertension | 180-209 mm Hg | 110-119 mm Hg | Evaluate and treat within 1 week |
| Stage IV hypertension | >210 mm Hg | >120 mm Hg | Evaluate and treat immediately |

## III. Correctable Causes of Hypertension

A. Clinical evaluation should include a search for causes of secondary hypertension including coarctation of the aorta, Cushing's syndrome, pheochromocytoma, primary aldosteronism from adrenal adenoma, and renovascular disease.

B. Secondary hypertension may be indicated by a sudden increase in previously normal BP, or by an increase in BP previously controlled by antihypertensive therapy.

C. **Findings That Suggest Secondary Hypertension:**
**Primary Aldosteronism:** Initial serum potassium <3.5 mEq/L on no medication.
**Aortic Coarctation:** Femoral pulse is delayed later than radial pulse, posterior systolic bruits below ribs.
**Pheochromocytoma:** Orthostatic hypotension, tachycardia, tremor, pallor
**Renovascular Stenosis:** Paraumbilical abdominal bruits
**Polycystic Kidneys:** Flank or abdominal mass
**Pyelonephritis:** Persistent urinary tract infections, costovertebral angle tenderness.
**Renal Parenchymal Disease:** Persistently increased serum creatinine >1.5 mg/dL, proteinuria

## IV. Assessment of Clinical Indicators of Target-Organ Disease

A. **Cardiac:** Evidence of coronary artery disease may be apparent based on clinical, electrocardiographic, or radiographic signs. Left ventricular hypertrophy or "strain" on electrocardiography or signs of cardiac failure should be sought.

B. **Cerebrovascular:** Previous transient ischemic attack, stroke.

C. **Peripheral Vascular:** Absence of one or more major pulses in extremities (except dorsalis pedis) with or without intermittent claudication.

D. **Renal:** Hypertensive nephropathy may be indicated by serum creatinine >1.5 mg/dL, proteinuria > 1 *, or microalbuminuria > 30 mg/24 hr.

E. **Retinal:** Hemorrhages or exudates with or without papilledema.

## V. Non-drug Treatment of Hypertension

A. The primary goal of antihypertensive therapy is to decrease systolic blood pressures below 140 mm Hg and diastolic blood pressures below 90 mm Hg.

B. Appropriate dietary sodium intake ranges from 1.5 to 2.5 g of sodium, or 4 to 6 g of salt. A 2-g sodium diet requires the omission of foods naturally high in sodium, as well as limitation of salt used in food preparation and seasoning. Prepackaged foods, fast-food restaurant products, or foods processed in brine are high in sodium.

C. Overweight hypertensive patients should be encouraged to lose weight. Patients should exercise at least three times a week for 20 to 45 minutes each session.

D. Alcohol intake should be limited to no more than 1 oz of ethanol a day (two 12-oz beers, two 4-oz glasses of wine or two 1-oz mixed drinks).

E. Patients who smoke cigarettes should be encouraged to quit smoking.

## VI. Pharmacologic Therapy of Hypertension

A. Pharmacologic therapy should be initiated if 3-6 months of diet and lifestyle modification fail to decrease blood pressure to below 140/90 mm Hg. A shorter follow-up interval is appropriate for persons with cardiovascular risk factors or evidence of target-organ disease.

B. **Patient Considerations in Choosing an Antihypertensive Agent:**
1. Unique demographic factors. The most important factor is race.
2. Concomitant diseases and drug-drug interactions.
3. Effect of therapy on patient's quality of life.
4. Effect of therapy on physiologic and biochemical values.
5. Medication cost and patient compliance.

C. **Treatment of Hypertension in Patients with Special Characteristics:**
1. **Elderly Patients:** Usually have low cardiac output, high systemic vascular resistance, reduced intravascular volume, and reduced renal function. Calcium channel blockers, ACE-inhibitors, and thiazide diuretics have the best efficacy and side effect profile.
2. **Young Hypertensive Patients:** Because of side effect profiles, the use of ACE inhibitors or calcium channel blockers is more favorable.
3. **Ischemic Heart Disease:**
   a. Beta blockers are preferred, and diuretics should be avoided. A calcium channel blocker may be used if a beta blocker is contraindicated.
   b. Nitroglycerin preparations may be used.
4. **Diabetes Mellitus and Dyslipidemia:** Beta blockers and diuretics should be avoided.
5. **Gout, Ventricular Ectopic Activity:** Diuretics should be avoided.
6. **Congestive Heart Failure:**
   a. An ACE-inhibitor is preferred, with or without a loop diuretic.
   b. CHF patients with diastolic dysfunction may respond well to beta-blockers.
7. **Asthma, Obstructive Airway Disease, or Claudication:** Should not receive a beta blocker.
8. **Renal Failure:** An ACE inhibitor may slow progression of renal failure, especially in the presence of diabetic nephropathy. Monitor closely for hyperkalemia and worsening of renal failure.
9. **African Hypertensive Patients:** Usually have lower cardiac output, expanded total blood volume, and high total peripheral resistance. These patients respond best to diuretics, calcium channel blockers, alpha blockers, central alpha agonists. African patients respond less well to ACE inhibitors and beta blockers.
10. **Gender:** Usually is not a factor in antihypertensive medication selection.

VII. **Individualized Approach to Initial Therapy**

| Patient Characteristics Demographic Features | Preferred Drugs | Less Preferred Drugs |
|---|---|---|
| Age below 50 | Calcium-Channel blocker, alpha blocker, ACE inhibitor | Diuretic |
| Age over 65 | Thiazide diuretic, calcium-channel blocker, ACE inhibitor | Alpha2-receptor agonist |
| African | Thiazide diuretic | Beta blocker, ACE inhibitor |
| European | Beta blocker, ACE inhibitor | |
| **Life-style** Physically active | Alpha blocker, ACE inhibitor, calcium-channel blocker | Beta blocker |
| Noncompliant | Once-a-day dosage | Alpha2-receptor agonist |
| **Concomitant Diseases** Coronary heart disease | Beta blocker, calcium-channel blocker | Direct vasodilator |
| Post-myocardial infarction | Beta blocker, ACE inhibitor | |
| Congestive heart failure | ACE inhibitor, direct vasodilator | Beta blocker, calcium-channel blocker |
| Supraventricular tachyarrhythmias | Verapamil, beta blocker | |
| Bradycardia, sick sinus | | Beta blocker, diltiazem, verapamil |
| Hypercholesterolemia | Alpha blocker, ACE inhibitor, calcium-channel blocker | Diuretic, beta blocker |
| Hypertriglyceridemia | Alpha blocker | Beta-blocker (non-ISA) |
| Migraine | Beta blocker | |
| History of depression | | Alpha2-receptor agonist, beta blocker |
| Peripheral vascular disease | ACE inhibitor, calcium-channel blocker, Alpha blocker | Beta blocker |

| Renal insufficiency | Loop diuretic, ACE inhibitor, minoxidil | Thiazide diuretic |
| Diabetes mellitus | ACE inhibitor, alpha2-receptor agonist, Alpha blocker | Thiazide diuretic, beta blocker |
| Gout | | Diuretic |
| Asthma | | Beta-blocker |

## VIII. Effects of Antihypertensive Drugs on Biochemical and Physiologic Measurements

| Pharmacologic class | Exercise capacity | Serum glucose | Left ventricular hypertrophy | Serum potassium | Lipids |
|---|---|---|---|---|---|
| ACE inhibitors | No change | Decrease | Decrease | Increase | No change |
| Alpha blockers | No change | Decrease | Decrease | No change | Decrease |
| Beta blockers | Decrease | Increase | Decrease | No change/increase | Increase* |
| Calcium blockers | No change | No change | Decrease | No change | Decrease |
| Diuretics | No change/decrease | Increase | Decrease | Decrease | Increases |

* Low-density lipoprotein (LDL) is not affected, but triglycerides and high-density lipoprotein (HDL) are adversely affected.

## IX. Dosages of Antihypertensive Agents

### A. Angiotensin Converting Enzyme Inhibitors:
-Ramipril (Altace) 2.5-10 mg PO qd, max 20 mg/day [1.25, 2.5, 5, 10 mg].
-Quinapril (Accupril) initial dose 10 mg PO qd; then 20-80 mg PO qd or in divided doses; max 80 mg/day [5, 10, 20, 40 mg].
-Lisinopril (Zestril, Prinivil) initial dose 5 mg PO qd; then 10-40 mg PO qd; max 80 mg/d [5, 10, 20, 40 mg].
-Benazepril (Lotensin) 10-40 mg PO qd, max 80 mg/day [5, 10, 20, 40 mg].
-Fosinopril (Monopril) 10-40 mg PO qd, max 80 mg/day [10, 20 mg].
-Enalapril (Vasotec) initial dose 2.5 mg, then 5-40 mg qd or in divided doses, max 40 mg/day [2.5, 5, 10, 20 mg].
-Captopril (Capoten) initial dose 6.25-12.5 mg PO x 1, then 25-150 mg PO bid-tid; max 450 mg/day [12.5, 25, 50, 100 mg].

### B. Calcium Antagonists:
-Diltiazem sustained release (Cardizem SR) initial dose 60 mg PO bid, then 60-120 mg PO bid; max 360 mg/d [60, 90, 120 mg] or Cardizem-CD 180-360 mg PO qd [180, 240, 360 mg] or (Cardizem) 30-90 PO qid [30, 60, 90, 120 mg].
-Nifedipine (Procardia) XL initial dose 30 mg PO qd, then 30-60 mg PO qd, max 120 mg/d [30, 60, 90 mg] or (Procardia) 10-30 mg PO bid-qid [10, 20 mg] .
-Verapamil sustained release, initial dose 180 mg PO qd, max 480 mg/d divided bid [240 mg] or (Calan, Isoptin) 80-120 mg PO tid-qid [40, 80, 120 mg].
-Amlodipine (Norvasc) 2.5-10 mg PO qd [2.5,5, 10 mg tabs].
-Felodipine (Plendil) 5-10 mg PO qd, max 20 mg/d [5, 10 mg].
-Bepridil (Vascor) 200 mg PO qd [200, 300, 400 mg].
-Isradipine (DynaCirc) 2.5-5 mg PO bid [2.5, 5 mg].
-Nicardipine (Cardene) 20-40 mg PO tid [20, 30 mg].

### C. Cardioselective Beta-Blockers (beta 1):
-Metoprolol (Lopressor) 50-100 mg PO bid [50, 100 mg].
-Atenolol (Tenormin) initial dose 50 mg PO qd, then 50-100 mg PO qd, max 200 mg/d [50, 100 mg].

### D. Non-Cardioselective Beta-Blockers (beta 1 & beta 2):
-Propranolol (Inderal-LA), 80-120 mg PO qd [60, 80, 120, 160 mg] or (Inderal) 40-160 mg PO bid; max 320 mg/day [10, 20, 40, 60, 80, 90 mg].
-Timolol (Blocadren) 5-10 mg PO bid [5, 10, 20 mg ].
-Nadolol (Corgard) 40-160 mg PO qd [20, 40, 80, 120, 160 mg].
-Pindolol (Visken) initial dose 5-20 mg PO qd, max 60 mg/d [5, 10 mg].

-Carteolol (Cartrol) 2.5-10 mg PO qd [2.5, 5 mg ].
-Labetalol (Trandate) 100-600 mg PO bid [100, 200, 300 mg].

E. **Alpha Blockers:**
   -Doxazosin (Cardura) initial dose 1 mg PO qd at bedtime; may double dose prn, max 16 mg/d [1, 2, 4, 8 mg].
   -Terazosin (Hytrin) initial dose 1 mg PO qd at bedtime; max 20 mg PO qd [1, 2, 5, 10 mg].
   -Prazosin (Minipress) initial dose 1 mg PO bid-tid; 6-20 mg/d PO bid-tid [1, 2, 5 mg].

F. **Diuretics:**
   -Hydrochlorothiazide (HCTZ, HydroDiuril) initial dose 12.5 mg PO qd; 25-100 mg PO qd-bid.
   -Chlorothiazide (Diuril) 250-500 mg PO qd-bid [250, 500 mg].
   -Indapamide (Lozol) 2.5-5 mg PO qd [2.5 mg].

G. **Diuretic Combinations:**
   -Moduretic (amiloride 5 mg, hydrochlorothiazide 50 mg) 1-2 tabs/d in 1-2 doses.
   -Maxzide (triamterene/hydrochlorothiazide 75/50 mg or 37.5/25 mg) 1-2 tabs PO qd.

## X. Monitoring of Pharmacologic Therapy
A. If adequate control is not achieved with a single agent, the dosage may be increased, another class of drug may be added, or another drug may be substituted for the initial agent.
B. Portable automated ambulatory monitoring is recommended only in specific situations such as in "Office" hypertension, nighttime blood pressure changes, episodic hypertension, or hypotensive episodes.
C. Refractory mild hypertension that remains above 140/90 mm Hg, although maximal doses of at least two appropriate antihypertensive agents have been taken, may be caused by secondary hypertension, over-the-counter medications, sclerotic arteries (pseudohypertension), inappropriate or inadequate treatment, or noncompliance.

## XI. Discontinuing Medication
A. In patients who have been taking monotherapy for at least 1 year and whose respective diastolic and systolic BPs are persistently below 85 and 130 mm Hg, it may be worthwhile to gradually decrease and discontinue drug treatment and to observe the BP at 6 week to 2 month intervals.
B. If a patient has target-organ damage (eyeground findings, renal involvement, LVH or more overt cardiovascular disease), discontinuation of antihypertensive therapy should probably not be considered, even if BP persists in the acceptable range.

# Hypertensive Emergencies

## I. Clinical Evaluation of Hypertensive Syndromes

A. Severe hypertension is characterized by diastolic blood pressure (BP) higher than 120 mmHg or systolic BP higher than 180 mmHg. Severe hypertension is subdivided into hypertensive emergencies and hypertensive urgencies.

B. **Hypertensive Emergency:** Defined by a diastolic blood pressure >120 mmHg with ongoing vascular damage. Symptoms or signs of neurologic, cardiac, renal, or retinal dysfunction are present.

Hypertensive emergencies include severe hypertension in the following settings:

Aortic dissection

Acute left ventricular failure and pulmonary edema

Acute renal failure or worsening of chronic renal failure

Hypertensive encephalopathy

Focal neurologic damage indicating thrombotic or hemorrhagic stroke

Pheochromocytoma, cocaine overdose, or other hyperadrenergic states

Unstable angina or MI

C. **Hypertensive Urgency:** Diastolic blood pressure >120 mmHg and no evidence of vascular damage; asymptomatic, no retinal lesions.

D. **Causes of Secondary Hypertension:** Renovascular hypertension, pheochromocytoma, cocaine use, withdrawal from alpha2 stimulants or beta blockers, or alcohol; noncompliance with antihypertensive medications.

## II. Initial Assessment of Severe Hypertension

A. When severe hypertension is noted, repeat the measurement in both arms with the arm resting on a flat surface, and note any significant differences; use an appropriate size blood pressure cuff.

B. Assess peripheral pulses for absence or delay. Look for evidence of pulmonary edema, and initially assess how ill the patient appears.

C. Target organ damage is evidenced by chest pain, neurologic signs, altered mental status, profound headache, dyspnea, abdominal pain, hematuria, focal neurologic signs (paralysis or paresthesia), and hypertensive retinopathy.

D. If focal neurologic signs are present, a CT scan may be required to differentiate hypertensive encephalopathy from a stroke syndrome. In stroke syndromes, hypertension may be transient and secondary to the neurologic event. The neurologic deficits are fixed and follow a predictable neuroanatomic pattern. By contrast, in hypertensive encephalopathy, the neurologic signs follow no anatomic pattern, and there is diffuse alteration in mental function.

E. Prescription drug use should be assessed, including the possibility of a missed dose of maintenance antihypertensive therapy. Ask about a recent history of cocaine or amphetamine use.

## III. Laboratory Evaluation

A. Complete blood cell count; urinalysis for protein, glucose, and blood; urine sediment examination for cells, casts, and bacteria; full chemistry panel (SMA-18).

B. If chest pain is present, order cardiac enzymes. If the history suggests a hyperadrenergic state, consider a 24 hour urine for metanephrines, and plasma catecholamines. Toxicology screen.

C. Electrocardiogram.

D. Begin a workup for secondary hypertension to rule out primary aldosteronism (24 hour urine potassium, plasma renin activity), or renal artery stenosis (captopril renography, intravenous pyelography).

## IV. Management of Hypertensive Emergencies

A. Hospitalize the patient for bed rest, intravenous access, continuous intra-arterial blood pressure monitoring, electrocardiographic monitoring. Assess volume status, urinary output.

B. A rapid, uncontrolled reduction in blood pressure may cause coma, stroke, myocardial infarction, acute renal failure, or death.

C. **Controlled BP Reduction:** A conservative strategy is to reduce BP by approximately 30% of its initial value in the first hour.

## V. Parenteral Antihypertensive Agents

A. **Nitroprusside:**
1. Drug of choice in almost all hypertensive emergencies (except myocardial ischemia or renal impairment). The starting dosage is 0.25-1.0 mcg/kg/min by continuous infusion with a range of 0.25-8 mcg/kg/min. Titrate to gradually reduce pressure.
2. Dilates both arteries and veins, and reduces preload and afterload.
3. Onset is nearly instantaneous, and effects disappear approximately 1-10 minutes after discontinuation.
4. When treatment is prolonged or with renal insufficiency, the risk of cyanide toxicity is increased. Thiocyanate toxicity signs include anorexia, disorientation, fatigue, hallucinations, nausea, and toxic psychosis.
5. Cyanide toxicity is unlikely to occur at doses less than 10 mcg/kg per minute; limit infusion to less than 6 hours. Clinical deterioration with metabolic acidosis and arrhythmias indicates cyanide toxicity;

B. **Nitroglycerine:**
1. Drug of choice for hypertensive emergencies with coronary ischemia. Should not be used with hypertensive encephalopathy because it increases intracranial pressure.
2. 15 mcg IV bolus, then 5-10 mcg/min (50 mg in 250 mL D5W). Titrate by increasing dose at 3-5-minute intervals up to 100 mcg/min.
3. Rapid onset of action of 2-5 minutes. Tolerance may occur within 24-48 hours.

C. **Labetalol IV (Normodyne)**
1. Good choice if BP elevation is associated with hyperadrenergic activity.
2. Its alpha-blockade reduces peripheral vascular resistance while its beta-blocking action prevents reflex tachycardia. Use 20 mg of labetalol slow IV over 2 mins; monitor BP q5min. Additional doses of 20-80 mg may be administered q5-10min to a maximum of 300 mg.
3. The onset of action is approximately 5 minutes, and maximum effect occurs 30 minutes after each dose. Effects persist for 3-6 hours.

D. **Nicardipine IV (Cardene I.V.):**
1. Increasingly used for emergent BP reduction; a fast-acting calcium channel blocker that shares many of the predictable antihypertensive qualities of nitroprusside.
2. Nicardipine infusion is started at 5 mg/h and may be increased to 15 mg/h; BP is usually controlled at 7.5 mg/h. Its onset of action is 5-10 minutes, and its effects cease 10-15 minutes after the infusion is discontinued.

E. **Phentolamine:** Used in excess catecholamine states such as pheochromocytoma. 2-5 mg boluses every 5-10 minutes. Nitroprusside is more titratable, and is a better choice than phentolamine.

F. **Trimethaphan:** Used for dissecting aortic aneurysms. Most physicians are unfamiliar with trimethaphan, therefore, nitroprusside is a better choice. Infusion (0.5 to 15 mg/min); use only after intravenous beta blocker has been given.

## VI. Treatment of Target Organ Damage

A. **Neurologic Syndromes:**
1. **Hypertensive Encephalopathy:**
   a. Subacute onset occurs over 24-48-hours. Mental status changes headache, nausea, vomiting, visual complaints, papilledema, focal neurologic deficits, or seizures; coma and death if untreated.
   b. Resolves with treatment of blood pressure.
2. **Cerebrovascular Accidents:**
   a. The presence of focal neurologic signs in a patient with severe hypertension calls for extreme caution. First, consider whether the BP elevation is the cause of the neurologic disturbance or a reaction to it. Often, BP begins to fall as the neurologic

event stabilizes.

b. If a stroke syndrome is suspected, order a CT of the head.

c. **Cerebral Thrombosis:** Only if the diastolic blood pressure exceeds 110 mm Hg should blood pressure be lowered gradually with nitroprusside while cautiously monitoring for worsening of neurologic deficits. Decrease infusion rate of hypotensive agents if neurologic status worsens. Rapid blood pressure reduction may cause infarct extension.

B. **Cardiovascular Syndromes:**

1. **Aortic Dissection:**

   a. Characterized by abrupt, severe, unremitting chest pain radiating to the intra scapular region that is maximal at onset. Pulse asymmetry may be detected, and a radial pulse may be absent; occurs in patients with a long history of hypertension.

   b. Asymmetric blood pressures in arms. Acute aortic insufficiency is manifest by soft S1 and A2 sounds, new S3 gallop, and soft diastolic murmur.

   c. Echocardiography and a CT scan with contrast will confirm the diagnosis.

   d. Lower systolic blood pressure to between 100 and 110 mm Hg with nitroprusside. Consult a cardiologist and thoracic surgeon.

2. **Unstable Angina:** Initiate oxygen, nitroglycerin drip, aspirin, and an intravenous beta blocker. Heparin should not be used until after the diastolic blood pressure is less than 110 mm Hg.

3. **Acute Myocardial Infarction:**

   a. Very high blood pressure may be reduced by treatment of pain and anxiety with nitrates, morphine, and a benzodiazepine.

   b. Nitroprusside is contraindicated in myocardial infarction because of coronary steal phenomenon.

   c. Therapy consists of oxygen, IV nitroglycerin; IV metoprolol or atenolol, aspirin. Thrombolytic therapy should not be started until the blood pressure has been lowered to less than 110 mmHg.

4. **Hypertension with Pulmonary Edema:** Treatment of systolic heart failure consists of IV furosemide, nitrates, digoxin, oxygen, nitroprusside, and an oral ACE-inhibitor.

C. **Renal Syndromes:**

1. **Hypertensive Nephropathy:** Serum creatinine levels >3 mg/dL, azotemia, and oliguria, and urine sediment accompanied by proteinuria and hyaline and red blood cell casts; hypertension may be related to a primary renal cause or may be secondary to hypertension induced renal injury.

2. Normalization of urinary findings and improvement in creatinine clearance with adequate control of blood pressure suggest malignant nephrosclerosis secondary to hypertension.

3. If the patient is not volume-depleted, initiate IV furosemide (Lasix). Avoid nitroprusside in patients with impaired renal function because of the risk of thiocyanate toxicity.

4. **Renal Ultrasound:** Useful to assess kidney size and exclude obstructive uropathy; renal atrophy indicates chronic renal failure.

5. **Bladder Outlet Obstruction** can cause hypertension, and relief of obstruction reduces blood pressure; avoid precipitous drops in blood pressure by clamping the urethral catheter after each 500-mL of urinary drainage.

D. **Hyperadrenergic States:**

1. **Signs of Catecholamine Excess:** Tachycardia, palpitations, sweating, pallor, headache, anxiety, dilated pupils.

2. **Differential Diagnosis:**

   a. Pheochromocytoma, sympathomimetic drug toxicity (amphetamine, pheniramine, phenylpropanolamine, ephedrine, phenylephrine).

   b. Withdrawal from clonidine (Catapres), or methyldopa (Aldomet), and cocaine use.

3. Labetalol or nitroprusside are the best choices because of simplicity of use even though phentolamine (2-5 mg IV) is more specific for alpha-receptor blockade.

4. Cocaine toxicity is an increasingly common cause of hypertensive emergencies. It responds well to IV labetalol.

     5. Before beginning labetalol, consider whether pheochromocytoma is a possibility. Urine for metanephrines must be obtained before initiating labetalol because it will affect urinary metabolites.

     6. If the BP elevation can be traced to withdrawal from clonidine (Catapres), the best option is to reinstitute the drug.

## VII. Treatment of Hypertensive Urgencies

  A. Patients with no evidence of target organ damage have hypertensive urgencies, and they do not require immediate normalization of blood pressure; initiation of therapy and early follow-up are important. Rapid normalization of blood pressure can have adverse consequences.

  B. Asymptomatic patients with diastolic BP that exceeds 130 mmHg may need acute treatment to bring BP into a safer range, even though they are not in immediate danger.

  C. **Acute Oral Therapy:**

     1. Patients with true hypertensive urgency usually may be managed acutely in the office.

     2. Oral Nifedipine (Adalat, Procardia) 10 mg PO may be used to reduce BP. Allowing the BP to fall too rapidly, increases the risk of cerebral hypoperfusion. Having the patient bite open a nifedipine capsule and either swallow it or squirt the contents under the tongue offers no advantage.

     3. Clonidine HCL (Catapres) may cause sedation and alter neurologic function. Consider the drug only for clonidine withdrawal. The initial dosage is 0.1-0.2 mg PO. Give additional 0.1-mg doses every hour until diastolic BP has been reduced to 110 mmHg or by 30% of pre-treatment levels.

# Hyperlipidemia

### Clinical Evaluation of Hyperlipidemia
A. Total cholesterol and HDL-cholesterol should be measured in all adults 20 years of age and over.
B. Testing should be repeated every 5 years; measurements may be made in the nonfasting state.

## I. Initial Classification Based on Total Cholesterol and HDL-Cholesterol
**Total Cholesterol**

| | |
|---|---|
| <200 mg/dL | Desirable Blood Cholesterol |
| 200-239 mg/dL | Borderline-High Blood Cholesterol |
| >240 mg/dL | High Blood Cholesterol |

**HDL-Cholesterol**

| | |
|---|---|
| <35 mg/dL | Low HDL-Cholesterol |

## II. Initial Management Based on Total Cholesterol and HDL-Cholesterol
A. Measure Nonfasting Total Blood Cholesterol and HDL-cholesterol and Assess Coronary Heart Disease Risk Factors.
B. Determine Cholesterol Level and Classify Patient as Follows:
  1. **Desirable Blood Cholesterol <200 mg/dL:**
    a. **Desirable HDL >35 mg/dL:** Repeat total cholesterol and HDL within 5 years.
    b. **Low HDL <35 mg/dL:** Obtain lipoprotein analysis, and determine LDL-cholesterol.
  2. **Borderline-high Blood Cholesterol 200-239 mg/dL:**
    a. **Desirable HDL >35 mg/dL AND Fewer than 2 Risk Factors:** Provide information on dietary modification, physical activity, and risk factor reduction. Reevaluate in 1-2 years.
    b. **Low HDL <35 mg/dL OR 2 or More Risk Factors:** Obtain lipoprotein analysis, and determine LDL-cholesterol.
  3. **High Blood Cholesterol >240 mg/dL:** Obtain lipoprotein analysis, and determine LDL-cholesterol.

## IV. Risk Factors for Coronary Heart Disease
A. **Positive Risk Factors:**
  1. **Age:** Male: age 45 and older. Women: 55 or older or menopause before age 55 without estrogen replacement therapy.
  2. **Family History of Premature Coronary Heart Disease:** Father or brother before age 55; mother or sister before age 65.
  3. **Cigarette Smoking**
  4. **Hypertension:** >140/90 mm Hg or currently taking antihypertensive medication
  5. **Low HDL-cholesterol level:** <35 mg/dL
  6. **Diabetes mellitus**
B. **Negative Risk Factor:**
  1. **High HDL** ≥ 60 mg/dL, subtract one risk factor from the total.

## V. Lipoprotein Analysis
Fasting plasma cholesterol, triglyceride, high-density lipoprotein (HDL) cholesterol.
**LDL-cholesterol is calculated as follows:**
LDL cholesterol = total cholesterol - HDL cholesterol - (triglyceride ÷ 5)

## VI. Primary Prevention of CHD
A. **Classification Based on LDL-Cholesterol:**
  1. **Obtain Lipoprotein Analysis After Fasting 9-12 hours.**
  2. **Use the average of two determinations 1-8 weeks apart, and manage patient as follows:**

3. **Diet Therapy:**
   a. **If patient without CHD and with fewer than 2 risk factors:**
      (1) If high LDL >160 mg/dL, initiate Diet Therapy to achieve goal LDL <160 mg/dL.
      (2) If desirable LDL <160 mg/dL, repeat total cholesterol and HDL within 5 years.
   b. **If patient without CHD and with 2 or more risk factors:**
      (1) If high LDL >130 mg/dL, initiate Diet Therapy to achieve goal LDL <130 mg/dL.
      (2) If desirable LDL <130 mg/dL, repeat total cholesterol and HDL within 5 years; provide education on diet and risk factor reduction.
   c. **If patient with CHD:**
      (1) If high LDL >100 mg/dL, initiate Diet Therapy to achieve goal LDL ≤100 mg/dL.
      (2) If desirable LDL <100 mg/dL, repeat total cholesterol and HDL within 5 years; provide education on diet and risk factor reduction.
4. **Drug Therapy (after no response to 6 months of dietary therapy):**
   a. **If patient without coronary heart disease and fewer than 2 risk factors:**
      (1) If LDL ≥ 190 mg/dL, initiate drug therapy to achieve goal of 160 mg/dL.
   b. **If patient without CHD but with 2 or more risk factors:**
      (1) If LDL > 160 mg/dL, initiate drug therapy with goal LDL < 130 mg/dL.
   c. **If patient has CHD:**
      (1) If LDL > 130 mg/dL, initiate drug therapy with goal LDL ≤ 100 mg/dL.

## VII. Summary of Treatment Decisions Based on LDL-Cholesterol

**Dietary Therapy**

| | Initiation Level | LDL Goal |
|---|---|---|
| Without CHD and with fewer than 2 risk factors | >160 mg/dL | <160 mg/dL |
| Without CHD and with 2 or more risk factors | >130 mg/dL | <130 mg/dL |
| With CHD | >100 mg/dL | ≤100 mg/dL |

**Drug Treatment**

| | Consideration Level | LDL Goal |
|---|---|---|
| Without CHD and with fewer than 2 risk factors | >190 mg/dL* | <160 mg/dL |
| Without CHD and with 2 or more risk factors | >160 mg/dL | <130 mg/dL |
| With CHD | >130 mg/dL | ≤100 mg/dL |

*In men under 35 years of age and premenopausal women with LDL-cholesterol levels 190-219 mg/dL, drug therapy should be delayed except in high-risk patients such as those with diabetes.

## VIII. Dietary Therapy and Physical Activity

A. Increased physical activity and dietary therapy should reduce intake of saturated fatty acids and cholesterol, and promote weight loss in overweight patients.

## IX. Assessment of Cholesterol Response to Dietary Therapy

A. After starting the diet, the serum total cholesterol level should be measured at 4-6 weeks and at 3 month intervals.
B. Six months of dietary therapy should be tried before adding drug therapy; shorter periods can be considered with severe elevations of LDL-cholesterol (>220 mg/dL).

## X. Drug Treatment of Hypercholesterolemia

A. **Pharmacologic Treatment Choices:**

| Drug: | LDL | HDL | Triglycerides |
|---|---|---|---|
| Bile acid sequestrants | ↓ 15-30% | ↑ 3-5% | ↑ 3% |
| Nicotinic acid | ↓ 10-25% | ↑ 15-35% | ↓ 20-50% |
| Statins (HMG CoA Reductase inhibitors) | ↓ 20-40% | ↑ 5-15% | ↓ 10-20% |
| Fibric acid | ↓ 10-15% | ↑ 10-15% | ↓ 20-50% |
| Probucol | ↓ 10-20% | ↓ 20-30% | |

* Combination therapy can decrease LDL by 40-50%

B. **Bile Acid Sequestrants:**
   1. The bile acid sequestrants, cholestyramine (Questran) and colestipol (Colestid), bind intestinal bile acids; drugs of first choice because of safety and efficacy.
   2. Can lower LDL by as much as 30%; minimal increase in HDL; triglycerides may increase.
   3. Start with 1 packet or scoop bid before, during, or after meals; increase up to 3 packets or scoops bid.
   4. **Common Side Effects:** Constipation, diarrhea, nausea, flatulence, abdominal pain. Constipation may be prevented by increasing dietary fiber or with stool softeners.
   5. Bile acid sequestrants bind anionic drugs (warfarin, thyroxin, digoxin, thiazides, beta blockers, statins). These agents should be taken 1 hour before or 4 hours after resin dose.

C. **Nicotinic Acid (Niacin):**
   1. Reduces LDL 20%, raises HDL 20% and reduces TG 40%.
   2. Effective, inexpensive, but side effects are often intolerable; exerts favorable effects on concentrations of all lipoproteins. Valuable in treating high blood cholesterol with low HDL-cholesterol levels, or elevated cholesterol and triglyceride.
   3. Start with low doses of 100-125 mg tid; taken with or after meals. Gradually increase total daily dose to 1 g/day in divided doses with meals, up to a daily dose of 4.5 g/day. Avoid taking with hot drinks.
   4. Take 1 aspirin or NSAID 30 minutes before each dose to prevent flushing.
   5. **Side Effects:** Common cutaneous flushing, nausea, abdominal discomfort, skin dryness; rarely blurred vision. Hepatitis, hyperglycemia, hyperuricemia and gout, peptic ulcer disease may occur.
   6. **Contraindications:** gout or hyperuricemia, liver disease, peptic ulcer disease, diabetes.
   7. Periodic monitoring of aminotransferases and alkaline phosphatase is required.
   8. Slow-release forms are not recommended because of decreased efficacy in raising HDL-cholesterol, and increased hepatic toxicity.

D. **Statins (HMG CoA Reductase Inhibitors):**
   1. The most effective and most potent drugs available for reducing LDL cholesterol; low incidence of side effects. Inhibits HMG CoA reductase and interferes with hepatic cholesterol synthesis.
   2. More effective than niacin in lowering LDL but less so for raising HDL. Reduces LDL cholesterol by 20-40%, decreases triglycerides by 5-15%. HDL cholesterol increases by 5-15%.
   3. HMG CoA reductase inhibitors may be used as first-line agents for lowering LDL-cholesterol. Useful for severe hypercholesterolemia and maximal lowering of LDL levels.
   4. **Dosages:**
      -Lovastatin (Mevacor) 20-40 mg PO qhs-bid with meals; max 80 mg/day [10, 20, 40 mg].
      -Pravastatin (Pravachol) 20 mg PO qhs with meals; max 40 mg /d [10, 20 mg tabs].
      -Simvastatin (Zocor) 10 mg PO qhs-bid with meals; max 40 mg /d [5, 10, 20, 40 mg tabs]; most potent agent.
      -Fluvastatin (Lescol) 20-40 mg PO qhs at bedtime, max 40 mg/d [20, 40 mg]; least expensive statin.
   5. **Side Effects:** Well tolerated; significant side effects are uncommon. Nausea, fatigue, insomnia, myalgias, headaches; changes in bowel function, skin rashes. Less commonly myopathy and elevations in liver enzymes. Contraindicated in hepatic disease.
   6. **Liver Function Tests:** Should be monitored at 6-8 week intervals during the first 6-12 months of therapy and 3-4 times per year thereafter.
   7. **Drug Interactions:** Warfarin, cimetidine, erythromycin, and gemfibrozil.

E. **Probucol:**
   1. Lowers LDL by 10% but decreases HDL by 17-33%; no effect on triglycerides.
   2. Not recommended because of HDL-cholesterol decrease and prolongation of QT

interval.
- F. **Fibrates:**
  1. Fibric acids are effective triglyceride-lowering drugs. Reduce triglycerides by 20-50% and increase HDL by 10-25% Activates lipoprotein lipase, suppresses fatty acid release from adipose tissue, inhibits hepatic triglyceride synthesis.
  2. Fibrates produce minimal reductions in LDL-cholesterol levels, and are not recommended as primary therapy to lower LDL-cholesterol.
  3. **Dosages:**
     - Gemfibrozil (Lopid) 600 mg PO bid 30 min before meals; max 1200 mg/d [600 mg tabs]
     - Clofibrate (Atromid-S) 500 mg PO qid or 1 gm PO bid [500 mg caps].
  4. **Side Effects:** Cholelithiasis, myositis, nausea, abdominal pain, decreased libido, weight gain, and drowsiness.
  5. Periodically monitor liver function tests. May potentiate the action of warfarin.
- G. **Hormone Replacement Therapy:** Hormone replacement therapy should be used to lower cholesterol in postmenopausal women. Hormone replacement decreases LDL-cholesterol and may increase HDL.

## XI. Monitoring of Drug Therapy
- A. After starting drug therapy, LDL-cholesterol level should be measured in 4-6 weeks, and then again in 3 months.
- B. Drug therapy is usually continued for many years or for life.
- C. If the response to initial drug therapy is not adequate, then switch to another drug, or to a combination of two drugs.
- D. **Combination Drug Therapy for Hypercholesterolemia:**
  1. Bile acid sequestrants may be combined with nicotinic acid, or statins to reduce LDL cholesterol by 40-50%.
  2. Bile acid sequestrants can bind to statins, and these drugs should be taken 2-3 hours after taking cholestyramine or colestipol.

## XII. Drug Treatment of Combined Hyperlipidemia (elevated LDL-cholesterol and elevated triglycerides)
- A. Aim of therapy is to reduce LDL cholesterol, triglycerides, and increase HDL cholesterol.
- B. The first-line drugs are nicotinic acid and the HMG CoA reductase inhibitors.
- C. Bile acid sequestrants are not recommended because they may increase triglycerides.

## XIII. Treatment of Low Plasma Concentrations of High-Density Lipoprotein Cholesterol
- A. Use of drugs solely to increase HDL cholesterol levels is not recommended; however, if low HDL cholesterol coexists with elevations of LDL or triglycerides, a lipid-lowering agent that concurrently raises HDL concentrations should be considered.
- B. **Drugs That Raise HDL Cholesterol:** Fibrates, nicotinic acid, and statins (HMG CoA reductase inhibitors).

## XIV. Drug Treatment of Hypertriglyceridemia
- A. Elevated serum triglycerides are positively correlated with risk for CHD. Triglyceride levels are classified as normal (<200 mg/dL), borderline-high (200-400 mg/dL), high (400-1,000 mg/dL), and very high (>1,000 mg/dL). Those with triglyceride levels in excess of 1,000 mg/dL are at increased risk for acute pancreatitis.
- B. Dietary therapy, weight reduction, alcohol restriction, and physical activity are recommended.
- C. Drug therapy should be considered when dietary therapy has failed to reduce triglycerides to less than 250-450 mg/dL.
- D. When triglycerides are elevated in association with high LDL-cholesterol, the chosen drug should lower LDL-cholesterol and triglycerides.
- E. In nondiabetic patients, nicotinic acid is the drug of first choice; fibrates (gemfibrozil) are a second choice.
- F. For severe hypertriglyceridemia, >800-1000 mg/dL, gemfibrozil is the drug of first choice.

# *Pulmonology*

---

# Asthma

## I. Steps in Asthma Management
A. Beta-agonists are now prescribed on an "as-needed" basis only.
B. Inhaled corticosteroids have a larger role as first-line therapy because of disease-modifying effects.
C. Nonsteroidal anti-inflammatory drugs such as inhaled cromolyn (Intal) are considered alternatives to corticosteroids or an additional safe medication for difficult cases.
D. Theophylline is a second-line therapy, but is still an option for nocturnal asthma and as a means to promote better patient compliance

## II. Treatment of Mild Asthma
A. Asthma is considered mild if cough and wheezing occur no more than 1-2 times a week.
B. **Primary Therapy** consists of as-needed use of inhaled beta agonists bronchodilators for occasional asthma attacks and training on use of inhaler devices.
C. More aggressive therapy with inhaled steroids should be started when patients need large daily doses of beta-agonists for symptomatic relief.
  -Albuterol (Ventolin) aerosol MDI 2 puffs bid-qid prn or powder 200 mcg/capsule inhaled bid-qid prn.
  -Metaproterenol (Alupent, Metaprel) 1-2 puffs bid-qid prn.
  -Pirbuterol (Maxair) MDI 1-2 puffs q4-6h prn.
  -Bitolterol (Tornalate) MDI 2-3 puffs q1-3min initially, then 2-3 puffs q4-8h prn.
  -Fenoterol (Berotec) MDI 3 puffs initially, then 2 puffs bid-qid prn.
  -Salmeterol (Serevent) 2 puffs bid; new long-acting agent prn.

## III. Treatment of Moderate Asthma
A. Asthma is considered moderate if cough and wheezing occur more than 2 times a week, or if there is exercise intolerance or if nocturnal asthma.
B. **First-line Therapy** consists of regular, frequent bronchodilator therapy combined with an anti-inflammatory drug such as an inhaled corticosteroid.
C. **Inhaled Corticosteroids:**
  1. Asthma is an inflammatory process; anti-inflammatory agents are a first line therapy. Steroids have disease-modifying activity, rather than simply promoting symptom control; minimum of side effects.
  2. All patients requiring a beta agonist more than occasionally should be treated with an inhaled corticosteroid agent.
  3. More potent than cromolyn; side effects: upper airway irritation, oropharyngeal Candida, dysphonia. Corticosteroids should be inhaled after bronchodilator.
  Beclomethasone (Beclovent) MDI 2-5 puffs bid-tid.
  Triamcinolone (Azmacort) MDI 2-4 puffs bid-tid.
  Flunisolide (AeroBid) MDI 2-4 puffs bid-tid.
  Budesonide MDI 1-4 puffs bid-tid.
D. **Nonsteroidal Agents:**
  1. Nonsteroidal drugs, such as Cromolyn (Intal), dampen the inflammatory response. Better for maintaining good control in asthma rather than improving uncontrolled attacks. May provoke cough or exacerbate an acute asthma attack.
  2. Nonsteroidal agents represent either an alternative to corticosteroid inhalers or a safe addition to the regimen in a difficult case.
  3. Cromolyn (Intal) diminishes the release of mediators from inflammatory cells and provides prophylaxis against bronchospasm. 2 puffs qid, or powder 20 mg/capsule inhaled qid, or 2 mL nebulized qid.
  4. Nedocromil (Tilade) is structurally unlike cromolyn but has similar and even broader anti-inflammatory effects; 2 puffs qid; dosage may be gradually reduced to bid-tid.

IV. **Treatment of Severe Asthma**
   A. Severe asthma is characterized by daily wheezing and/or a tendency for severe exacerbations (more than three urgent physician or emergency department visits per year).
   B. Maximal doses of inhaled bronchodilating agents plus aerosol corticosteroids or cromolyn should be used; may need to use home nebulized bronchodilator therapy.
   C. **Long-Term, Systemic Corticosteroids:**
      1. Use in the lowest effective dosage (alternate days when possible).
      2. Short-term oral therapy is the most effective method of treating refractory asthma; more effective when instituted early.
      3. Prednisone 40 mg PO qd for one week, followed by tapering over 7-14 days. [5, 10, 20, 50 mg].
   D. **Theophylline:**
      1. Theophylline is a second-line therapy with only mild bronchodilating properties.
      2. **Side Effects:** Nausea, headache, insomnia, tremor, arrhythmias, and seizures.
      3. Serum levels are affected by cimetidine, ciprofloxacin, erythromycin, and calcium channel blockers. Increasing age increases risk for toxicity.
      4. Theophylline sustained release (Theo-Dur, Elixophyllin, Uniphyl) PO 100-400 mg PO bid [100, 200, 300, 450 mg].
   E. **Nontraditional Agents:**
      1. **Antihistamines:** Newer, more potent antihistamines such as terfenadine (Seldane) and astemizole (Hismanal) inhibit bronchospasm, and may be useful for seasonal, allergic type asthma.
      2. **Calcium Channel Blockers:** May reduce bronchoconstriction after exercise, and should be considered for hypertension control in asthmatic patients (in whom beta-blockers are contraindicated).
      3. **Cytotoxic Agents:** Methotrexate may be considered as additional therapy for severe asthma when large doses of prednisone have been unable to control the disease.

V. **Emergency Treatment of Asthma**
   A. Albuterol (Ventolin) nebulized, 2.5 mg in 3 mL saline q20min initially, then q2-8h.
   B. Administer every 20 minutes for one hour, then clinically assess with a portable peak flow meter.
   C. If no improvement within one hour, administer an intravenous corticosteroid. Methylprednisolone (Solu-Medrol) 40-125 mg IV q6h.

VI. **Other Factors Affecting Response to Therapy**
   A. **Allergies** contribute to asthma in many patients. Allergy shots are effective in selected patients.
   B. **Environmental Irritants:** Second-hand tobacco smoke; wood-burning stoves, perfume, room deodorizers, insect sprays, cooking odors, household cleaning products; outdoor air pollutants (ozone and sulfur dioxide).
   C. **Chronic Sinusitis** may be an asthma trigger. Computed tomographic (CT) scans of the sinuses are superior to standard sinus radiographs.
   D. **Gastroesophageal Reflux** may exacerbate asthma by stimulating parasympathetic output. Theophylline may exacerbate gastroesophageal reflux.
   E. **Viral infections** often trigger asthma exacerbations; early aggressive treatment of asthma exacerbations lessens severity.
   F. **Spacer Devices** (Aerochamber, InspirEase) may dramatically improve the effectiveness of inhaler therapy by increasing the amount of drug reaching the lungs. Rinsing the mouth and throat with water after inhaling corticosteroids reduces candida infections.
   G. **Portable Peak Flow Meters:** Used for monitoring asthma status in the office and in the home. A drop in peak flow to less than 80% of the patient's personal best indicates less than optimal control. A peak flow rate that is below 50% of patient's personal best requires urgent medical attention. Pulmonary function testing should also be used to document airway disease.

# Chronic Obstructive Pulmonary Disease

## Pathogenesis

A. Emphysema and chronic bronchitis are the main disease states in chronic obstructive pulmonary disease, although there is usually significant overlap between the two conditions. Smoking is the single overwhelming risk factor for the development of COPD.

B. **Emphysema** is characterized by permanent enlargement of alveolar air spaces with destruction of the alveolar walls.

C. **Chronic Bronchitis** is defined as chronic sputum production and variable degrees of airway obstruction for more than 3 months in each of 3 successive years.

## Diagnosis of Chronic Obstructive Pulmonary Disease

A. Symptoms are often insidious and may be manifest early by exercise intolerance only; later symptoms include wheezing, dyspnea, chronic cough, sputum production, recurrent pneumonias, bronchitis.

B. **Signs:** Wheezing, decreased air movement in the chest, hyperinflation, prolonged expiratory time, barrel chest, and supraclavicular retractions.

C. **Pulmonary Function Testing:**

1. Significant airway obstruction is present when the forced expiratory volume in 1 sec (FEV1) is less than 80% of predicted, and the FEV1/Forced Vital Capacity ratio is less than 70% of predicted.

2. Hyperinflated lungs are indicated by increased total lung capacity and residual volume, and by loss of alveolar surface area and decreased diffusing capacity.

## Management Of Chronic Obstructive Pulmonary Disease

A. **Smoking Cessation** is effective in halting the progression of chronic obstructive pulmonary disease.

B. **Beta Agonists:**

1. **Beta2-adrenergic Agonist** should be used for occasional "as needed" use for symptom relief.

2. **Side Effects:** Tremor, nervousness, tachycardia, hypokalemia in higher doses.

3. **Dosages:**

   a. Albuterol (Ventolin), aerosol MDI 2-3 puffs tid-qid prn, or powder 200 mcg/capsule inhaled qid prn.

   b. Metaproterenol (Alupent, Metaprel) 2-3 puffs tid-qid prn.

   c. Pirbuterol (Maxair) MDI 1-2 puffs tid-qid prn.

   d. Bitolterol (Tornalate) MDI 2-3 puffs tid-qid prn.

   e. Fenoterol (Berotec) MDI 3 puffs initially, then 2 puffs bid-qid prn.

   f. Salmeterol (Serevent) 2 puffs bid; long-acting agent; useful for nocturnal COPD; not effective for acute exacerbates because of slow onset of action.

4. **Technique for Usage of Metered Dose Inhalers:**

   a. Invert and shake inhaler briskly with the opening downward.

   b. Hold inhaler 2 fingerbreadths in front of open mouth.

   c. Exhale normally to functional residual capacity.

   d. Inhale slowly and deeply to total lung capacity.

   e. Hold breath for 10 seconds.

   f. Exhale slowly. Wait 3-5 minutes and repeat.

C. **Anticholinergic Agent:**

1. **Ipratropium bromide (Atrovent):** 2-6 puffs qid or nebulized qid. Does not have systemic, atropine-like side effects because it is not absorbed from the respiratory mucosa

2. Should be used regularly with a beta agonist for most patients with COPD.

D. **Corticosteroids:**

1. Effect in COPD is less pronounced than in asthma. Most beneficial during exacerbations; only a small percentage (10-20%) of outpatients with COPD respond to corticosteroids.

2. Aerosolized corticosteroids provide the benefits of oral corticosteroids with fewer side effects. Oropharyngeal candidiasis can be prevented by using proper technique and by rinsing throat with water after use.
   Beclomethasone (Beclovent) MDI 2-5 puffs tid-qid.
   Triamcinolone (Azmacort) MDI 2-4 puffs bid-qid.
   Flunisolide (AeroBid, AeroBid-mint) MDI 2-4 puffs bid.
   Budesonide MDI 1-2 puffs bid.
   Dexamethasone Sodium Phosphate (Decadron Respihaler) 1-3 puffs q6-8h.
3. Oral steroids are warranted in severe COPD. Prednisone 0.5-1.0 mg/kg or 40 mg may be given qAM. An improvement in FEV1 of 20% after a 2 week trial is indicative of enough improvement to warrant long-term treatment. The dose should be tapered over 1-2 weeks following clinical improvement.
4. **Side Effects of Corticosteroids:** Cataracts, osteoporosis, sodium and water retention, hypokalemia, muscle weakness, aseptic necrosis of femoral and humeral heads, peptic ulcer disease, pancreatitis, endocrine and skin abnormalities, muscle wasting.

E. **Theophylline:**
   1. Theophylline is not a potent bronchodilator, and probably offers little additional bronchodilation when added to inhaled agents; should be used only after adequate doses of beta2-agonists, ipratropium, and corticosteroids have been tried.
   2. Narrow therapeutic range. Adverse drug interactions occur with ciprofloxacin, erythromycin, cimetidine, calcium channel blockers.
   3. **Side Effects:** Nausea, restlessness, ventricular arrhythmias, seizures, insomnia, headaches. Avoid caffeine because it may contribute to side effects.
   4. **Usual starting dose of long-acting theophylline:** 200-300 mg bid. Theophylline preparations with 24 hour action may be administered once a day in the early evening Useful for nocturnal or morning dyspnea.

IV. **Treatment of Complications of COPD**
   A. **Infection:**
      1. Infection frequently causes bronchitis exacerbations, and is associated with increased or purulent sputum, increased cough, chest congestion and discomfort, and increased dyspnea and wheezing. Chills and fever suggest pneumonia. Acute bacteria episodes tend to be seasonal, appearing more frequently in winter.
      2. **Gram's Stain:**
         a. Gram stain is a useful guide in the selection of an empiric antibiotic.
         b. First confirm that the specimen is sputum and not saliva; the presence of more than 25 neutrophils and fewer than 10 epithelial cells per low-power field is indicative of sputum.
         c. The presence of bacteria on high-power examination of such a specimen is presumptive evidence of infection. Although patients with COPD can be colonized by influenzae and pneumoniae, these organisms should not be present in sufficient numbers to be seen on a Gram stain.
      3. Sputum culture and sensitivity testing are generally not necessary but may be required if the patient is very ill or if the infection is hospital-acquired.
      4. A chest film is helpful in ruling out pneumonia or other disorders.
      5. The primary pathogens for COPD exacerbations include H influenzae, parainfluenzae, S pneumoniae, and Moraxella catarrhalis. Other less common pathogens are staphylococci, Neisseria, Klebsiella, and Pseudomonas.
      6. **Treatment of Exacerbations of COPD:**
         a. The selected antimicrobial agent should have good in vitro activity against the primary causative pathogens: Haemophilus species, S pneumoniae, and M catarrhalis, and not be hydrolyzed by beta-lactamase.
         b. Treat 7-10 days.
            Trimethoprim/Sulfamethoxazole (Septra DS) 160/800 mg PO bid.
            Amoxicillin/clavulanate (Augmentin) 500 mg PO tid [250, 500 mg]; stable against beta lactamases; gastrointestinal side effects (diarrhea) are common.

Cefuroxime axetil (Ceftin), 250-500 mg bid; good activity against primary pathogens; stable to beta lactamase.

Cefixime (Suprax), 400 mg qd; stable to beta lactamase, lacks Staphylococcus aureus coverage.

Loracarbef (Lorabid), 400 mg bid; moderate activity against beta-lactamase-producing strains of H influenzae.

Doxycycline (Vibramycin), 100 mg bid; not affected by beta-lactamase producers, S pneumoniae resistance in 10%-20%.

Azithromycin (Zithromax), 500 mg on day 1, then 250 mg PO qd; reserved for treatment of infections due to Mycoplasma, Chlamydia, Legionella species.

Clarithromycin (Biaxin), 250-500 mg bid; moderate activity against H influenzae.

Erythromycin, 250-500 mg qid; inexpensive; poor activity against H influenzae; raises theophylline levels.

## B. Preventive Care:

1. Evaluate tuberculosis exposure status using PPD skin testing, and treat if positive. Future corticosteroid therapy may activate latent tuberculosis.

2. Influenza therapy should be given promptly after influenza exposure; Amantadine (Symmetrel) 100 mg PO bid (qd if >65 years old). Rimantadine (Flumadine) 100 mg PO bid (qd if >65 years old).

3. **Long-Term Antibiotic Therapy** should be considered in patients with repeated respiratory infections. Rotating antibiotics may be helpful in decreasing bacterial resistance.

4. **Immunization:** Pneumococcal vaccination every six years, and yearly influenza vaccinations should be provided.

## C. Cor Pulmonale:

1. Severe COPD may cause right-sided heart failure secondary to pulmonary hypertension resulting from chronic hypoxia. Patients with moderate to severe airflow obstruction (FEV1 <1.25 L) should have an arterial blood gas measurement on room air.

2. Diuretics are used to decrease edema. Ischemia and other causes of heart failure should be excluded.

3. **Oxygen Therapy:**
   a. Reduces dyspnea and hypoxia; prolongs life and prevents complications.
   b. Criteria for Long-Term Oxygen Therapy:
      (1) Resting pAO2 of 55 mm Hg or less **or** pAO2 level between 56-59 mm Hg and secondary changes of tissue hypoxemia, such as a hematocrit level >55%, or cor pulmonale are present.
      (2) COPD confirmed by pulmonary function tests.
      (3) Maximal medical therapy in a stable outpatient.
   c. Use the lowest oxygen liter flow possible to raise pAO2 to 60-65 mm Hg or oxygen saturation to 90-94%; increase baseline flow by one liter per minute during exercise and sleep. Oxygen should be administered at least 12 hours daily, but continuous use is more effective.

## D. Breathing Training:

1. **Diaphragmatic Breathing:** The patient places one hand on the abdomen and inhales. Diaphragmatic contraction during inspiration causes the abdomen to move outward.

2. **Pursed-lip Breathing:** Exhale slowly for 10 seconds against the slight resistance created by tightly pursing the lips. Oxygenation may be improved; dyspnea is reduced in about 50%.

3. Daily stationary cycling or walking should be advised. Patients may need increased oxygen supplementation during activity.

## E. Surgical Options:

1. Single or bilateral lung transplantation has proven to be effective therapy for severe emphysema.

2. Surgical removal of an emphysematous bulla occupying one-third or more of the hemithorax can ameliorate symptoms and improve pulmonary function.

# Bronchitis

## I. Pathogenesis of Acute Bronchitis
  A. Acute Bronchitis is an inflammatory reaction of the tracheobronchial tree usually caused by viral infection.
  B. Usually a self-limiting illness that lasts 1-2 weeks, occurring mostly during the winter months. Environmental factors, such as cold and damp weather, pollution, cigarette smoke may worsen attacks.
  C. Acute bronchitis is usually caused by viruses, and it is only occasionally caused by bacteria. The most common viral causes are influenza virus, adenovirus, rhinovirus, coronavirus, parainfluenza virus, respiratory syncytial virus, and coxsackievirus.
  D. Bacteria that may rarely cause acute bronchitis include Mycoplasma pneumoniae, Chlamydia pneumoniae (TWAR), Streptococcus pneumoniae, H influenzae, and Moraxella catarrhalis.

## II. Diagnosis
  A. Acute bronchitis usually presents as an acute productive cough, low-grade temperature, and no evidence of pneumonia.
  B. Sputum culture is rarely indicated.

## III. Treatment of Acute Bronchitis
  A. Although acute bronchitis is usually a self-limiting disease, antimicrobial treatment may be justified in some high risk patients to avoid disease progression. Drug selection should be based on coverage of M pneumoniae, S pneumoniae, and H influenzae.
  B. **Treatment of Acute Bronchitis:**
    1. Erythromycin base (Eramycin) 250-500 mg PO qid [250, 500 mg].
    2. Trimethoprim/Sulfamethoxazole (Septra DS) 160/800 mg PO bid.
    3. Doxycycline (Vibramycin) 100 mg PO bid [50, 100 mg].
    4. Azithromycin (Zithromax) and clarithromycin (Biaxin) have enhanced activity against H influenzae and are active against atypical pathogens that cause lower respiratory tract infections, such as Mycoplasma, Chlamydia, and Legionella.
       a. Clarithromycin (Biaxin) 250-500 PO bid 7-10 days [250, 500 mg].
       b. Azithromycin (Zithromax) 500 mg PO x 1 dose, then 250 mg PO qd x 4 days [250, 500 mg].
    5. The newer beta-lactam antibiotics, such as amoxicillin/clavulanate (Augmentin), are not active against Mycoplasma pneumoniae.
    6. Fluoroquinolones have a relatively poor coverage against S pneumoniae making them a poor choice for first-line therapy.

# Allergic Rhinitis

## I. Clinical Evaluation of Allergic Rhinitis

A. **Signs and Symptoms:** Allergic rhinitis is characterized by repetitive sneezing, rhinorrhea, nasal congestion, pruritic eyes, ears, nose, or throat. Chronic cough (postnasal drip) and sinus headaches may occur. Symptoms may be perennial and/or seasonal in onset.

B. **Aggravating Factors** may include freshly cut grass, dust, dampness, leaves, animals. Precipitating factors at home, work or school may be present.

C. **Physical Examination:**
1. Thoroughly examine eyes, ears, nose, throat, neck, and lungs.
2. **Nasal Mucosa** will appear pale and boggy, with serous secretions, edematous turbinates.
3. Patients may exhibit darkening under their eyes (allergic shiners) or a nasal crease under nose from rubbing.

## II. Diagnostic Testing

A. Skin testing with the prick method can confirm allergic rhinitis. Long-acting antihistamines will interfere with skin testing.

B. IgE levels are not helpful in the diagnosis of allergic rhinitis.

C. Sinus X-rays may be necessary to exclude sinusitis.

## III. Differential Diagnosis of Rhinitis

A. **Allergic Rhinitis:** Seasonal or perennial

B. **Vasomotor Rhinitis:** Vasoconstriction mediated

C. **Infectious Rhinitis:** Viral, bacterial, fungal

D. **Rhinitis Medicamentosa:** Topical decongestant overuse, beta blockers

E. **Anatomic Obstructive Rhinitis:** Septal deviation, tumors, nasal polyps, adenoid hypertrophy

## IV. Treatment of Allergic Rhinitis

A. **Allergen Avoidance Measures:**
1. Close windows and use air conditioners, and avoid lawn mowing or leaf raking. Place dust-proof covers over pillows and mattress; dust frequently with a damp cloth and frequently clean flooring. Maintain indoor humidity below 50%.
2. Killing of dust mites with acaricides is effective. Animals should be kept outdoors; indoor pets should be bathed once a week.
3. High-efficiency particulate air (HEPA) cleaners are effective. Electronic cleaners are less expensive and are installed in central furnace.

B. **Antihistamines:**
1. Second-generation agents have few side effects and are non-sedating. Rarely may cause Torsade de pointes ventricular tachycardia, leading to cardiac arrest. Concurrent administration with ketoconazole or macrolides causes prolongation of QT interval and should be avoided.
2. Patients with impaired liver function, known cardiac arrhythmias, or those taking erythromycin, clarithromycin (Biaxin), azithromycin (Zithromax), fluconazole (Diflucan), or ketoconazole (Nizoral), should avoid using second-generation antihistamines.
3. Terfenadine (Seldane), 60 mg PO bid [60 mg] or Seldane-D (terfenadine/pseudoephedrine) one tab bid.
4. Astemizole (Hismanal) 30 mg PO qd x 1 day, then 20 mg PO qd x 1 day, then 10-20 mg PO qd [10 mg]. Onset of effect may be delayed by 2-3 days.
5. Loratadine (Claritin) one tab PO qd [10 mg]. Not associated with Torsades de Pointes arrhythmias.

C. **Decongestants:**
1. Frequent administration of topical decongestants may result in tachyphylaxis and

decreased efficacy. If used for a week or longer, rebound nasal congestion results when discontinued (rhinitis medicamentosa). Rarely, exacerbation of hypertension, cardiac arrhythmias, or urinary obstruction can occur. Use of topical decongestants is appropriate only on a short-term basis to "open up" the nasal passages to allow other topical medications access into the nasal cavity.

-Pseudoephedrine (Sudafed) 60 mg PO tid [tabs: 30, 60 mg; sustained release caps: 120 mg] **OR** topical spray 0.25-0.5% 1-2 sprays q4h.

-Phenylpropanolamine (Entex) 25 mg PO q4h [25, 50 mg] or Entex SR 75 mg PO q12h [75 mg].

-Oxymetazoline (Nafrine) (0.5%) 2-3 drops or sprays in each nostril qd-tid.

D. **Topical Nasal Corticosteroids:**
1. Topical nasal steroids are comparable in efficacy. Aqueous solutions, such as Vancenase AQ or Beconase AQ, may be more soothing to nasal tissues and cause less irritation and epistaxis.

   -Nasalide (flunisolide): Two sprays bid

   -Nasacort (triamcinolone acetonide): Two sprays qd-bid

   -Vancenase AQ (beclomethasone): Two sprays bid

   -Vancenase Pocket haler (beclomethasone): 1 spray tid

   -Beconase AQ (beclomethasone): 2 sprays bid

   -Beconase aerosol (beclomethasone): 1 spray tid

2. Corticosteroids are safe and effective, but may occasionally cause nasal irritation, burning, bloody nasal discharge. If nosebleeds occur, the patient should discontinue the steroid nasal spray for a week, substitute a saline spray, and apply petroleum jelly with a cotton swab. An aqueous preparation should be used if nosebleeds occur. Rare but serious complications include nasal septal perforation, candidiasis, and cataracts.

E. **Nasal Cromolyn:**
1. Delayed onset of action, short duration of activity (used four times or more a day), high cost, and inferior efficacy compared with steroids are disadvantages.

   -Cromolyn (Nasalcrom) 1 puff in each nostril q3-4h.

   -Cromoglycate (Rynacrom) 1 spray in each nostril 4-6 x daily.

F. **Saline nose sprays** such as Ocean Nasal Mist and NaSal can be helpful in moisturizing nasal tissues and dislodging mucus.

G. **Immunotherapy with Allergy Injections:**
1. **Indications for Immunotherapy:** Severe symptoms present for more than a few months of the year when medication and avoidance measures have not been effective.

2. Allergy injections reduce symptoms in 90%; however, they are expensive and inconvenient.

# Infectious Diseases

## Pneumonia

I. **Diagnostic Evaluation**
   A. Attempt to categorize the illness as a Typical bacterial pneumonia or an Atypical pneumonia based on history, physical exam, and x-ray changes. Gram's stain of expectorated sputum should be completed.
   B. **Atypical Pneumonia** is defined as pneumonia for which none of the usual bacterial causes are evident. Systemic complaints are more prominent than respiratory complaints, especially gastrointestinal symptoms. The patient does not appear acutely ill, there is an insidious onset rather than abrupt onset, and a non-productive cough. Hilar or segmental lower lobe infiltrates are seen on chest films.
   C. **Typical vs. Atypical Community-Acquired Pneumonia:**

| | Typical | Atypical |
|---|---|---|
| Symptom Onset | Sudden | Gradual |
| Rigors | Common | Uncommon |
| Fever | High | Low-grade |
| Cough | Productive | Paroxysmal, nonproductive |
| Sputum | Purulent | Mucoid (if present) |
| Chest congestion | Common | Uncommon |
| Sputum | Neutrophils | Mononuclear cells |
| Gram's stain | Abundant bacteria | Rare bacteria |
| White blood cell count | Elevated, left shift | Normal |
| Chest x-ray | Consolidation | Patchy infiltrate |

   D. **Pathogens Causing Community Acquired Pneumonia in Adults:**
      1. Streptococcus pneumoniae (most common cause), H. influenzae (especially if underlying lung disease), Mycoplasma pneumoniae, oral anaerobes (aspiration pneumonia), and, less commonly, Staphylococcus aureus and gram negative bacilli or viruses.
      2. Moraxella catarrhalis may cause respiratory infection. Legionella species and Chlamydia pneumoniae (TWAR) are linked to a significant number of cases.
      3. P carinii pneumonia and other opportunistic pathogens are often associated with HIV infection. Tuberculosis has been seen increasingly (especially in AIDS).
      4. **Conditions Predisposing to Specific Pathogens:**

| Condition | Common Pathogens: |
|---|---|
| Alcoholism | Oral anaerobes, gram-negative bacilli, S pneumoniae |
| Nursing home residency | S pneumoniae, gram-negative bacilli, H influenzae |
| COPD | H influenzae, S pneumoniae, Moraxella catarrhalis |
| Influenza | Influenza virus, S pneumoniae, Staph aureus |
| Poor dental hygiene | Oral anaerobes |
| Travel | Endemic mycoses |
| Exposure to birds | Chlamydia psittaci |
| HIV infection | Pneumocystis carinii, S pneumoniae, H influenzae, M tuberculosis |

II. **Diagnostic Studies**
   A. **Chest Radiography:**
      1. Useful for differentiating bronchitis and pneumonia, outpatients should receive an x-ray if they have an ill appearance, immunocompromised, failure to respond to initial treatment, or if diagnostic precision is required.
      2. If no infiltrate is seen on x-ray, pneumonia is virtually excluded, even for dehydrated, elderly patients. Infiltrates may not be detected in 10-15% of AIDS patients with P carinii pneumonia.

B. **Gram's Stain and Culture:**
1. Squamous epithelial cells in large numbers suggests that the specimen is contaminated with upper respiratory secretions; specimen should have <10 squamous epithelial cells per low power field. WBC's indicate a lower respiratory source of sputum.
2. Sputum culture reports should always be interpreted in light of the Gram stain results.

C. **Blood Cultures** can occasionally provide additional diagnostic information in hospitalized patients, particularly in HIV infected patients.

D. **Specialized Tests:**
1. Acid-fast stain and culture for tuberculosis.
2. Specific tests for Legionella pneumophila, fungi, viruses
3. **Serologic tests:** Complement fixation (M pneumoniae), ELISA (IgM and IgA) for M pneumoniae.
4. Indirect fluorescent antibody test (L pneumophila); microimmunofluorescence (Chlamydia pneumoniae)
5. Testing for viruses, fungi, Coxiella burnetii, Chlamydia psittaci, direct special stains (Pneumocystis carinii).
6. Urinary antigen test (L pneumophila)

## III. Outpatient Management of Pneumonia

A. **Treatment of Atypical Pneumonia:**
Erythromycin, 500 mg PO qid; not effective for pneumonia caused by H influenzae.
Clarithromycin (Biaxin), 500 mg bid
Azithromycin (Zithromax), 500 mg PO x 1 dose, then 250 mg PO qd x 4 days [250, 500 mg].
Ofloxacin (Floxin), 200-400 mg PO bid
Doxycycline (Vibramycin, Vibra-Tabs), 100 mg PO bid; most strains of S pneumoniae and H influenzae are susceptible to doxycycline.

B. **Treatment of Typical Pneumonia:**
Community-acquired pneumonia is more likely to be caused by H influenzae or S pneumoniae and less likely to be caused by M pneumoniae.
Cefuroxime axetil (Ceftin), 500 mg PO bid.
Cefpodoxime (Vantin), 200 mg q12h
Loracarbef (Lorabid), 400 mg PO bid.
Amoxicillin/clavulanate (Augmentin) 500 mg tid, plus erythromycin or other macrolide. Amoxicillin/clavulanate is effective against S pneumoniae, H influenzae, and M catarrhalis. Erythromycin is necessary because ampicillin/clavulanate does not cover M pneumoniae, L pneumophila, and C pneumoniae.
**Allergy to Penicillin:** Trimethoprim-sulfamethoxazole (TMP-SMZ) one DS tab bid or doxycycline 100 mg bid.

## IV. Inpatient Management

A. **Hospitalized Patients with Community-Acquired Pneumonia** should receive a second or third-generation cephalosporin or beta-lactam/beta-lactamase inhibitor (Unasyn) plus erythromycin. If methicillin-resistant S aureus is prevalent, vancomycin may be added.

B. The beta-lactamase inhibitor combinations, ampicillin/sulbactam (Unasyn) or ticarcillin clavulanate (Timentin), provide excellent coverage for anaerobes as well as traditional bacterial pathogens.
-Erythromycin 500 mg IV q6h **AND/OR**
-Cefuroxime (Zinacef) 1.5 gm IV q8h **OR**
-Cefotaxime (Claforan) 1-2 gm IV q8 **OR**
-Ceftriaxone (Rocephin) 1-2 gm IV q12h **OR**
-Ceftizoxime (Cefizox) 1-2 gm IV q8-12h **OR**
-Cefuroxime (Zinacef) 0.75-1.5 gm IV q8h **OR**
-Trimethoprim/Sulfamethoxazole (Septra DS) 6-10 mg TMP/kg/d IV in 2-3 divided doses **OR**
-Ampicillin/Sulbactam (Unasyn) 1.5 gm IV q6h. **OR**

-Ticarcillin/clavulanate (Timentin) 3.1 gm IV q4-6h (200-300 mg/kg/d). **OR**
-Piperacillin/Tazobactam (Zosyn) 3.375 gm IV q6h. **OR**
-Imipenem/cilastatin (Primaxin) 0.5-1.0 gm IV q6-8h.

# Tuberculosis

## I. Pathophysiology of Tuberculosis

A. In most individuals initially infected with mycobacterium tuberculosis (usually b respiratory aerosols), the primary pulmonary infection occurs early in life, and th organism is contained by host defenses. The primary infection usually resemble pneumonia or bronchitis, and the infection usually resolves without treatment.

B. Later in life, the organism may escape immunological control and cause reactivatic disease, usually pulmonary, but many anatomic sites can be involved (genitourinar system, bones, joints, meninges, brain, peritoneum, and the pericardium).

## II. Risk Factors for Tuberculosis

A. Infection with human immunodeficiency virus (HIV) is the most important risk factor f development of tuberculosis.

B. Elderly residents of long-term care facilities are at risk for reactivation of tuberculosis an for primary tuberculosis from nosocomial transmission.

C. Household and close contacts of TB infected patients and recent PPD converters are risk.

D. Prolonged steroid therapy, immunosuppressive therapy, diabetes mellitus, silicosis, rap weight loss or malnutrition, malignancy, hemodialysis also are risk factors.

## III. Diagnosis of Active Tuberculosis

A. Diagnosis of active tuberculosis rests upon sputum examination for acid fast bacilli an subsequent culture of the specimen to identify antibiotic sensitivities. This proces requires 4-6 weeks for identification and another 4-6 weeks for sensitivity testing.

B. Sensitivity testing is more rapid with DNA polymerase chain reaction (PCR); however, thi test is not yet available.

C. Tuberculosis is often the initial manifestation of HIV infection; serologic testing for HIV i recommended in all tuberculosis patients. Tuberculosis in HIV-infected patients characterized by extrapulmonary disease in 70% of patients.

## IV. Treatment of Active Tuberculosis

A. Suspected TB should be treated with a 4 drug combination as empiric therapy due to th high rates of drug resistance.

B. The four-drug regimen consists of Isoniazid (INH), rifampin, pyrazinamide (PZA), an either ethambutol or streptomycin. A modified regimen is recommended for patient known to have INH-resistant TB.

C. All patients diagnosed with TB now must be treated with the four-drug regimen for weeks, followed by 18 weeks of INH and rifampin.

D. The same approach should be used in both HIV-positive and HIV-negative patients.

E. If multi-drug resistant TB (resistant to both INH and RIF) is encountered, therapy shoul be more prolonged and guided by antibiotic sensitivities and repetitive sputum culture:

F. Vitamin B6 (pyridoxine) should be added for malnourished patients taking INH.

G. Directly observed therapy, usually on a twice per week basis, should be instituted situations where compliance is questioned.

## H. Drugs Used in Chemotherapy of TB

| | | |
|---|---|---|
| Isoniazid | 5-10 mg/kg (300 mg) | hepatitis, peripheral neuropathy |
| Rifampin | 10-15 mg/kg (600 mg) | hepatitis, purpura |
| Pyrazinamide | 25 mg/kg (max 2 g) | hepatotoxicity, skin rash |
| Ethambutol | 15-25 mg/kg (max 2.5 g) | Retrobulbar neuritis, skin rash |

I. Rifamate is a combination capsule of 150 mg of isoniazid and 300 mg of rifampin.

J. **Monitoring During Therapy:**

1. Symptoms improve within 4 weeks, and sputum cultures become negative within months in patients receiving effective antituberculosis therapy. Delayed resolution symptoms or persistently positive cultures indicate noncompliance or drug-resistance

2. Sputum cultures should be obtained monthly until they are negative and also after completion of therapy. Obtain a chest x-ray after 2-3 months, and after completion of treatment to assess efficacy and to provide a baseline for comparison in the event of relapse.

K. **Monitoring for Drug Toxicity:**
   1. Isoniazid, rifampin, and pyrazinamide are potentially hepatotoxic.
   2. If transaminase levels increase to more than 5 times the upper limit of normal, isoniazid, rifampin, and pyrazinamide should be discontinued and alternative agents substituted.
   3. Optic neuritis can result from ethambutol.

## Skin Testing for Tuberculosis

A. Skin testing with purified protein derivative (PPD) has limited usefulness in determining the presence of active disease, but is more useful in detecting patients who are harboring latent tuberculosis who may need "prophylactic" therapy.

B. A reactive tuberculin skin test supports the diagnosis of tuberculosis, but it is not specific.

C. The skin test should be performed with controls and should utilize 5 tuberculin units in an intradermal injection. The test is read at 48 hrs and must be interpreted in combination with clinical and historical information. For example, a HIV positive individual has a positive PPD if 5 mm of induration is present, while a patient without other risk factors has a positive PPD only if 15 mm or more of induration is present.

D. If fluid leaks out of the blister, the test should be repeated. A ball point pen may be used to assess the amount of induration by tracing inward until the induration is encountered.

E. **The booster phenomenon** is seen in older individuals who may have been PPD positive for many years, but whose reaction wanes with time. If the individual is tested now, the PPD may be falsely negative, but if this patient is immediately retested, the immune system will have been boosted, and the true PPD positive status will become apparent. This phenomenon can be obviated by re-testing PPD negative individuals in 1-4 weeks. A positive test at that time interval could be attributed to the booster phenomenon and is indicative of infection with tuberculosis.

F. A history of vaccination with bacille Calmette-Guerin should be ignored in interpreting the results of tuberculin skin testing, because skin test reactivity from the vaccine declines by adulthood.

G. A negative tuberculin skin test and a positive control skin test makes the diagnosis of tuberculosis unlikely. Failure to react to control skin tests suggests anergy.

## Chemoprophylaxis

A. Chemoprophylaxis with isoniazid (INH) greatly decreases the likelihood of progression of latent tuberculous infection to active disease.

B. Before administration of chemoprophylaxis, active tuberculosis must be excluded clinically and by chest x-ray because inadvertent use of isoniazid alone in active tuberculosis may induce drug resistance.

C. Prophylaxis with 6-9 months of INH should be considered in the following patients:
   1. Recent skin test converters (within the past 2 years) and close household contacts (who can then be re-tested at 3 months).
   2. Patients with a positive PPD and an abnormal CXR (suggesting latent tuberculosis), patients with a positive PPD who are less than 35 years of age.
   3. Patients who are PPD positive with one of the following:
      a. Prolonged high dose steroid therapy
      b. Immunosuppressive disease
      c. Insulin dependent diabetes mellitus
      d. Rapid weight loss or malnutrition
      e. IV drug use
      f. Dialysis for chronic renal failure.

D. In situations of exposure to INH resistant organisms, prophylaxis may be attempted with RIF and EMB for 12 months.

E. If age greater than 35, liver function tests should be measured initially and monthly wh
on INH.

# Pharyngitis

I. **Prevalence of Pharyngitis**
   A. Group A beta-hemolytic streptococcus (GABHS) is responsible for 10-30% of sore throat cases; typically occurs in patients age 5-11 years and is uncommon in children under 3.
   B. Acute rheumatic fever is a complication of GABHS pharyngitis. Severe infections may cause a toxic-shock-like illness (toxic strep syndrome), GABHS bacteremia, streptococcal deep tissue infections (necrotizing fascitis), and streptococcal cellulitis.

II. **Clinical Evaluation of Sore Throat**
   A. **Etiologic Causes of Sore Throat:**
      1. **Viral:** Common cold, influenza, Epstein-Barr
      2. **Bacterial:** Streptococcal (S. pyogenes, S. pneumoniae), Haemophilus influenzae, M. catarrhalis, Staphylococcus aureus, anaerobes, Mycoplasma, fungal, candida albicans
   B. In patients who present with pharyngitis, the major goal is to detect GABHS infection, which has potentially serious medical sequelae.
   C. **Presentation:** Sudden onset of sore throat, fever, and tender swollen anterior cervical lymph nodes, typically in a child 5-11 years of age. Headache, abdominal pain, nausea and vomiting may occur; cough, rhinorrhea and hoarseness are generally absent.
   D. Similar symptoms are often present within the family or in the community.

III. **Physical Examination**
   A. Assess vital signs, especially temperature.
   B. Examine for tympanic membrane erythema and middle ear effusion.
   C. Purulent nasal discharge, especially from the middle meatus, implies sinusitis. Viral infections may cause oral vesicular eruptions.
   D. Streptococcal infection is suggested by erythema and swelling of the pharynx, enlarged and erythematous tonsils, tonsilar exudate, and palatal petechiae.
   E. Unilateral inflammation and swelling suggests peritonsillar abscess. Distortion of the posterior pharyngeal wall indicates retropharyngeal abscess. Corynebacterium diphtheriae is indicated by a dull membrane that bleeds on manipulation.
   F. Palpate the neck for lymph node enlargement; tender nodes usually occur in an acute infection, whereas nontender enlargement indicates chronic infection or tumors.
   G. Auscultate the lungs because viral infection occasionally causes pneumonia.
   H. Examine skin for rashes and petechiae associated with viral infections. Rash of scarlet fever is characterized by a fine, blanching appearance, sandpaper texture; circumoral pallor and hyperpigmentation in the skin creases.
   I. The clinical diagnosis of GABHS infection is correct in only 50-75% of cases when based on clinical criteria alone.

IV. **Diagnostic Testing**
   A. **Rapid Streptococcal Test:** Specificity 90%; sensitivity is 50-90%. A dry swab should include both the posterior wall and the tonsillar fossae, especially erythematous or exudative areas.
   B. **Throat Culture:** Most accurate test available for the diagnosis of GABHS pharyngitis.
   C. If indicated by history, test for Neisseria gonorrhoeae or Corynebacterium diphtheriae.

V. **Diagnosis**
   A. Patients presenting with an acute, severe episode of pharyngitis should receive a rapid streptococcal antigen test, and if negative, a culture should be done.
   B. If the rapid test is positive, treatment with an antibiotic should be initiated for 10 days.
   C. The presence of physical and historical findings suggesting GABHS infection may also prompt the initiation of antibiotic therapy despite a negative rapid strep test.
   D. After throat culture, presumptive therapy should be initiated, pending culture results. If the culture is positive for GABHS, a 10-day course of therapy should be completed. If the

culture is negative, antibiotics may be discontinued. Patients with negative throat cultures should be offered symptomatic measures to alleviate symptoms.

E. Indiscriminate antibiotic use increases the incidence of allergic reactions to antibiotics, and many viral exanthems will be incorrectly attributed to allergic responses to antibiotics. Increased antibiotic use may lead to the emergence of resistant bacterial strains.

F. Starting antibiotic therapy within the first 24-48 hours of illness decreases the duration of sore throat, fever and adenopathy by 12-24 hours, and treatment minimizes risk of transmission and of rheumatic fever.

VI. **Antibiotic Therapy**

A. Penicillin is the antibiotic of choice for GABS. Dosing with oral penicillin twice daily or four times daily is effective. A 10-day regimen is necessary if oral therapy is used. 250 mg PO qid or 500 mg PO bid x 10 days [250, 500 mg].

B. Penicillin G benzathine (Bicillin L-A) may be used as one-time therapy when compliance is a concern. 1.2 million units IM x 1 dose.

C. **Penicillin Allergic Patients:**
-Erythromycin base 250 mg PO qid; or enteric coated delayed release tablet 333 mg PO tid or 500 mg PO bid [250, 333, 500 mg]
-Erythromycin ethyl succinate (EES) 400 PO qid or 800 mg PO  bid [400 mg].

D. **Alternative Agents:**
-Amoxicillin 250-500 mg PO tid
-Clarithromycin (Biaxin), 500 mg PO bid; bacteriologic efficacy similar to that of penicillin VK and may be taken twice a day.
-Cephalexin (Keflex) 250-500 mg PO qid [250, 500 mg].
-Amoxicillin/clavulanate (Augmentin) 250-500 mg PO tid  [250, 500 mg].
-Dicloxacillin 250-500 mg PO qid [125, 250, 500 mg].
-Sulfonamides, trimethoprim, and the tetracyclines are not acceptable for the treatment of GABHS pharyngitis.

VII. **Complications**

A. Complications of GABHS include otitis media, sinusitis, cervical adenitis, retropharyngeal or peritonsillar abscess, acute glomerulonephritis, and acute rheumatic fever.

B. Acute rheumatic fever occurs about 18 days after GABHS pharyngitis in 3% of untreated patients. This illness has not been associated with GABHS skin infections. Antibiotic treatment minimizes the risk of acute rheumatic fever. Therapy may be initiated as late as 9 days after the onset of pharyngitis and still be effective.

C. The development of acute glomerulonephritis can follow GABHS pharyngitis after 10 days or can follow GABHS skin infections after three weeks. Antibiotic treatment does not prevent acute glomerulonephritis.

# Otitis Media

## I. Predisposing Factors for Otitis Media
A. **Biologic Factors:** Adenoid hypertrophy; male gender; family history; congenital anomalies (cleft palate); prematurity or low birth weight.

B. **Environmental:** Exposure to passive smoke; frequent upper respiratory infections.

## II. Pathogenesis and Epidemiology
A. The first episode of otitis media usually occurs after 6 months of age, with the loss of maternal antibody protection. The incidence is highest between 6 months and 3 years of age. Uncommon after age 8.

B. More common among boys. Incidence rises during winter and falls during summer.

C. **Common Pathogens:** Most common bacterial pathogen in all age groups is Streptococcus pneumoniae, causing 40% of effusions. Next most common is non-typable Haemophilus influenzae, causing 20% of effusions; incidence declines with age. Anaerobic bacteria, Chlamydia or Mycoplasma cause less than 2-5%. Viruses are rarely a direct cause of otitis, but may permit bacterial colonization

D. **Pathophysiology:** Recurrent otitis is sometimes the result of eustachian tube dysfunction, which prevents effective drainage. Native Americans have extremely patent tubes and a high incidence of otitis media.

## III. Treatment
A. **First-line Antibiotics:**
1. Oral antibiotics should be prescribed for 10-14 days.
2. **Amoxicillin** is the standard initial treatment for infants and children with acute otitis media; 40 mg/kg/day in divided doses q8h.
3. **Trimethoprim/sulfamethoxazole** (Bactrim, Septra) 8-10 mg/kg/day in divided doses q12h; provides reasonable coverage for S. pneumoniae and H. influenzae, but is less effective against S. pyogenes; toxic reactions include Stevens-Johnson syndrome, renal tubular acidosis, growth failure; may cause rash. Useful if allergic to penicillin.
4. **Erythromycin/sulfisoxazole (Pediazole):** Coverage against H. influenzae and other common pathogens. 50 mg/kg of erythromycin component in 4 divided doses qid; may cause gastric upset and bone marrow suppression.
5. **Oral Cephalosporins** cover beta-lactamase-producing, ampicillin-resistant organisms; highest percentage of complete resolution.
   a. **Cefuroxime axetil (Ceftin)** <2 y: 125 mg PO bid; 2-12 yrs: 250 mg PO bid **OR** >12 yrs: 250-500 mg PO bid, max 500 mg/dose.
   b. **Cefixime (Suprax):** 8 mg/kg in one dose (max 400 mg); pneumococcus response rate is somewhat lower than with other agents.
6. An antipseudomonal antibiotic is the agent of choice for malignant otitis media (caused by Pseudomonas aeruginosa), and for persistent cases of chronic infection.

B. **Second-line Antibiotics:**
1. Second line agent may be used in patients who do not improve within a few days of treatment or if eardrums are still inflamed at 2-4 weeks follow-up.
2. **Amoxicillin/clavulanate (Augmentin)** is useful in settings where B-lactamase organisms are common. 40 mg/kg/day in divided doses q8h.
3. **Loracarbef (Lorabid):** 30 mg/kg in 2 divided doses (max 800 mg) in children 6 months to 12 years; only the liquid form should be used, due to its increased rate of absorption.

C. **Treatment of Difficult Cases:**
1. A 5- to 7-day trial of prednisolone sodium phosphate (Pediapred), 0.5-1.0 mg/kg qd, combined with a 30-day regimen of trimethoprim-sulfamethoxazole may resolve up to 70% of chronic cases. Amoxicillin/clavulanate may also be used.
2. Myringotomy may be used for treatment of otitis media with effusion in both acute and chronic situations. Tubes are reserved for children with bilateral effusions that persist for longer than 90 days with hearing loss and for those with recurrent otitis media,

defined as 3 episodes in 6 months or 4 episodes in 1 year.

D. **Pain Control:** Auralgan Otic Solution with benzocaine and antipyrine helps relieve pain.

E. **Topical Antibiotics:** Tympanic membrane perforation may be treated with topical neomycin sulfate, polymyxin B, and hydrocortisone (Cortisporin Otic) suspensions; neomycin is toxic to the cochlea.

F. **Antibiotic Prophylaxis:**
  1. **Indication:** 3 or more episodes of acute otitis media within a 6 month period or 4 episodes within 12 months.
  2. **Antibiotics of Choice:**
     Amoxicillin, 20 mg/kg qd, or
     Sulfisoxazole (Gantrisin), 75 mg/kg qd at bedtime.
     Trimethoprim-sulfamethoxazole (Bactrim) 5 mg/kg qhs.
  3. Prophylaxis is given for 3-6 months. If seasonally frequent respiratory infections cause otitis, give prophylactic antibiotics during the season.

# Sinusitis

**Clinical Evaluation**

A. **Acute Sinusitis in Adults** is characterized by colored nasal discharge, unilateral facial pain, headache, and cough. Pain associated with acute maxillary sinusitis may radiate to the upper teeth and worsens when the patient bends over.

B. High fever and signs of acute toxicity are unusual except in the most severe cases.

C. Rhinoscopy with a nasal speculum frequently reveals erythematous, swollen, mucous membranes and purulent secretions on the floor of the nasal vault. The presence of mucopus in the external nares or posterior pharynx is highly suggestive of sinusitis. Blockage of sinus drainage may prevent visualization of purulent drainage.

D. Facial tenderness, elicited by percussion, is an unreliable sign of sinusitis.

E. **Transillumination:**
   1. Can help in diagnosing maxillary and frontal sinusitis.
   2. In a completely darkened room, the maxillary sinuses are transilluminated by placing the light over the middle of the inferior orbital rim and watching for transmission of light through the hard palate. The frontal sinuses are visualized by directing the light upwards toward the medial border of the supraorbital ridge and assessing light transmission into the lower forehead.

F. **Complications:** Orbital cellulitis, periorbital abscess, meningitis, chronic otitis media, exacerbation of bronchial asthma; cavernous sinus thrombosis; osteomyelitis, oroantral fistula.

**Chronic Sinusitis**

A. Sinusitis is considered chronic if it persists for longer than 3 months.

B. Present with indolent symptoms of chronic nasal congestion, postnasal drip, and cough. Facial fullness and headache may occur. Reduced taste and smell, and bad breath are frequent.

**Management of Sinusitis**

A. Empiric antibiotic therapy for acute sinusitis should be directed against common sinus pathogens. Streptococcus pneumoniae and Haemophilus influenzae account for more than half of all cases. Moraxella catarrhalis is also an important pathogen in up to 23% of children.

B. Cultures of nasal secretions correlate poorly with results of antral aspiration.

C. **Antibiotic Therapy for Sinusitis**

Amoxicillin (Amoxil): Adults: 500 mg tid orally for 14 days. Children: 40 mg/kg/d in 3 divided doses

Amoxicillin/clavulanate (Augmentin): Adults: 500 mg tid. Children: 40 mg/kg/d in 3 divided doses

Cefuroxime axetil (Ceftin): Adults: 250-500 mg bid. Children: 125-250 mg bid

Cefixime (Suprax): Adults: 200 mg bid. Children: 8 mg/kg/d bid

Loracarbef (Lorabid): Adults: 400 mg bid

Clarithromycin (Biaxin): Adults: 500 mg bid

Erythromycin/sulfisoxazole (Pediazole): Children: 50/150 mg/kg/d qid (maximum: 6 g/d)

Trimethoprim/sulfamethoxazole (Bactrim, Septra): Adults: 160/800 mg bid. Children: 8/40 mg/kg/d bid

D. **Refractory or Difficult Cases:** If response to antibiotics is unsatisfactory, beta-lactamase-producing bacteria are likely to be present, and amoxicillin/potassium clavulanate, erythromycin/sulfisoxazole, trimethoprim-sulfamethoxazole, cefixime, and cefuroxime axetil or newer broad spectrum macrolide antibiotics should be used.

E. **Chronic Sinusitis:** Commonly caused by anaerobic organisms. At least 3 weeks of therapy is required.

F. **Ancillary Treatments:**
   1. **Steam and Saline** improves drainage of mucus. Spray bottle saline (NaSal, Ayr, Ocean, Salinex) or bulb syringe method with saline (1 tsp of salt in 1 qt of warm

water).
2. **Decongestants:**
   a. Topical or systemic decongestants may be used in acute or chronic sinusitis. Prolonged use may result in rhinitis medicamentosa (rebound vasodilation); therefore they should not be used for longer than 3-5 days. Phenylephrine (Neo-Synephrine) or oxymetazoline (Afrin) nasal drops or sprays.
   b. Oral decongestants such as phenylephrine or pseudoephedrine are active in areas not reached by topical agents.

# Infectious Conjunctivitis

I. **Clinical Evaluation of Conjunctivitis**
   A. Infectious conjunctivitis is one of the most common causes of red eye. Infectious conjunctivitis may be sight threatening, such as with infection with herpes simplex or in gonococcal keratoconjunctivitis.
   B. **Symptoms:** Redness, foreign body sensation, itching, burning, tearing, discharge, and eyelid heaviness.
   C. **Significant Visual Loss, Photophobia, or Pain** suggests corneal or intraocular involvement.
   D. **Exposure History:** Recent contact with an individual with red eye indicates possible adenoviral conjunctivitis.
   E. **Systemic Illnesses or Symptoms** suggests viral conjunctivitis (adenovirus, herpes simplex, or infectious mononucleosis).

II. **Examination of the Eye**
   A. Visual acuity for each eye should be tested before examination. Check for eyelid swelling, erythema, discharge. Examine lids, conjunctiva, and cornea. Lid vesicles or ulcers indicate primary herpes simplex conjunctivitis. Examine cornea for poor surface light reflex, infiltrate, ciliary or limbal injection.
   B. **Conjunctivitis with Follicles** suggests viral etiology, usually adenovirus and, occasionally, primary herpes simplex or chlamydia.
   C. **Fluorescein:** Place in the eye following the instillation of a topical anesthetic. Use cobalt blue light to examine the cornea for apple-green areas of fluorescence, indicating abrasion, corneal ulcer, or herpes simplex dendritic corneal lesions.
   D. **Preauricular and Submandibular adenopathy** indicates viral conjunctivitis (adenovirus or herpes simplex), or bacterial conjunctivitis.

III. **Physical Signs of Conjunctivitis**
   **Conjunctival Papillae:** Nonspecific inflammatory response appearing as fine, elevated, polygonal areas of hyperemia.
   **Chemosis:** Swelling of the conjunctiva and hyperemia.
   **Follicles:** Smooth, opalescent elevations of the conjunctival surface, usually 1-2 mm in diameter, with a pebbly appearance; indicative of certain types of viral conjunctivitis.
   **Bacterial Conjunctivitis:** Pseudomembrane or a membrane of exudate may be present.
   **Viral Conjunctivitis:** Almost always accompanied by preauricular adenopathy. The only bacterial agents commonly causing preauricular adenopathy are chlamydia and Neisseria.

IV. **Laboratory Studies**
   A. **Cultures and Gram Stain:** Cultures and gram stain should be performed for neonatal conjunctivitis, and in severe conjunctivitis.
   B. **Normal Flora of the Conjunctiva:** Staphylococcus epidermidis, Diphtheroids, and Staphylococcus aureus may be present on routine culture. Other organisms include S viridans, S pneumoniae, Moraxella, Propionibacterium acnes, Lactobacillus, Eubacterium, and Peptostreptococcus.

V. **Treatment of Bacterial Conjunctivitis**
   A. Bacterial conjunctivitis is characterized by conjunctival hyperemia, lid edema, moderate-to-copious purulent discharge, chemosis, discomfort, and possibly pain. Pseudomembrane or membrane may be present.
   B. Abrupt in onset; symptoms are usually present for less than a week.
   C. **Topical Antibiotics:**
   Bacitracin ointment, apply into affected eye 1-3 times daily.
   Sulfacetamide (Bleph-10, Sulamyd), apply ointment to affected eyes qid and hs or 2 drops into eyes q2h.

Tobramycin (Tobrex), 1-2 drops into affected eyes q1-4h.
Erythromycin, apply ointment to affected eyes q4-6h.
Ciprofloxacin, 1-2 drops into affected eyes q2h while awake for 2 days, then the q4h.
Norfloxacin, 1-2 drops qid.

D. Conjunctivitis due to H. influenzae, N. gonorrhoeae, and N. meningitidis requires systemic antibiotic therapy in addition to topical treatment.

E. **Topical steroids** are not recommended in conjunctivitis because of the risk of potentiating infection.

F. Topical anesthetic agents should not be prescribed for ocular pain because they may cause severe local reactions, permanent scarring, and corneal damage.

G. **Contact Lenses:** Discontinue use of lenses until symptoms and signs have completely resolved. All ocular solutions should be discarded and lenses disinfected. The lenses, or lens solution, may be cultured.

H. **Staphylococcus and Streptococcus:**
   1. Most common pathogen in bacterial conjunctivitis. Infection is common at any age. Characterized by stickiness of the lids on awakening, redness, and foreign body sensation; hyperemia, mild-to-severe papillary response, scant discharge, and fibrin deposits at the base of the lashes.
   2. **Treatment:**
      a. Place warm compresses over the eyes 3-4 times a day for 10 minutes, followed by gentle cleaning of the eyelid crusting with a diluted baby shampoo or eyelid scrub.
      b. **Antibiotic ointments or drops:** Bacitracin, erythromycin, or sulfacetamide applied 4 times daily.

I. **Hemophilus influenzae:**
   1. Common cause of conjunctivitis in children but also occurs in adults.
   2. **Clinical Findings:** Chemosis, hyperemia, and a mucopurulent discharge. In children a bluish periorbital discoloration and swelling may be present. Corneal opacities preseptal or orbital cellulitis may occur. Risk of meningitis.
   3. **Diagnosis:** Gram stain and culture.
   4. **Therapy:** Systemic and topical antibiotics. Topical ciprofloxacin or trimethoprim-polymyxin eye drops. Cool compresses.

J. **Neisseria sp:**
   1. Uncommon cause of conjunctivitis in developed countries. Neisseria gonorrhoeae is the most common pathogen. Often associated with concomitant genital infection, or acquired during birth.
   2. **Symptoms:** Abrupt onset of redness, lid swelling, marked hyperemia, chemosis, and purulent discharge. Membrane or pseudomembrane may be present. Penile or vaginal discharge may be present.
   3. **Diagnosis:** Gram stain (Gram-negative intracellular diplococci) and culture or chocolate agar.
   4. **Systemic and Topical Therapy:**
      **Adults:** Ceftriaxone, 1 g intramuscularly, with frequent topical saline irrigation.
      **Neonates:** Cefotaxime, 25 mg/kg every 8-12 hours for 7 days.
      Also treat presumed chlamydial infection with doxycycline or erythromycin. Rule out genital infection by cultures. Sexual partners and mothers of neonates should be treated.

K. **Chronic Bacterial Conjunctivitis:**
   1. Conjunctivitis has been present for more than 1 month and has an indolent course. S. aureus and Moraxella are frequent pathogens.
   2. Treatment includes lid hygiene, topical antibiotic ointments, and tetracycline, 500 mg tid, or doxycycline, 100 mg PO daily for 1 month.

L. **Chlamydial Conjunctivitis:**
   1. One of the most common causes of blindness worldwide; usually with a concomitant genital infection.
   2. **Symptoms:** Mild-to-moderate lid swelling, mucopurulent discharge, redness, and irritation. Chlamydia may be cultured from scrapings.
   3. **Treatment:** Oral tetracycline 500 mg tid, doxycycline 100 mg bid, or erythromycin 250

mg qid for 3 weeks.

M. **Adenoviral Conjunctivitis:**
  1. Most common type of acute viral conjunctivitis; itching, moderate-to-severe tearing, redness, photophobia; foreign body sensation. Symptoms of upper respiratory tract infection.
  2. Unilateral or bilateral. Recent exposure to red eye at home, school, or work.
  3. **Examination:** Preauricular adenopathy, hyperemia, watery discharge, lid edema, ptosis, follicles, and fine papillae (more commonly lower lid); pseudomembrane or membrane.
  4. **Treatment:** No antiviral agents are effective. Use ice cold compresses and lubricants, such as artificial tears. Topical vasoconstrictors should not be used due to rebounding of symptoms and hypersensitivity. Excuse from work or school for up to 2 weeks to prevent spread.

N. **Herpes simplex:**
  1. A common cause of conjunctivitis in children but rare in adolescents and adults. Usually follicular; less often causing membrane or pseudomembrane. Significant preauricular adenopathy; lid vesicles or ulcers, upper respiratory infection, and gingivostomatitis.
  2. **Topical Antiviral Agents:**
    Idoxuridine solution (Herplex Liquifilm), 1 drop in each infected eye q1h during day and q2h at night.
    Vidarabine ointment (Vira-A), apply ½ inch into lower conjunctival sac 5 times a day at 3 hour intervals.
    Trifluridine solution (Viroptic), 1 drop into affected eyes q2h while awake.

O. **Varicella-zoster Virus:**
  1. Can infect the conjunctiva during chickenpox causing conjunctival ulcerations, or may be a part of herpes zoster ophthalmicus; conjunctivitis always occurs with cutaneous lesions in the trigeminal dermatome; corneal involvement and iritis are frequent.
  2. **Treatment:** Acyclovir, 800 mg PO 5 times daily for 7-10 days.

# Septic Shock

## I. Classification of Sepsis
A. **Sepsis** is a Systemic Inflammatory Response Syndrome (SIRS) in the presence of infection; increases occur in temperature, heart rate, respiratory rate, and white cell count.
B. **Severe Sepsis** is associated with hypoperfusion or hypotension.
C. **Septic Shock** is characterized by hypoperfusion and hypotension that is not responsive to fluids, and requires the use of drugs to maintain arterial pressure.

## II. Clinical Features
A. **Fever** is common, although hypothermia may be observed. Tachypnea and tachycardia occur initially.
B. **Changes in mental status** may be prominent, particularly in the elderly; hypoperfusion is manifested by oliguria, hypoxemia, and lactic acidosis.
C. The majority of patients with septic shock survive their initial resuscitation. Mortality is related to the development of multiple organ failure.
D. Resolution of septic shock is associated with normalization of the hyperdynamic state, marked by an increase in systemic resistance and decreases in heart rate, cardiac output, and arterial lactic acid level.

## III. Labs
A. Leukocytosis or leukopenia, thrombocytopenia; arterial blood gases show mild hypoxemia with a respiratory alkalosis. A metabolic acidosis unrelated to lactic acid accumulation may be present. Hyperglycemia often occurs and may require insulin.
B. Hyperbilirubinemia, minimal transaminase, and alkaline phosphatase elevations are often present due to intrahepatic cholestasis.
C. Cardiac output usually is increased and maintained by an increase in heart rate in the early stages. Systemic vascular resistance is decreased, reflecting decreased arteriolar and venular tone.

## IV. Clinical Approach to Septic Shock
### A. Resuscitation:
1. **Large volumes of fluid** are required to maintain effective venous return. Resuscitation should be guided by hemodynamic measurements. The optimal pulmonary artery wedge pressure is 10-15 mm Hg. Colloid solutions may be associated with a reduced incidence of pulmonary edema.
2. Significant hemodilution may result from the large volumes of fluids, compromising systemic oxygen delivery. A hemoglobin level of 10 g/dL should be maintained. With myocardial ischemia or failure, higher levels of hemoglobin are required.

### B. Vasoactive Drugs:
1. Frequently are required due to myocardial depression and persistent hypotension.
2. **Dopamine** is an inotropic and vasopressor drug used in hypotension; may be used to protect renal flood flow. If hypotension does not respond adequately to dopamine or responds with excessive tachycardia, norepinephrine, a more potent adrenergic agent, may be used to enhance organ perfusion and elevate arterial pressure.
3. **Dobutamine**, a beta1, beta2 adrenergic agent, is an inotrope and vasodilator used primarily to augment cardiac output when hypoperfusion is present.

### C. Oxygenation and Ventilation:
1. The increased work of breathing and respiratory muscle fatigue during sepsis often necessitates ventilatory support.
2. Early initiation of mechanical ventilation enhances peripheral perfusion.

### D. Treatment of Infection:
1. The use of appropriate antibiotics should be dictated by the presumed site of infection.
2. Two drugs should be used, including an aminoglycoside, because of the high incidence of gram-negative infection. There is an increased incidence of gram-positive bacteria in septic shock, particularly with intravascular devices.

3. Failure to respond to appropriate antibiotics may suggest an occult or undrained site of infection.

-Ampicillin 2 gm IV q4h **OR**

-Piperacillin, ticarcillin or mezlocillin 3 gms IV q4-6h **AND**

-Gentamicin or tobramycin 5 mg/kg IV qd; or 100-120 mg (1.5-2 mg/kg) IV, then 80 mg IV q8h (3-5 mg/kg/d) **AND**

-Clindamycin 600-900 IV q8h (15-30 mg/kg/d) **OR**

-Metronidazole 500 mg (7.5 mg/kg) IV q6h **OR**

-Piperacillin/tazobactam (Zosyn) 3.375 gm IV q6h **OR**

-Ticarcillin/clavulanate (Timentin) 3.1 gm IV q4-6h (200-300 mg/kg/d) (with gent/tobramycin). **OR**

-Ampicillin/Sulbactam (Unasyn) 1.5-3.0 gm IV q6h (with gent/tobramycin) **OR**

-Imipenem/cilastatin (Primaxin) 0.5-1.0 gm IV q6-8h (with gent/tobramycin).

-Vancomycin 500 mg IV q6h, or 1 gm IV q12h.

-Ceftazidime (Fortaz) 1-2 g IV q8h **OR**

-Ceftizoxime (Cefizox) 1-2 gm IV q8h **OR**

-Cefotaxime (Claforan) 2 gm q4-6h **OR**

-Ceftriaxone (Rocephin) 1-2 gm IV q12h (max 4 gm/d). **OR**

-Cefoxitin (Mefoxin) 1-2 gms q6-8h **OR**

-Cefotetan (Cefotan) 1-2 gms IV q12h

# Diverticulitis

## I. Pathogenesis

A. By age 50 one third of the patients have diverticulosis coli, and approximately two thirds have diverticulitis by age 80. 10-20% of patients with diverticulosis will have complications of diverticulitis or diverticular hemorrhage.

B. **Causes of Diverticulosis:** Aging, elevation of colonic intraluminal pressure, and decreased dietary fiber. Diverticuli occur where nutrient arteries penetrate the muscularis propria. Eighty-five percent are found in the sigmoid colon.

## II. Clinical Presentation of Diverticulitis

A. Usually >60 years of age; abrupt onset of unremitting left-lower quadrant abdominal pain, fever, alteration in bowel pattern. Diverticulitis of the transverse colon may simulate ulcer pain; diverticulitis of the cecum and redundant sigmoid may resemble appendicitis. Right sided diverticulosis is more common among Asians (>75%) than among Europeans.

B. Frank rectal bleeding is usually not seen with diverticulitis.

C. **Physical Exam:** Left-lower quadrant tenderness. Abdominal examination is often deceptively unremarkable in the elderly and in persons taking corticosteroids. Leukocytosis may occur.

D. **Differential Diagnosis:**

| Elderly: | Middle Aged and Young: |
|---|---|
| Ischemic colitis | Appendicitis |
| Carcinoma | Salpingitis |
| Volvulus | Inflammatory bowel disease |
| Colonic Obstruction | Penetrating ulcer |
| Penetrating ulcer | Urosepsis |
| Nephrolithiasis/urosepsis | |

## III. Diagnostic Evaluation

A. **Plain X-rays** may show ileus, obstruction, mass effect, ischemia, perforation.

B. **CT scan** is the test of choice to evaluate acute diverticulitis; used for staging the degree of complications and ruling out other diseases.

C. **Contrast Enema:** Water soluble contrast is safe, and useful in mild-to-moderate cases of diverticulitis when the diagnosis is in doubt.

D. **Endoscopy:** Acute diverticulitis is a relative contraindication--exclude perforation first. Used when the diagnosis is in doubt to exclude the possibility of ischemic bowel, Crohn's disease, or carcinoma.

E. **Ultrasound:** May be a helpful to evaluate acute diverticulitis. Intestinal gas often interferes with the exam.

F. **Complete Blood Count:** May show leukocytosis

## IV. Treatment

A. **Outpatient Treatment:**
   1. **Clear liquid diet**
   2. **Oral antibiotics:**
      Trimethoprim/SMX (Bactrim DS) 160/800 mg DS PO bid or Ciprofloxacin (Cipro) 250-500 mg PO bid or 200-300 mg IV q12h **AND**
      Metronidazole (Flagyl), 500 mg PO 2 times a day.

B. **Inpatient Treatment:**
   1. Severe cases should be hospitalized for gastrointestinal tract rest (NPO), intravenous fluids, antibiotics; initiate nasogastric suction if the patient is vomiting or if abdominal distention.
   2. Antibiotic coverage for enteric gram-negative and anaerobic organisms:
      Ampicillin 1-2 gm IV q4-6h **AND**
      Gentamicin or tobramycin 100-120 mg IV (1.5-2 mg/kg), then 80 mg IV tid (5 mg/kg/d) **AND**

Cefoxitin (Mefoxin) 2 g IV q8h **OR**
Metronidazole (Flagyl) 500 mg q6-8h (15-30 mg/kg/d) or Clindamycin (Cleocin) 600-900 mg IV q8h for more severe disease.

C. Frequently reassess for the first 48-72 hours. Improvement should occur over 48-72 hours with decreased fever, leukocytosis, and abdominal pain. Failure to improve or deterioration are indications for reevaluation and consideration of surgery.

## Complications of Diverticulitis

A. **Fistula:**
1. With repeated attacks of diverticulitis, a fistulous tract can form between bowel, urinary bladder, integument, pelvic floor, or vagina.
2. Colovesicular fistula is the most common. Pneumaturia and recurrent urinary tract infections, characterized by multiple organisms may occur. Reflux of contrast into the urinary bladder during contrast enema confirms the diagnosis.

B. **Intestinal Obstruction:** After repeated episodes of diverticulitis, the colon becomes fixed, fibrotic, stenosed, and obstruction may result. Surgical resection is indicated.

C. **Abscess:**
1. If no response to medical therapy within 24-48 hours, or of if an abdominal mass is palpable, consider the possibility of an intra-abdominal abscess, and obtain an abdominal CT scan.
2. Obtain early surgical consultation for percutaneous drainage followed by surgical drainage.

D. **Perforation and Peritonitis:**
1. Diverticular perforation will result in peritonitis.
2. Pain becomes severe, with peritoneal signs (guarding, rebound tenderness, rigidity), fever, tachycardia, elevation of white blood count. Most patients are toxic and require prompt surgical intervention.
3. Perforation is indicated by free peritoneal air that may be visible below diaphragm on a chest x-ray. Perforated viscus from an ulcer is a much more common cause of free air.

# Urinary Tract Infection

I. **Clinical Evaluation**
  A. **Acute Uncomplicated Upper Tract Infection** is associated with Dysuria, urgency, and frequency without fever or back pain. Most common in women in their childbearing years. Internal dysuria indicates bladder infection, external dysuria indicates vaginitis.
  B. **Acute Pyelonephritis** is associated with fever and costovertebral angle pain and tenderness with frequency, urgency, and dysuria. Leukocytosis is often present; urinalysis reveals pyuria and bacteriuria. White blood cell and bacterial casts confirm parenchymal invasion. Blood cultures may be useful, particularly in older patients.

II. **Pathogenesis of Urinary Tract Infection**
  A. Enterobacteriaceae are the bacteria most often responsible. Escherichia coli causes 80% of urinary tract infections. Staphylococcus saprophyticus (Gram-positive, coagulase-negative) is the second most common, particularly in young women; the diagnosis is often missed due to low urine colony counts and negative nitrite screening.
  B. Chlamydia trachomatis infection may cause dysuria, urgency, frequency, pyuria, and sterile bacterial cultures; diagnosed by cell culture or monoclonal antibody techniques of cellular material from urethral or cervical exudate. It is a major sexually transmitted cause of prostatitis, epididymitis, and nongonococcal urethritis in men under age 40.
  C. **Risk Factors for Urinary Tract Infection**: Diaphragm or spermicide use (alters vaginal pH), sexual intercourse, elderly, acquired anatomic abnormality, calculi, gynecologic abnormalities, prostatic obstruction, confinement in bed, urinary tract instrumentation.

III. **Laboratory Evaluation**
  A. Microscopic pyuria is a nonspecific indicator of inflammation; bacteriuria confirms the diagnosis. Bacteria on microscopic examination of unspun urine correlates well with UTI.
  B. Positive nitrite reading on reagent stick examination is useful, but false-negatives occur. False-negative and false-positives may also be seen with leukocyte esterase.
  C. Culture and sensitivity testing is indicated if there is failure to respond to therapy, suspected acute pyelonephritis, or complicated infections (calculi, obstruction, diabetes, immunosuppression).
  D. Follow-up post treatment culture is indicated in pyelonephritis or complicated infections. Recurrence or persistence of the same organism indicates a residual focus of infection that may respond to long-term (4-6-week) therapy.

IV. **Treatment of Acute, Uncomplicated Lower Urinary Tract Infection**
  A. **A 3-day course** is now recommended because of greater initial success in eliminating infection. A 7 day course is indicated if diabetes, symptoms >7 days, or elderly.
    Trimethoprim-sulfamethoxazole (Septra) 1 double strength tab (160/800 mg) PO bid
    Amoxicillin 500 mg PO tid
    Norfloxacin (Noroxin) 400 mg PO bid
    Ciprofloxacin (Cipro) 250 mg PO bid
    Ofloxacin (Floxin) 400 mg PO bid
    Lomefloxacin (Maxaquin) 400 mg PO qd
    Enoxacin (Penetrex) 200-400 mg PO q12h; 1h before or 2h after meals
    Cefadroxil (Duricef) 500 mg PO bid
    Nitrofurantoin (Macrodantin) 100 mg PO qid or Macrobid 100 mg PO bid
    Amoxicillin/clavulanate (Augmentin) 250 mg PO tid
  B. **Urinary Analgesia:**
    Phenazopyridine (Pyridium) 100-200 mg PO tid [100 mg]

V. **Treatment of Acute Pyelonephritis**
  A. Parenteral antibiotics are usually indicated in older patients, coexistent illness (diabetes, heart disease), or for ill appearing patients.
  B. Outpatient oral therapy is indicated in young patients with community-acquired infection

without complications, who are reliable, compliant, and without signs of sepsis.

C. Coverage should include gram-negative organisms and enterococci. For hospital-acquired infections, evaluate local resistance patterns of common gram negative organisms; E coli resistance to ampicillin and trimethoprim/sulfamethoxazole is increasing.

D. Parenteral therapy should be continued for 24 hours after afebrile; oral agents should be used to complete a 10-14 day course. If fever does not respond within 72 hours, an underlying factor should be suspected. Imaging studies should be obtained to exclude obstruction, calculi, or abscesses.

E. **Antibiotic Therapy for Acute Pyelonephritis:**

Trimethoprim-sulfamethoxazole (Septra) 1 double strength tab (160/800 mg) PO bid or 10 mLs in 100 mLs D5W IV over two hours q12h

Amoxicillin 500 mg PO tid

Norfloxacin (Noroxin) 400 mg PO bid

Ofloxacin (Floxin) 400 mg PO or IV bid

Lomefloxacin (Maxaquin) 400 mg PO qd

Enoxacin (Penetrex) 200-400 mg PO q12h; 1h before or 2h after meals

Cefadroxil (Duricef) 500 mg PO bid

Nitrofurantoin (Macrodantin) 100 mg PO qid or Macrobid 100 mg PO bid

Amoxicillin/clavulanate (Augmentin) 500 mg tab PO tid

Ampicillin 1 gm IV q4-6h **AND** Gentamicin or tobramycin - loading dose of 100-120 mg IV (1.5-2 mg/kg); then 80 mg IV q8h (2-5 mg/kg/d).

Ceftizoxime (Cefizox) 1 gm IV q8h.

Ceftazidime (Fortaz) 1 gm IV q8h.

Ticarcillin/clavulanate (Timentin) 3.1 gm IV q6h

## I. Recurrent Urinary Tract Infections

A. If recurrent UTI's occur, use of a diaphragm and spermicide should be discontinued. Postcoital voiding and long-term, single-dose, antimicrobial therapy may be used.

B. **Long-term Suppressive Therapy:** Trimethoprim/sulfamethoxazole (Bactrim, Septra), one-half of single-strength tablet 3 times weekly.

C. Self administration of single-dose or short-term antibiotic such as trimethoprim/sulfamethoxazole may be prescribed.

## II. Urinary Tract Infections in Men

A. Etiologic agents are the same as for women, and the same antibiotics may be used.

B. Antibiotics should be administered for a prolonged, 7-14 day course. Obtain a pretreatment culture.

## III. Indwelling Catheters

A. Antibiotic prophylaxis is not recommended while the catheter is in place; antibiotics should be reserved for symptomatic infection or other evidence of sepsis.

B. Bacteriuria that is acquired after short-term catheter use should be treated.

# Syphilis

## I. Clinical Evaluation

### A. Primary Syphilis:

1. The incubation period for syphilis is 10-90 days; 21 is average.
2. Begins as a painless, solitary nodule that becomes an indurated ulceration (chancre) with a ham-colored, eroded surface, and a serous discharge. 95% of primary lesions are found on or near the genitalia. Atypical lesions are frequent an may take the form of small multiple lesions.
3. Usually accompanied by painless, enlarged regional lymph nodes.
4. Untreated lesions heal in 1-5 weeks.
5. The diagnosis is made by the clinical appearance and a positive darkfield examination; the serologic test (VDRL, RPR) is often negative in early disease.

### B. Secondary Syphilis:

1. 25% of untreated patients progress to secondary syphilis 2-6 months after exposure, and secondary syphilis lasts 4-6 weeks.
2. Bilateral, symmetrical, macular, papular, or papulosquamous skin lesions are widespread and non-pruritic, and frequently involve the palms, soles, and face, in addition to the trunk and extremities. Condyloma lata consists of rash and moist lesions. Secondary syphilis is highly infectious.
3. Mucous membranes are often involved; white patches in the mouth, nose, vagina, rectum.
4. Generalized nontender lymphadenopathy. Patchy alopecia sometimes occurs. A small percentage have iritis, hepatitis, meningitis, fever, and headache.
5. The serologic test (VDRL. RPR) is positive in >99 % of cases; the test may be falsely negative because of the prozone phenomenon caused by high antigen titer Retesting of a diluted blood sample may be positive. No culture test is available.

### C. Latent Syphilis consists of the interval between secondary syphilis and late syphilis. Patients have no signs or symptoms, only positive serological tests.

### D. Late Syphilis: Characterized by destruction of tissue, organs, and organ systems.

1. **Late Benign Syphilis:** Gummas occur in skin or bone and do not result in severe incapacity or death.
2. **Cardiovascular Syphilis:** Medial necrosis of the aorta with dilation of the ascending aorta may lead to aortic insufficiency or saccular aneurysms of the thoracic aorta.
3. **Neurosyphilis:**
   a. Spinal fluid shows elevated WBCs, increased total protein, and positive serology.
   b. Pupillary changes are common; Argyll Robertson pupil accommodates but does not react to light.
   c. Can result in general paresis or tabes dorsalis--degeneration of the ascending sensory neurons in the posterior columns of the spinal cord.

## II. Serology

### A. Nontreponemal Tests:

1. Complement fixation tests (VDRL or RPR) are used for screening; become positive 4-6 weeks after infection. They start in low titer and, over several weeks, may reach 1:32 or higher. After adequate treatment of primary syphilis, the titer falls and, in most cases, is nonreactive within 9-18 months.
2. False positive tests occur in hepatitis, mononucleosis, viral pneumonia, malaria, varicella, autoimmune diseases, diseases associated with increased globulins, narcotic addicts, leprosy, or old age.

### B. Treponemal Tests:

1. Treponemal tests include the FTA-ABS test, TPI test, and microhemagglutination assay for T. pallidum (MHA-TP). A treponemal test should be used to confirm a positive VDRL or RPR.

2. Treponemal tests are specific to treponema antibodies, and will remain positive after treatment.

C. All patients with syphilis should be tested for HIV.

## III. Treatment of Primary or Secondary Syphilis

A. **Nonallergic Patients with Primary or Secondary Syphilis:** Benzathine penicillin G, 2.4 million units IM in a single dose.

B. Treatment of HIV infected patients with syphilis requires consultation with a specialist.

C. Patients who have syphilis, and who also have symptoms or signs suggesting neurologic disease (meningitis) or ophthalmic disease (uveitis), should be fully evaluated for neurosyphilis and syphilitic eye disease (CSF analysis and ocular slit-lamp examination).

D. Unless clinical signs or symptoms of neurologic involvement are present (auditory, cranial nerve, meningeal, or ophthalmic manifestations), lumbar puncture is not recommended for routine evaluation of primary or secondary syphilis.

E. **Penicillin Allergic Patients:** Doxycycline 100 mg orally 2 times a day for 2 weeks or Tetracycline 500 mg orally 4 times a day for 2 weeks contraindicated in pregnancy.

F. **Follow-Up and Retreatment:**
   1. Early syphilis--repeat VDRL at 3, 6, and 12 months; ensure that titers are declining.
   2. Syphilis >1 year--also repeat VDRL at 24 months.
   3. Neurosyphilis-- also repeat VDRL for 3 years.
   4. **Indications for Retreatment:**
      a. Clinical signs or symptoms persist or recur.
      b. 4-fold increase in the titer of a nontreponemal test (VDRL).
      c. Failure of an initially high titer nontreponemal test (VDRL) to show a 4-fold decrease within a year.
   5. Sex Partners should be evaluated and treated.

## IV. Treatment of Latent Syphilis

A. Patients who have latent syphilis who have acquired syphilis within the preceding year are classified as having early latent syphilis. Nearly all others have latent syphilis of unknown duration and should be managed as late latent syphilis.

B. These treatment regimens are for nonallergic patients with normal CSF examination (if performed).

C. **Treatment of Early Latent Syphilis:** Benzathine penicillin G, 2.4 million units IM in a single dose.

D. **Treatment of Late Latent Syphilis or Latent Syphilis of Unknown Duration:** Benzathine penicillin G, 7.2 million units total, administered as 3 doses of 2.4 million units IM each, at 1-week intervals.

E. All patients should be evaluated clinically for evidence of late (tertiary) syphilis (aortitis, neurosyphilis, gumma, iritis). The recommended therapy for patients with latent syphilis is not optimal for persons with late syphilis or asymptomatic neurosyphilis.

F. **Indications for CSF Examination Before Treatment:**
   1. Neurologic or ophthalmic signs or symptoms
   2. Other evidence of active syphilis (aortitis, gumma, iritis)
   3. Treatment failure
   4. HIV infection
   5. Serum nontreponemal titer >1:32, unless duration of infection is known to be <1 year
   6. Nonpenicillin therapy planned, unless duration of infection is known to be <1 year.

G. **CSF Examination** includes cell count, protein, and CSF-VDRL. CSF examination may be completed for persons who do not meet the criteria listed above. If a CSF examination is performed and the results are abnormal, the patient should be treated for neurosyphilis.

**V. Treatment of Late Syphilis**
   A. Benzathine penicillin G, 7.2 million units total, administered as 3 doses of 2.4 million units IM, at 1-week intervals.
   B. Patients with late syphilis should undergo CSF examination before therapy. Infectious disease consultation is recommended.

**VI.  Treatment of Neurosyphilis**
   A. Central nervous system disease can occur during any stage of syphilis.  Clinical evidence of neurologic involvement (e.g., ophthalmic or auditory symptoms, cranial nerve palsies) warrants a CSF examination.  Syphilitic eye disease should be treated as neurosyphilis.
   B. Patients  with CSF abnormalities should have follow-up CSF examinations to assess response to treatment.
   C. **Treatment of Neurosyphilis:**  12-24 million units aqueous crystalline penicillin G daily, administered as 2-4 million units IV every 4 hours, for 10-14 days.
   D. **Follow-Up:**  If CSF pleocytosis was present initially, CSF examination should be repeated every 6 months until the cell count is normal. Follow-up CSF examinations also may be used to evaluate changes in the VDRL-CSF or CSF protein in response to therapy.

# Gastroenterology

## Peptic Ulcer Disease

I. Clinical Evaluation
   A. Of the three well-identified causes of peptic ulcer disease--Helicobacter pylori, nonsteroidal anti-inflammatory drugs (NSAIDs), and pathologically high acid-secreting states (Zollinger-Ellison syndrome)--H pylori is the most frequent cause.
   B. H2 blockers, sucralfate (Carafate), omeprazole (Prilosec) only temporarily heal ulcers. However, eradication of H pylori permanently cures peptic ulcer disease, eliminating the need for long-term therapy.
   C. H pylori is found in almost all cases of chronic duodenal ulcers, and in the majority of cases of gastric ulcers that are not caused by use of an NSAID.
   D. **Nonendoscopic Tests for Helicobacter pylori:**
      1. If the patient has documented peptic ulcer disease and is having recurrent symptoms, it is reasonable to treat with antibiotics without further study if serologic tests are positive for H pylori. Eradication is usually assessed clinically by alleviation of symptoms. If symptoms recur, a breath test or endoscopic biopsy is necessary to confirm eradication.
      2. A reliable urea breath test is available, in which the patient ingests a capsule containing urea with radiolabeled carbon. The urea is broken down by the H pylori present, and the tagged carbon dioxide is expired via the lungs.
   E. **Endoscopic biopsy** and histologic examination are still the primary means of H pylori diagnosis.

II. Treatment of Peptic Ulcer Disease
   A. **Eradication of H pylori Infection:**
      1. Treat duodenal and gastric ulcers, new ulcers, recurrent ulcers, and maintained ulcers with antimicrobials.
      2. **Triple Drug Therapy:**
         -Bismuth Subsalicylate (Pepto-Bismol) 2 tabs or 30 mLs PO qid **AND**
         -Metronidazole (Flagyl) 250 mg qid x 14 days **AND**
         -Tetracycline 500 mg qid x 14 days.
      3. **Omeprazole and Antibiotic Therapy:**
         -Omeprazole (Prilosec), 40 mg qd **AND** tetracycline 500 mg qid or amoxicillin, 500 mg PO qid, for 14 days.
      4. **Omeprazole and Clarithromycin Therapy:**
         -Clarithromycin (Biaxin) 250-500 mg PO bid x 14 days **AND**
         -Omeprazole (Prilosec) 40 mg PO qd x 14 days, then 20 mg PO qd x 14 days.
   B. **H2 Blockers:** H2 blockers may be used in either twice-daily or single night-time doses.
      1. **Dosages for Acute Therapy:**
         Cimetidine (Tagamet), 400 mg bid or 800 mg hs
         Ranitidine (Zantac), 150 mg bid or 300 mg hs
         Famotidine (Pepcid), 20 mg bid or 40 mg hs
         Nizatidine (Axid Pulvules), 150 mg bid or 300 mg hs
      2. Side effects are uncommon; occasionally drug interactions, neurologic symptoms.
   C. **Proton Pump Inhibitors:**
      1. **Omeprazole (Prilosec):** Reserved for ulcers refractory to H2 blockers and sucralfate. 20 mg qd. Side effects are rare.
      2. **Lansoprazole (Prevacid):** 15 mg before meals [15, 30 mg]
   D. **Mucosal Protective Agents:**
      1. **Sucralfate (Carafate):**
         a. Aluminum-containing, mucosal, protective agent; 1 gm before meals and hs.
         b. Constipation is a common. Can bind with other drugs.

2. **Misoprostol (Cytotec):**
   a. 200 mcg PO qid; prostaglandin E1 analogue; mucosal protective.
   b. Not a first-line agent.
   c. Effective in healing peptic ulcer disease; side effects are significant; 25% experience diarrhea that resolves by reducing the dosage to 200 mcg bid. Can cause spontaneous abortion.

## III. Maintenance Therapy for Peptic Ulcer Disease

A. If H. pylori therapy has been completed, most ulcers will not recur, and maintenance therapy will not be required.

B. **Maintenance dose is half of the standard therapeutic dose:**

   Cimetidine (Tagamet), 400 mg hs
   Ranitidine (Zantac), 150 mg hs
   Famotidine (Pepcid), 20 mg hs
   Nizatidine (Axid Pulvules), 150 mg hs
   Sucralfate (Carafate), 1 g bid

# Gastroesophageal Reflux Disease

**I. Clinical Evaluation of Gastroesophageal Reflux Disease (GERD)**
  A. The most common symptom is heartburn, a burning sensation in the epigastric or retrosternal area, rising toward the throat, often occurring postprandially.
  B. Regurgitation, dysphagia, and belching may occur.
  C. Hoarseness, nocturnal cough and wheezing may be caused by chronic reflux. Asthma may be exacerbated by gastroesophageal reflux.
  D. Chronic reflux may cause Barrett's esophagus (columnar metaplasia of esophageal mucosa), and may predispose to esophageal adenocarcinoma.
  E. GERD is associated with decreased lower esophageal sphincter pressure caused by inappropriate relaxation of the lower esophageal sphincter, low basal sphincter pressure, or increases in intra-abdominal pressure. Sphincter tone can be impaired by consumption of fatty foods and anticholinergic medications.

**II. Antireflux Therapy**
  A. **Empiric Therapy:** With classic symptoms (heartburn, regurgitation), and no evidence of complications or systemic illness, a presumptive diagnosis of reflux disease may be made. An H2 receptor blocker and prokinetic drug may be prescribed.
  B. If reflux symptoms persist after 8-12 weeks of treatment, endoscopy is indicated.
  C. Severe or atypical symptoms occurring many times a week warrant early diagnostic evaluation with esophagoscopy. 24-hour ambulatory esophageal pH monitoring is the "gold standard" of testing.

**III. Non-Pharmacologic Therapy for Gastroesophageal Reflux Disease**
  A. **Inclined Bed:** Place blocks (6 inches high) under head of bed or support patient's upper body with a foam wedge.
  B. **Dietary Modifications:**
    1. Avoid foods that reduce lower esophageal sphincter pressure, impair gastric emptying, or that irritate mucosal lining. Chocolate and carminatives (spearmint, peppermint), fatty foods, onions may exacerbate reflux. Coffee and tomato-based products irritate the esophageal mucosa.
    2. Refrain from overeating, and avoid eating before bedtime.
    3. **Avoid causative medications** such as anticholinergic drugs, potassium chloride, nonsteroidal anti-inflammatory drugs, theophylline, calcium channel blockers, and progesterone. Prolonged contact of the esophagus with corrosive drug tablets or capsules may irritate mucosa. When taking medications, patients should consume ample liquid.
  C. **Pharmacologic Treatment of Gastroesophageal Reflux Disease**

| Agent: | Dosage: | Mechanism of action: |
|---|---|---|
| **Histamine-2 blockers**<br>Cimetidine (Tagamet)<br>Famotidine (Pepcid)<br>Nizatidine (Axid Pulvules)<br>Ranitidine (Zantac) | Up to 800 mg bid<br>20-40 mg bid<br>150 mg bid<br>150 mg bid | Inhibit gastric acid secretion |
| **Prokinetic drugs**<br>Bethanechol chloride | Up to 25 mg qid | Increase lower esophageal sphincter pressure, increase peristalsis |
| Metoclopramide (Reglan) | 10 to 15 mg up to four times daily | Neurologic and psychotropic side effects. |
| Cisapride (Propulsid) | Up to 20 mg qid [10 mg] | Does not have neurologic or psychotropic side effects |

| H+,K+-ATPase (proton-pump) inhibitors Omeprazole (Prilosec) Lansoprazole (Prevacid) | 20 mg qd or bid 30 mg qd | Inhibit gastric acid secretion |
| --- | --- | --- |

IV.   **Refractory Cases**
   A. Doubling the standard dose or the dose frequency of medications may provide greater symptomatic relief and a higher rate of healing.
   B. Consider substituting omeprazole (Prilosec), which profoundly inhibits gastric acid production.
   C. **Anti-Reflux Surgery:**  A small minority of patients with truly intractable disease should be considered for antireflux surgery to reestablish a competent lower esophageal sphincter.  Antireflux surgery has shown disappointing long-term results, and is indicated only on rare occasions.

# Viral Hepatitis

I. **Clinical Manifestations of Viral Hepatitis**
   A. **Acute Viral Hepatitis:**
      1. **Symptoms of Acute Hepatitis:** Anorexia, fatigue, myalgias, and nausea which usually develop 1-2 weeks prior to the onset of jaundice. Weight loss and distaste for food and cigarettes may occur early in the illness, followed by headaches, arthralgias, vomiting, and right upper quadrant tenderness. Diarrhea often occurs in children but is unusual in adults.
      2. Symptoms of hepatitis A, B, and C are indistinguishable, except that patients with hepatitis A are more frequently febrile. A few patients will develop a serum-sickness syndrome following infection with HBV, which occurs in 5-10%, and which is characterized by fever, rash, and arthralgias that precedes the onset of jaundice.
      3. **Less Common Manifestations of Acute Viral Hepatitis:** Cough, pharyngitis, rash, arthritis, and glomerulonephritis. Dark brown urine and clay colored stools sometime occur during the icteric phase.
      4. **Physical Examination:**
         a. Jaundice, hepatomegaly, and/or splenomegaly may be present.
         b. Jaundice can be observed clinically when the bilirubin is greater than 2.5 mg/dL and is most easily observed under the tongue or in the sclerae. The absence of jaundice does not rule out the diagnosis of hepatitis.
         c. Jaundice occurs in less than one-half of hepatitis patients. Patients with acute hepatitis may present merely with flu-like symptoms or malaise.
         d. Fulminant hepatic failure may result from hepatitis, and is manifested by signs and symptoms of severe liver dysfunction, associated with encephalopathy, developing within 8 weeks of the acute illness.
         e. Lymphadenopathy is not a clinical feature of HAV, HBV, or HCV, and its presence suggests infection with another virus such as EBV, CMV, HIV.
   B. **Chronic Hepatitis:**
      1. The clinical presentation of patients with chronic hepatitis is varied. The most frequent symptom is fatigue; jaundice is rarely present. The major difference between chronic hepatitis caused by HBV compared to HCV is a higher rate of cirrhosis that develops with HCV. Additionally, it is common for patients with chronic hepatitis C to have fluctuating levels of aminotransferases.
      2. Hyperbilirubinemia usually does not occur until late. There is no correlation between the aminotransferase level and disease severity; up to one-third of patients with normal aminotransferases have evidence of chronic hepatitis on biopsy.
      3. Chronic Hepatitis requires performance of a liver biopsy to confirm the diagnosis and to assess severity so as to determine whether treatment is needed.
      4. In both hepatitis B and hepatitis C, evidence of chronic liver disease may be present, such as amenorrhea, muscle wasting, gynecomastia, and spider angiomata. As the disease progresses, asterixis, ascites, hepatic encephalopathy, peripheral edema, easy bruisability, testicular atrophy, bleeding, and esophageal varices may develop.
      5. A major complication of chronic hepatitis is hepatocellular carcinoma.

II. **Diagnosis of Acute Hepatitis**
   A. **Laboratory Findings in Acute Hepatitis:**
      1. Aspartate aminotransferase (AST) and alanine aminotransferase (ALT) enzymes increase proportionally during the prodromal phase in patients with hepatitis and may reach 20 times normal. The peak usually occurs when the patients are jaundiced, then rapidly falls during recovery.
      2. Alkaline phosphatase and lactate dehydrogenase are normal or only mildly elevated.
      3. In icteric patients, the bilirubin continues to increase as the aminotransferases decline and may reach 20 mg/dL. There are equal proportions of direct and indirect bilirubin in patients with hepatitis.
      4. The prothrombin time is usually normal in acute hepatitis, but can become prolonged in patients with severe hepatitis; PT can serve as a marker of prognosis.

5. Hemoglobin and white blood cell count are usually normal. Platelet count is normal except in fulminant hepatic failure where it may be decreased.

6. If acute viral hepatitis is suspected then appropriate serologic tests should include IgM anti-HAV, IgM anti-HBc, HBsAg, and anti-HCV. In patients with fulminant hepatic failure or known previous infection with HBV, an anti-HDV can also be ordered.

7. **Hepatitis Panels and Tests**

| Panel | Marker Detected |
|---|---|
| Acute hepatitis panel | IgM anti-HAV, IgM anti-HBc, HBsAg, anti-HCV |
| To monitor HBV | HBsAg, HBeAg, anti-HBe, HBsAg, HBeAg, total anti-HBc |
| HBV immunity panel | Anti-HBs, total anti-HBc (if anti-HBc positive and anti-HBs negative, reflex to HBsAg to rule out chronic carrier |

| Individual Tests | |
|---|---|
| Immunity to HBV | Anti-HBs (post-vaccination) |
| Immunity to HAV | Total anti-HAV |
| To screen for HBV infection | HBsAg for pregnant women |
| To monitor HCV infection | Anti-HCV |

B. **Clinical Evaluation of Acute Hepatitis:**

1. Initially, patients should be evaluated for other etiologies of liver disease that can cause elevated liver enzymes.

2. **Common Causes of Elevated Aminotransferase Levels:**
   a. Infection:Pneumococcal bacteremia, sepsis, Epstein-Barr virus, cytomegalovirus, herpes simplex virus, Varicella-zoster virus, yellow fever, virus, syphilis tuberculosis, mycobacterium avium complex.
   b. **Drugs and Toxins:** Acetaminophen, benzenes, carbon tetrachloride, halothane, isoniazid, ketoconazole, 6-Mercaptopurine, methyldopa, phenytoin, propylthiouracil, rifampin. In patients taking these medications, discontinuation of therapy usually results in normalization of liver enzymes.
   c. **Vascular Anoxia:** Budd-Chiari syndrome, congestive heart failure, veno-occlusive disease.
   d. **Metabolic:**alpha1 anti-trypsin deficiency, hereditary hemochromatosis, Wilson's disease.
   e. **Others:**Alcoholic liver disease, choledocholithiasis, nonalcoholic steatohepatitis, malignancy shock.
   f. **Autoimmune Hepatitis:** Occurs primarily in young women with systemic manifestations of autoimmune phenomena. These patients have positive tests for antinuclear antibody and anti-smooth muscle antibody.
   g. **Wilson's disease** is an autosomal recessive condition that results in toxic copper accumulation in the liver as well as other organs. Diagnosis can be made by identifying the characteristic Kayser-Fleischer rings in the eyes, documenting an elevated urinary copper, or low serum ceruloplasmin.

3. **Blood Studies Useful in Evaluating Patients With Chronic Elevations of Serum Liver Enzyme Levels:**

| Disease to be Ruled Out | Suggested Blood Test |
|---|---|
| alpha1 -antitrypsin deficiency | alpha1 -antitrypsin |
| Autoimmune chronic hepatitis | ANA, anti-smooth muscle antibody |
| Hemochromatosis | Serum iron, TIBC, ferritin |
| Hepatitis B | HBsAg, HBeAg, anti-HBc |
| Hepatitis C | Anti-HCV |
| Primary biliary cirrhosis | AMA |
| Wilson's disease | Ceruloplasmin |

III. **Hepatitis A Virus (HAV)**

A. Hepatitis A is usually an acute, self-limited infection that does not result in a chronic carrier state. Fulminant hepatic failure resulting in encephalopathy or death is rare.

B. Hepatitis A should be suspected if infection occurs following ingestion of contaminated food or shellfish, following natural disasters (floods, earthquakes), in institutionalized persons, children or families of children in day care centers, or if travel to an endemic area.

C. Generally a mild disease (frequently asymptomatic and anicteric) in children.

D. The diagnosis is confirmed by the presence of IgM anti-HAV in serum during the acute illness. The IgM anti-HAV titer decreases over several months and the IgG anti-HAV rises and persists indefinitely and affords immunity to subsequent HAV exposure.

E. Transmission--fecal-oral.

F. Incubation period--2-6 weeks.

G. Low grade fever (< 101 F) is common at onset, with malaise, anorexia, dark urine, pale stools.

H. **Treatment:**
   1. Symptomatic treatment for acute illness with antipyretics.
   2. Over 99% of symptomatic adult acute hepatitis A will resolve without any serious sequelae.

IV. **Hepatitis B**

A. Hepatitis B is difficult to distinguish from hepatitis A clinically, but usually has a more protracted course. The diagnosis of acute hepatitis B is made by the demonstration of HBsAg in the serum, and IgM antibody to hepatitis B core antigen (anti-HBc IgM) which appears approximately the same time as symptoms. Anti-HBc IgM gradually declines during recovery.

B. **Transmission:**
   1. Parenteral (needlestick, transfusion).
   2. Sexual (heterosexual, anal intercourse).
   3. Maternal-fetal (perinatal): associated with HBeAg (marker for infectivity) in the 3rd trimester. Most transmission occurs at the time of birth rather than in utero.
   4. Oral transmission (inefficient).

C. **Incubation period:** 50-160 days.

D. Fulminant hepatic failure occurs in approximately 1% of cases.

E. Asymptomatic acute illness probably accounts for 40-50% of all infections. These patients are often recognized later in life as either HBsAg carriers with anti-HBs and anti-HBc antibodies.

F. **Laboratory Diagnosis of Hepatitis B:**
   1. Antibody to HBsAg (anti-HBs) develops after active infection and serves as an indicator of immunity. Anti-HBs alone is also detectable in the serum of individuals who have been vaccinated against HBV or who have passive immunity from hepatitis B immune globulin (HBIG).
   2. IgM anti-HBc indicates recent infection with HBV, usually within the preceding 4-6 months.
   3. Presence of HBeAg indicates active viral replication and high infectivity. Antibody to HBeAg (anti-HBe) develops in most people infected with HBV and indicates decreasing replication and infectivity of the virus.
   4. The persistence of HBsAg for six months after the diagnosis of acute HBV is indicative of progression to chronic hepatitis B.

G. **Management of Acute Hepatitis B:**
   1. **Indications for Hospitalization:**
      a. Inability to maintain intake of nutrition and fluids.
      b. Complications of severe hepatitis (encephalopathy, bleeding, prothrombin time >50%)
   2. **Bed rest** is not mandatory in uncomplicated cases.
   3. **Diet** should be free of fried or fatty foods.
   4. **Corticosteroids** are not indicated even in severe disease.
   5. Over 90% of adult patients with acute hepatitis B recover uneventfully. The mortality rate from acute hepatitis B is 1-2%.
   6. **Chronic hepatitis** will develop in 6-10% in varying degrees of severity, manifested by persistent HBsAg positivity.
   7. **Fulminant hepatic failure** occurs in <1% of patients following HBV infection, and is characterized by prolongation of the prothrombin time, hyperbilirubinemia, and

encephalopathy. Prolongation of the international normalized ratio (INR) > 1.5, accompanied by an altered mental status with hepatic encephalopathy, predicts a poor prognosis unless transplantation is successfully performed. Without urgent transplantation, mortality is very high primarily due to gastrointestinal hemorrhage, sepsis, adult respiratory distress syndrome (ARDS), and renal failure.

H. **Management of Chronic Hepatitis B:**
1. Alpha-interferon has been shown to be effective in the treatment of certain cases of chronic hepatitis B. A liver biopsy is required to determine who should be treated.
2. Usual dosage of interferon alpha-2b is 5 million units SQ daily (or 10 million units 2 times a week) for 16 weeks. 37% of patients will become HBeAg-negative with improvement in ALT level; over 10% of patients may eventually lose HBsAg and become anti-HBs positive.

## V. Hepatitis C

A. At present there are no serologic tests that can detect HCV antigen or IgM; therefore, diagnosis is based on the absence of serologic markers for hepatitis A and B, as well as the lack of clinical manifestations of other etiologies causing hepatitis. Anti-HCV antibody is positive in 70-90% of patients with hepatitis C, although there is a prolonged interval between onset of illness and seroconversion. The test does not distinguish acute from chronic infection; it has a sensitivity of about 90%.

B. Clinical features of acute hepatitis C are indistinguishable from those of other viral hepatitides. Clinically recognized acute hepatitis C infection occurs less commonly than HAV or HBV and the majority of patients are asymptomatic.

C. Multiple transfusions, injection drug use, or high-risk sexual activity increase the index of suspicion for HCV.

D. Perinatal transmission can occur in the 3rd trimester only; may require high levels of virus; in HIV and HCV-infected mothers, offspring infected 50% of time.

E. **Heterosexual or household contacts** have a 1-14% prevalence of anti-HCV. Between homosexuals, the attack rate is 2.9% per year.

F. **Epidemiology:** Approximately 50% of patients with acute hepatitis C will progress to chronic liver disease, and 20% of these will develop cirrhosis. Patients with chronic hepatitis C are also at risk for the development of hepatocellular carcinoma.

G. **Incubation period:** mean is 7.8 weeks (range 2-26 weeks).

H. Between 40-50% of cases will progress to chronic NANB hepatitis.

I. **Treatment of Hepatitis C:**
1. **Acute hepatitis C** is infrequently identified, it usually is not severe, and it only requires symptomatic and supportive therapy.
2. **Chronic HCV infection:**
   a. Interferon in a dose of 3 million units SQ 3 times weekly for 24 weeks has resulted in improved ALT levels in 50% of treated patients. However, ½ of these patients will relapse following discontinuation of treatment.
   b. A liver biopsy is necessary to determine who should be treated.

## VI.    Hepatitis D

A. Hepatitis D occurs in patients who are coinfected with HBV and HDV, or infect in a patient already infected with HBV who becomes superinfected with HDV. Infection can result in acute or chronic hepatitis.

B. The clinical manifestations of HDV infection are indistinguishable from HBV alone; however, coinfected patients are at higher risk for fulminant hepatic failure.

C. Cirrhosis may develop in up to 70%, with rapid progression to cirrhosis occurring within two years in 10-15%.

D. Hepatitis D should be suspected in patients with fulminant hepatitis or in a patient who is known to be HBsAg positive who suffers a clinical deterioration. An anti-HDV test should be ordered.

E. If the patient has Acute HBV and the anti-HDV test is positive, then he is coinfected with HDV. If the patient has Chronic HBV and the anti-HDV test is positive, then he is superinfected. In patients with superinfection, a high titer (> 1:100) of anti-HDV indicates chron.ic delta hepatitis.

F. **Epidemiology:** Relatively high incidence in drug addicts, hemophiliacs.

## VII. Hepatitis E

A. **Acute hepatitis E** is difficult to diagnose because there are no commercially available tests. The clinical course of HEV is similar to that of HAV, and this infection should be suspected in individuals recently returning from underdeveloped countries.

B. **Epidemiology:** Associated with waterborne epidemics in India, Southeast Asia, Middle East, North Africa, and Mexico.

C. **Incubation period** 30-40 days. Causes a self-limiting infection in young adults. Occasionally causes a severe disease in pregnant women with a 10-20% maternal mortality.

D. **Diagnosis:** Immune electron microscopy of stool filtrates. A serologic test is not yet available.

E. **Treatment:** Supportive care.

## VIII. Prevention of Hepatitis

A. **Prevention of Hepatitis A:**

1. Employees of child care facilities and travelers to undeveloped areas of third world countries should consider vaccination against hepatitis A (Havrix), and they should avoid eating uncooked shellfish, fruits, vegetables or water that may be contaminated.

2. Vaccination is given 2 weeks prior to exposure, and a booster dose anytime between 6 and 12 months. Children and adults exposed to hepatitis A at home or in child care facilities should receive immune globulin (0.02 mg/kg).

B. **Prophylactic Therapy for Hepatitis B:**

1. Passive immunization with hepatitis B immune globulin (HBIG) is recommended for:
   a. Accidental needlestick or mucosal exposure to HBsAg.
   b. Accidental transfusion of HBSAG-positive blood products.
   c. Spouses and/or sexual contacts of acute cases.
   d. Infants born to HBSAG-positive mothers.

2. **Active immunization (Hepatovax-B, Engerix, Recombivax-B vaccines) recommendations:**
   a. **Pre-exposure:** All infants and children, high-risk health care workers and hospital staff, clients and staff of institutions for mentally retarded, hemodialysis patients and staff, homosexual males, illicit drug abusers, recipients of multiple blood products, sexual and household contacts of HBV carriers, prison inmates, heterosexually active persons with multiple partners, travelers to HBV-endemic areas.
   b. **Post-exposure (in conjunction with HBIG):** Infants born to HBsAg positive mothers; sexual contacts of acute hepatitis B cases; needlestick exposure to HBV; vaccine recipients with inadequate anti-HBs and needlestick exposure.

3. There are two hepatitis B vaccines available. Recombivax HB and Engerix-B. The vaccine is given as a series of three injections. Protective antibody against HBV occurs in 90-95% of vaccinated individuals.
   a. If doses are inadvertently missed, the second and third dose should be administered 3-5 months apart.
   b. Currently, there are no recommendations for postvaccination testing in normal hosts except for health-care workers who are at risk for occupational exposure to hepatitis B.
   c. In immunocompromised patients, consideration should be given to documentation of immunity. For nonresponders, some clinicians administer a fourth dose, while others repeat the entire series.

4. Infants born to HBsAg-positive women should receive HBIg (0.5 mL) and hepatitis B vaccine.

5. Postexposure prophylaxis following sexual exposure to HBV: HBIG and simultaneous hepatitis B vaccination with completion of the vaccine series at 1 and 6 months.

C. **Hepatitis C:**
  1. Available data do not support the use of immune globulin for postexposure prophylaxis of hepatitis C.
  2. No vaccine against hepatitis C is available.

IX. **Unusual Viral Causes of Hepatitis**
  A. **Herpes Viruses:**
    1. **Herpes simplex (HSV)** may rarely cause severe hepatitis in immunocompromised individuals. Often with mucocutaneous vesicles.
    2. **Cytomegalovirus (CMV):** Hepatitis typically seen in immunocompromised individuals, particularly transplant recipients. Fever, pneumonia, colitis may be seen.
    3. **Epstein-Barr virus (EBV):** Rare cause of hepatitis, associated with infectious mononuclear cells in sinusoids.
    4. **Varicella-Zoster Virus:** Rarely a cause of mild-moderate liver cell inflammation, usually in association with skin lesions.
  B. **Other Rare Causes of Hepatitis:** Measles, rubella, yellow fever, Lassa fever, Rift Valley fever, Marburg virus, Ebola virus, adenovirus.

# Acute Pancreatitis

### Diagnosis of Acute Pancreatitis

A. Pancreatitis usually presents as abdominal pain associated with elevated pancreatic enzymes. Pain is typically epigastric or in the left upper quadrant, and described as constant, dull, or boring; radiation of the pain to the mid-back and worsening in the supine position may occur.

B. Low-grade fever to 101 F is common. Higher temperature may indicate infectious complications. May present with volume depletion, manifesting as hypotension or shock, due to vomiting, hemorrhage, or third spacing of fluid into the retroperitoneum.

C. Patients may have a distended abdomen, and bowel sounds may be absent. Epigastric tenderness and localized rebound may be elicited.

D. Bleeding into the pancreatic bed rarely manifest as ecchymoses of the flanks (Grey Turner's Sign) or as periumbilical bleeding (Cullen's sign).

### Etiology

Identification of the etiology of an attack of pancreatitis is essential to prevent recurrences.

A. **Alcohol:** Alcoholic pancreatitis can develop after an alcohol binge.

B. **Gallstones:**
   1. Ultrasonography is the procedure of choice to visualize gallstones. 65-75% of patients with "idiopathic" acute pancreatitis have occult gallstones or biliary sludge.
   2. **Conditions that Predispose to Biliary Stones:** Prolonged fasting (total parenteral nutrition, very low calorie weight loss diet), pregnancy.

C. **Hypertriglyceridemia:**Pancreatitis is associated with triglyceride levels >1000 mg/dL; lipid-reducing therapy will prevent recurrences.

D. **Abdominal Trauma:** Trauma such as an automobile accident can result in acute pancreatitis.

E. **Postoperative:**Pancreatitis may occur after upper abdominal, renal, or cardiovascular surgery.

F. **Hypercalcemia:** Pancreatitis has been reported with hypercalcemia.

G. **Pregnancy:**Acute pancreatitis is most likely during the third trimester and in the 6 weeks postpartum. Usually related to alcohol abuse or gallstone disease.

H. **Anatomic Causes:** May be caused by duodenal diverticula, choledochoceles, pancreatic or ampullary strictures, pancreas divisum, tumors of the pancreas.

I. **Infections Associated with Acute Pancreatitis:** Viruses, parasites, and bacteria may cause pancreatitis.

J. **Vasculitis:** Pancreatitis may be an initial manifestation of systemic vasculitis.

K. **Drugs:**Nonsteroidal anti-inflammatory drugs, erythromycin, thiazides can induce severe pancreatitis. Dideoxyinosine (ddI), pentamidine, sulfonamides, 5-aminosalicylate (5-ASA) have been associated with pancreatitis.

L. **Other Causes:** Acute pancreatitis may occur as a complication of endoscopic retrograde cholangiopancreatography, hereditary pancreatitis, scorpion stings (found in Trinidad), organophosphate insecticides, and other toxins.

## II. Laboratory Evaluation

A. Elevated amylase is not pathognomonic for pancreatitis. Ruptured ectopic pregnancy, tubo-ovarian abscess, ovarian cysts, duodenal perforation, and mesenteric infarction may result in moderate hyperamylasemia. Clearance of amylase is reduced in renal failure, resulting in up to a threefold elevation.

B. In acute pancreatitis the amylase elevation is generally more pronounced than in other settings; values are usually at least 3 times normal. Mild hyperamylasemia may be seen in asymptomatic alcoholics and in acute cholecystitis or cholangitis.

C. An elevated WBC count is common in pancreatitis.

D. **Isoamylase Determination:** Distinguishes pancreatic amylase from salivary amylase. Elevation of salivary isoamylase occurs with mumps, pneumonia, lung tumors; breast, prostate cancers.

E. **Macroamylasemia:**
1. An elevation of serum amylase results from low renal excretion of amylase. Not a[n] unusual finding in the normal population.
2. Macroamylasemia occurs in 1% of all healthy persons and in 2.5% of patients with hyperamylasemia. Diagnosis is through detection of a low amylase clearance rati[o] (ACR).
   ACR = Urine Amylase x Serum Creatinine ÷ Serum Amylase x Urine Creatinine x 10[0]
   With macroamylasemia, the ACR is less than 0.2%.
3. Patients with macroamylasemia and pancreatitis may be diagnosed on the basis of a[n] elevated serum lipase activity.

F. **Lipase:**
1. Lipase is more pancreas specific than amylase.
2. May increase due to chemotherapy, radiotherapy, alcohol, bile induced enteritis; extrahepatic biliary obstruction; hepatic failure or necrosis; chronic active hepatitis; alcoholic cirrhosis. In these disorders, the lipase level seldom exceeds the upper lim[it] of normal by more than 3 times.

IV. **Imaging Studies**
A. **Radiographic Studies:**
1. Flat and upright films of the abdomen help exclude perforated viscus (free air under diaphragm).
2. **Nonspecific Findings of Acute Pancreatitis:** Adynamic ileus or a sentinel loop (localized jejunal ileus). Pancreatic calcifications may be found with chronic pancreatitis.

B. **Ultrasonography:**
1. Useful for evaluation of the biliary tract for gallstones, increased gallbladder wall thickness, and pericholecystic fluid associated with cholecystitis, or bile duct dilation due to obstruction.
2. Acute pancreatitis is indicated by reduced pancreatic echogenicity, enlargement, o[r] ductal dilation. The pancreas cannot be visualized in 40% due to overlying bowel gas.

C. **Computed Tomography (CT) Scanning:**
1. Contrast-enhanced CT scans have a sensitivity of 90% and a specificity of 100% for the diagnosis of acute pancreatitis.
2. **Indications for CT Scan:** Patients with acute pancreatitis who are seriously ill or uncertain diagnoses.

D. **Endoscopic Retrograde Cholangiopancreatography (ERCP):** Not routinely indicated during an attack of acute pancreatitis. Important role in specific situations:
1. Preoperative evaluation of suspected traumatic pancreatitis.
2. Suspected biliary pancreatitis with severe disease that is not improving and may need sphincterotomy and stone extraction.
3. In patients older than 40 years with no identifiable cause, ERCP is indicated once the attack of pancreatitis has subsided to determine the etiology.

V. **Assessment of Prognosis**
A. **Ranson's Criteria:**
1. Used to assess prognosis early in the course of acute pancreatitis.
2. Overall, mortality from acute pancreatitis is approximately 1% in patients with less than 3 signs, 15% with 3 or 4 signs, 40% with 5 or 6 signs, and 100% with 7 or more signs.

**Ranson's Criteria for Alcoholic Pancreatitis:**

| At Admission: | During Initial 48 Hours: |
|---|---|
| 1. Age over 55 years | 1. Hematocrit drop >10% points |
| 2. WBC >16,000/mm³ | 2. BUN rise >5 mg/dL |
| 3. Blood glucose >200 mg/dL (in a nondiabetic) | 3. Arterial PO2 <60 mm Hg |
| 4. Serum LDH >350 IU/L | 4. Base deficit >4 mEq/L |
| 5. AST >250 U/L | 5. Serum calcium <8.0 mg/dL |

6. Estimated fluid sequestration >6 L

**Ranson's Criteria for Nonalcoholic Pancreatitis:**

| Admission | Initial 48 hours |
|---|---|
| 1. Age over 70 years | 1. Hematocrit drop > 10% points |
| 2. WBC > 18,000/mm3 | 2. BUN rise > 2 mg/dL |
| 3. Blood glucose > 220 mg/dL (in a nondiabetic) | 3. Base deficit > 5 mEq/L |
| 4. Serum LDH > 400 IU/L | 4. Serum calcium < 8.0 mg/dL |
| 5. AST > 250 U/L | 5. Estimated fluid sequestration > 4 L |

I. **Complications**
  A. **Pseudocyst** is a pancreatic fluid collection that may regress or progress to a mature pseudocyst. Treated expectantly; monitor for infection or growth associated with increasing symptoms. If pseudocyst does not resolve by 6 weeks or if complications occur, drainage is indicated either percutaneously or surgically.
  B. **Necrotizing pancreatitis** occurs after infection of the necrotic pancreatic tissue, often within 6 days after the episode begins.
  C. Systemic complications include shock, adult respiratory distress syndrome (ARDS), renal failure, gastrointestinal bleeding.

II. **Treatment of Pancreatitis**
  A. **Supportive Medical Care for Local and Systemic Complications:** The majority of patients (>80%) have rapid resolution of the inflammatory process and a noncomplicated course.
  B. **Replace Intravascular Volume**, and maintain adequate urine output. Monitor central venous pressure and replace of calcium and magnesium deficits.
  C. **Pancreatic Rest:** No oral feeding until clinical symptoms of nausea, vomiting, and abdominal pain have subsided. Thereafter, feeding may be started, with gradual progression from liquids to a regular diet.
  D. **Nasogastric Suction** is not indicated routinely, and should be used only if severe nausea, vomiting or ileus.
  E. **Antibiotics:** Use prophylactic antibiotics only in patients with a temperature greater than 101.5°F, suspected cholangitis, or severe pancreatitis. Cefoxitin (Mefoxin) 1-2 gm IV q6-8h.
  F. **Analgesics:** Meperidine (Demerol) should be used; morphine may cause spasm of the sphincter of Oddi.
  G. **Necrotizing Pancreatitis:** Severe pancreatitis requires necrosectomy to remove necrotic pancreatic tissue and septic material, followed by local lavage and open drainage with surgically placed drains.
  H. **Cholecystectomy:** Should be performed early after an attack of biliary pancreatitis to prevent recurrences.

# Lower Gastrointestinal Bleeding

## I. Pathogenesis

A. Most acute LGI bleeding originates from the colon; however, 15-20% of episodes aris
from the small intestine and the upper gastrointestinal tract.

B. 80% of acute bleeding episodes stop spontaneously; bleeding is recurrent in 25%. N
source of bleeding can be identified in 12%.

## II. Initial Clinical Evaluation

A. Assess severity of blood loss and hemodynamic status; resuscitate with fluids and packe
red blood cells.

B. Perform an initiate diagnostic evaluation while the patient is being resuscitated t
determine the source of bleeding.

C. **Elderly Patients:** Diverticulosis and angiodysplasia are the most common causes c
lower GI bleeding.

D. **Younger Patients:** Hemorrhoids, anal fissures, and inflammatory bowel disease (IBC
are more common causes.

E. **Hematochezia:** Bright red or maroon blood per rectum suggests a lower GI source
however, 11-20% of patients with an upper GI bleed will have hematochezia as a resu
of rapid blood loss (these patients are usually in shock).

F. **Melena:** Sticky, black, foul-smelling stools suggest a source proximal to the ligament c
Treitz, but can result from bleeding in the small intestine or proximal colon. Melena i
often confused with clotted blood; however, melena is black and does not turn toilet wate
red, whereas clotted blood does. Iron and bismuth can turn stools black but not melanoti
(shiny and tarry).

G. **Causes of Acute Lower GI Bleeding:**

| | | | |
|---|---|---|---|
| Upper GI tract | 10% | Colon | 85% |
| Small intestine | 5% | | Diverticulosis |
| | Neoplasm | | Angiodysplasia |
| | Crohn's disease | | Neoplasms |
| | Aortoenteric fistula | | Inflammatory bowel disease |
| | Angiodysplasia | | Ischemia |
| | Meckel's diverticulum | | Colitis (radiation/infectious) |
| | | | Hemorrhoids |
| | | | Undiagnosed (10%) |

H. **Associated Findings:**

1. Abdominal pain may result from ischemic bowel, inflammatory bowel disease, or ruptured aortic aneurysm.
2. Painless, massive bleeding often indicates vascular bleeding from diverticul angiodysplasia, or hemorrhoids.
3. Bloody diarrhea suggests inflammatory bowel disease or an infectious origin.
4. Bleeding with rectal pain is seen with anal fissures, hemorrhoids, and rectal ulcers
5. Chronic constipation suggests hemorrhoidal bleeding; new onset constipation or thi stools suggests a left-sided, colonic malignancy.
6. Blood on the toilet paper or dripping into the toilet water after a bowel movemer usually indicates a perianal source.
7. Blood coating the outside of a normal stool suggests a lesion in the anal canal.
8. Blood streaking or mixed in with the stool may result from a polyp or malignancy i the descending colon.
9. Maroon colored stools often indicate small bowel and proximal colon bleeding.

## III. Physical Examination

A. **Postural Hypotension** suggests a 20% blood volume loss, whereas signs of shoc
pallor, hypotension, and tachycardia indicate a 30-40% blood loss.

B. **Digital Rectal Examination** should be performed on all patients, even in presumed UG bleeding. Check for anal fissures, hemorrhoids, and rectal masses. Examine the color and character of the stool, and test for occult blood to be certain that what is being reported as melena is not ingested iron or bismuth, or dark colored feces.

C. **Nasogastric (NG) lavage** is helpful if grossly positive; however, a negative lavage occurs in up to 16% of patients with a significant UGI bleeding. A negative lavage may often occur with a duodenal ulcer and pylorospasm that prevents regurgitation of blood into the stomach.

D. **Occult Blood Testing** of lavage fluid is useless because mild trauma from tube placement may cause a positive result.

E. Lower GI bleeding is usually intermittent, regardless of cause. Bleeding has usually ceased by the time the patient presents to the emergency room, although copious amounts of blood and clots may continue to be passed from the rectum.

IV. **Diagnostic Modalities**

A. **Anoscopy/Sigmoidoscopy:** Anoscopy and sigmoidoscopy should be done for all patients with acute LGI bleeding. Anoscopy should seek anal fissures and hemorrhoids. Sigmoidoscopy may reveal mucosal abnormalities, mass lesions in the rectum, sigmoid, and descending colon.

B. **Colonoscopy:** If large volume LGI hemorrhage has stopped, the colon can be prepared before colonoscopy. Active bleeding may impair visualization.

C. **Barium enema** has no role in the evaluation of acute LGI bleeding because it interferes with colonoscopy and angiography.

D. **Radionuclide Scanning:**
   1. Radionuclide scanning is used for localization of GI bleeding; they are noninvasive and relatively sensitive.
   2. **Technetium 99m-labeled Red Blood Cell Scan:** Autologous RBC's are labeled in vitro with technetium and injected. Can scan several times over 24 hours to detect intermittent bleeds; localizes the site of bleeding in 97%; specificity 83%. Only able to localize the bleeding to an area of the abdomen. Best used to determine which patients are bleeding sufficiently to undergo angiography.

E. **Angiography:**
   1. Extravasation of contrast material occurs if the arterial bleeding is >0.5 mL/min; does not require bowel preparation; anatomic localization is precise. Infusion of vasopressin and transcatheter embolization may be performed. Vasopressin is 90% successful in stopping colonic bleeding from diverticula or angiodysplasia.
   2. **Disadvantage:** Bleeding must be active; relatively high complication rate. Complications occur in 9%, including arterial thrombosis, embolization, renal failure. Success rate is 14-72%.

V. **Diagnostic Approach to Lower GI Bleeding**

A. **Resuscitation** should be performed before diagnostic or therapeutic studies are attempted. Provide intravenous fluids, blood transfusions, and correct coagulopathy.

B. **If Moderate-Severe Bleeding Has Stopped:**
   1. Examine with anoscopy/sigmoidoscopy for source of bleeding. If there is clinical suspicion of an upper GI source, initiate nasogastric lavage.
   2. If lavage is unrevealing, colonoscopy should be done.
   3. It may be difficult to make a definitive diagnosis of diverticular or angiodysplastic bleeding unless there is actively bleeding. Diagnosis of these disorders may often be presumptive because bleeding usually stops spontaneously.

C. **If Bleeding Continues at a Slow but Significant Rate:**
   1. A tagged RBC scan should be done.
   2. If this is unrevealing, endoscopy or mesenteric angiography should be considered.

D. **Severe, Continuous, or Recurrent Bleeding:**
   1. **Nasogastric lavage:** If lavage reveals signs of bleeding or is inadequate, perform an upper endoscopy.
   2. **If No Obvious Upper GI Bleeding Site Is Found:** Anoscopy/sigmoidoscopy should be done.

3. If no bleeding site is found, perform colonoscopy or a tagged RBC scan (followed by an angiogram if the tagged RBC scan is positive).

## VI. Therapeutic Options for Lower GI Bleeding

A. If the active bleeding site is identified at colonoscopy or angiography, the bleeding may be cauterized during the exam. Complications include bleeding and perforation.

B. Most patients will not require therapy because 80% of acute LGI bleeding episodes stop spontaneously.

C. Urgent therapy should be considered in patients with recurrent or continuous bleeding who require more than 3 units of blood.

D. Surgery should be considered in any patient requiring 6 or more units of blood.

E. **Angiographic Intra-arterial Vasopressin and Embolization:** Intra-arterial vasopressin is effective in up to 90% of patients bleeding from either angiodysplasia or diverticula Rebleeding occurs in about 50%, and complications occur in 5-15%. Selective arterial embolization should be reserved for patients who have failed intra-arterial vasopressin and who are not surgical candidates.

F. **Indications for Surgery:**
   1. Large-volume blood loss, or recurrent bleeding after colonoscopic and angiographic therapy.
   2. Angiodysplasia that are not controlled with electrocoagulation.
   3. Numerous angiodysplasia, making electrocoagulation unfeasible.

## VII. Common Causes of Lower GI Bleeding

A. **Diverticulosis:**
   1. Present in more than 50% of persons over 60 years old. The most common cause of acute LGI bleeding. Bleeding stops spontaneously in 80-90%; 10-25% will have recurrent episodes.
   2. Most are in the sigmoid colon; however, 35% of patients with diverticulosis have involvement of the ascending, transverse, or descending colon. Despite the greater involvement of the left colon, 50-70% of bleeding diverticula occur in the right colon
   3. Bleeding is sudden in onset, painless, and massive. Color is bright red or maroon but can be melanotic if bleeding occurs in the right colon.
   4. **Diagnosis:** Colonoscopy, tagged RBC scanning, and angiography.
   5. **Treatment:** Most cases of diverticular bleeding resolve spontaneously; however intra-arterial vasopressin or surgery may be needed.

B. **Angiodysplasia:**
   1. Angiodysplasia are mucosal vascular ectasia that develop as a process of aging.
   2. Angiodysplastic lesions occur in 25% of elderly. Most common after 50 years although they can occur at any age. Frequently multiple, <5 mm in diameter primarily involve the cecum and right colon (55%).
   3. Less than 10% of patients with angiodysplasia will bleed. May cause intermitten hemoccult positive stools, iron-deficiency anemia, melena, or hematochezia. 15-20% of patients present with an acute GI hemorrhage. Bleeding stops spontaneously in 80%; rebleeding occurs in 25-50%.
   4. **Diagnosis:** Colonoscopy is highly sensitive and can provide definitive therapy with electrocoagulation.
   5. **Treatment:** Recurrent bleeding requiring transfusion or causing anemia should be treated with electrocoagulation or surgical resection.

C. **Colon Polyps and Colon Cancers:**
   1. Rarely cause significant acute LGI hemorrhage.
   2. Left-sided and rectal neoplasms are more likely to cause gross bleeding than right sided lesions. Right sided lesions are more likely to cause anemia and occult bleeding.
   3. **Diagnosis:** Colonoscopy or barium enema.
   4. **Treatment:** Colonoscopic excision or surgery.

D. **Inflammatory Bowel Disease:**
  1. Ulcerative colitis can occasionally cause severe GI bleeding associated with abdominal pain and diarrhea.
  2. **Diagnosis:** Colonoscopy and biopsy.
  3. **Treatment:**Medical treatment of the underlying disease; surgery is required on rare occasions.

E. **Ischemic Colitis:**
  1. Seen in elderly patients with known vascular disease; abdominal pain may be postprandial, and is associated with bloody diarrhea or rectal bleeding. Severe blood loss is unusual but can occur.
  2. **Diagnosis:** Abdominal films may reveal "thumbprinting", caused by submucosal edema. Colonoscopy reveals a well-demarcated area of hyperemia, edema, and mucosal ulcerations. The splenic flexure and descending colon are the most common sites.
  3. **Treatment:** Most episodes resolve spontaneously; however, vascular bypass or resection may be required.

F. **Hemorrhoids:**
  1. Rarely cause massive acute blood loss requiring transfusion. In patients with portal hypertension, rectal varices must be sought.
  2. **Diagnosis:** Anoscopy and sigmoidoscopy.
  3. **Treatment:** High fiber diet, stool softeners, or hemorrhoidectomy.

G. **Small-Bowel Sources of Bleeding:**
  1. Account for only 5% of LGI bleeding and include malignancy, vascular lesions, Crohn's disease, and aortoenteric fistula. Meckel's diverticulum bleeding usually occurs in children but has been reported in adults.
  2. **Diagnosis:**Endoscopy, enteroclysis, angiography, and intraoperative enteroscopy.

H. **Uncommon Causes of Acute LGI Bleeding:** Infectious colitis, radiation colitis, and colonic ulcers.

# Acute and Chronic Diarrhea

I. **Clinical Evaluation of Acute Diarrhea**
   A. Assess the nature of onset, duration, frequency, and timing of the diarrheal episodes. Determine the stool's appearance, quantity, buoyancy; presence of blood or mucus; vomiting, pain, weight loss.
   B. Determine if contact with a potential source of infectious diarrhea has occurred.
   C. **Drugs That May Cause Diarrhea:** Laxatives, magnesium-containing compounds, sulfa drugs, antibiotics, alcohol.

II. **Physical Examination**
   A. **Assess Volume Status:** Dehydration is suggested by dry mucous membranes, orthostatic hypotension, tachycardia, mental status changes, and acute weight loss.
   B. **Abdominal tenderness,** mild distention, and hyperactive bowel sounds are common in acute infectious diarrhea. However, the presence of peritoneal signs or rigidity suggests toxic megacolon or perforation, requiring radiologic examination of the abdomen.
   C. **Evidence of systemic atherosclerosis** suggests ischemia. Lower extremity edema suggests malabsorption or protein loss.
   D. **Examination of a fresh stool** sample for color, consistency, buoyancy, and smell may provide evidence of steatorrhea.

III. **Acute Infectious Diarrhea**
   A. **Infectious diarrhea** is usually classified as noninflammatory or inflammatory, depending on whether the infectious organism has invaded the intestine.
   B. **Noninflammatory** infectious diarrhea is caused by organisms that produce a toxin (enterotoxigenic E coli strains, Vibrio cholerae). Noninflammatory infectious diarrhea is usually self-limiting and lasts less than 3 days.
   C. **Blood or mucus** in the stool suggests inflammatory disease, usually caused by bacterial invasion of the mucosa (enteroinvasive E coli, Shigella, Salmonella, Campylobacter) Patients usually appear to have sepsis and fever; some have abdominal rigidity and severe abdominal pain.
   D. **Vomiting out of Proportion to Diarrhea** is usually related to a neuroenterotoxin-mediated food poisoning from Staphylococcus aureus or Bacillus cereus, or from an enteric virus such as rotavirus (in an infant) or a small round virus such as Norwalk virus (in older children or adults). The incubation period for neuroenterotoxin food poisoning is less than 4 hours, while that of a viral agent is more than 8 hours.
   E. **Traveler's Diarrhea:** The most common type of acute infectious diarrhea. Typically, three or four unformed stools are passed per 24 hours, usually starting on the third day of travel and lasting 2-3 days. Accompanying symptoms may include anorexia, nausea, vomiting, abdominal cramps, abdominal bloating, and flatulence.
   F. **Antibiotic-Related Diarrhea:**
      1. Diarrhea ranges from mild illness to life-threatening pseudomembranous colitis.
      2. Overgrowth of Clostridium difficile causes pseudomembranous colitis. Ampicillin or amoxicillin, cephalosporins, and clindamycin have been implicated most often, but almost all antibiotics can cause this complication.
      3. Patients with pseudomembranous colitis have high fever, cramping, leukocytosis, and severe, watery diarrhea. Sigmoidoscopy reveals colitis, possibly with pseudomembranous plaques.
      4. Bacterial culture for C difficile requires 48 hours for results. Latex agglutination testing requires only 30 minutes.

IV. **Diagnostic Approach to Acute Infectious Diarrhea**
   A. Attempt to obtain a pathologic diagnosis in patients who give a history of recent ingestion of seafood (Vibrio parahaemolyticus), travel or camping, antibiotic use, homosexual activity, or who complain of fevers and abdominal pain.
   B. Determine if blood or mucus is visible in the stools, indicating the presence of Shigella

Salmonella, Campylobacter jejuni, enteroinvasive E. coli, C. difficile, or, less likely, Yersinia enterocolitica.
C. Most cases of mild diarrheal disease do not require laboratory studies to determine etiology.
D. In moderate to severe diarrhea with fever or pus in stools, submit a liquid stool culture for bacterial pathogens (Salmonella, Shigella, or Campylobacter). If a history of recent antibiotic use, stools should be sent for Clostridium difficile toxin.

## V. Laboratory Tests and Procedures for Acute Diarrhea
A. **Fecal Leukocytes:** Used as a screening test in moderate to severe diarrhea. Numerous leukocytes indicates Shigella, Salmonella, and C jejuni.
B. **Stool Cultures for Bacterial Pathogens:** Should be obtained if high fevers, severe or persistent (>14 d) diarrhea, dysentery, severe illness, bloody stools, or leukocytes.
C. **Examination for Ova and Parasites:** Indicated for persistent diarrhea (>14 d), travel to high-risk region, gay male, infant in day care center, dysentery with negative stool culture or with sparse fecal leukocytes.
D. **Blood Cultures:** Should be obtained prior to starting antibiotics if severe diarrhea and high fever.
E. **E coli 0157:H7 Cultures:** Hemorrhagic E coli should be suspected if bloody stools with minimal fever, or when diarrhea follows hamburger or fast food consumption, or when hemolytic uremic syndrome is diagnosed.
F. **Clostridium difficile Cytotoxin:** If diarrhea follows use of an antimicrobial agent, fecal samples should be tested for C difficile cytotoxin.
G. **Rotavirus Antigen Test (Rotazyme):** Indicated for hospitalized children <2 years old with gastroenteritis. The finding of rotavirus eliminates the need for antibiotics.

## VI. Treatment of Acute Diarrhea
A. **Fluid and Electrolyte Resuscitation:**
1. **Oral Rehydration:** For cases of mild to moderate diarrhea, administer Pedialyte or Ricelyte. For adults with travelers' diarrhea, flavored soft drinks augmented with saltine crackers are usually adequate.
2. **Intravenous Hydration:** Should be used in patients with contraindications to oral rehydration; potassium and sodium bicarbonate may be added.
B. **Diet:**
1. **Infants:** Breast milk or lactose-free formula should be continued.
2. **Older Children and Adults:** Boiled starches (potatoes, noodles) and cereals (rice, wheat) with some salt. Crackers, bananas, soup and boiled vegetables. Milk products are excluded until clinically well.
3. Diet may return to normal when stools become formed.
4. The recommendation that clear liquids only be ingested during diarrhea is incorrect. Clear fluids can lead to an osmotic diarrhea and electrolyte imbalance.

## VII. Antimicrobial Treatment of Acute Diarrhea
A. **Empiric Drug Therapy:**
1. **Febrile Dysenteric Syndrome:**
   a. If diarrhea is associated with high fever and stools with mucus and blood, empiric antibacterial therapy may be given for Shigella or Campylobacter jejuni.
   b. **Children:** Trimethoprim/sulfamethoxazole and erythromycin. **Adults:** Norfloxacin (Noroxin) 400 mg bid, ciprofloxacin (Cipro) 500 mg bid, ofloxacin (Floxin) 300 mg bid, or fleroxacin 400 mg qd for 3-5 days.
2. **Travelers' Diarrhea:**
   a. **Acute Travelers' Diarrhea:** Children with severe cases: TMP/SMX and erythromycin. Adults: Norfloxacin 400 mg bid, ciprofloxacin 500 mg bid, ofloxacin 300 mg bid, or fleroxacin 400 mg qd for 3 days. Loperamide is added if no fever or dysentery.
   b. **Persistent Travelers' Diarrhea** lasting longer than 2 weeks and nonresponsive to antibiotics, treat with metronidazole (Flagyl), 250 mg qid for 7-10 days.

B. **Agent-specific Therapy:**
   1. When culture identifies an etiologic agent in stool, specific antimicrobial therapy may be used.
   2. **Shigella:** TMP/SMX DS bid PO for 3-5 d
   3. **Salmonella:**Only toxic and febrile patients require antimicrobial therapy. Children, TMP/SMX for 2 weeks. Adults, ciprofloxacin 500 mg bid or ofloxacin 300 mg bid for 10 days. For milder forms of disease, antibacterials should be withheld to prevent prolongation of illness.
   4. **Campylobacter jejuni:** Children: Erythromycin for 5 days. Adults: Erythromycin 250 mg PO qid for 5 days.
   5. **Aeromonas, Plesiomonas, Shigelloides:** Treat as for Shigella infection.
   6. **Enteropathogenic E coli:** Susceptibility testing is needed to determine optimal drug because of antimicrobial resistance.
   7. **Enterohemorrhagic E coli (0157:H7):** Antibiotics are not used to treat hemorrhagic E coli colitis.
   8. **Clostridium difficile colitis:** Metronidazole, 250 mg PO qid.
   9. **Giardiasis:**Children: Quinacrine or furazolidone for 7 d. Adults: Quinacrine 100 mg tid or metronidazole 250 mg PO qid for 7 d.
   10. **Amebiasis:** A trophozoite-active drug (metronidazole) is indicated to treat the symptoms, and a cyst-active drug (diiodohydroxyquin) is needed to prevent relapses. Adults: Metronidazole 750 mg PO tid for 5 d and diiodohydroxyquin 650 mg PO tid for 20 d.
   11. **Cryptosporidiosis:** No treatment is indicated in children; adults may be treated in severe cases with paromomycin 500 mg PO qid for 7-10 days.

C. **Symptomatic Treatment of Acute Diarrhea:**
   1. **Attapulgite (Kaopectate):** Adults: 3 tablespoonfuls initially, repeat after each unformed stool.
   2. **Antimotility Drugs:**
      a. Should not be used if fever or dysentery; should not be used for more than 48 hours.
      b. **Diphenoxylate (Lomotil):** 1-2 tabs PO qid, max 12 tabs/day. Diphenoxylate has greater overdose liability for children; anticholinergic side effects.
      c. **Loperamide (Imodium):** 4 mg initially, followed by 2 mg after each unformed stool, max 16 mg/d.

VIII. **Clinical Evaluation of Chronic Diarrhea**
   A. Diarrhea is considered chronic if it occurs acutely, subsides, and then returns, or if it lasts longer than 2 weeks.
   B. Determine characteristics of diarrhea, including volume, mucus, blood, flatus, cramps, tenesmus, duration, frequency, effect of fasting, stress, effect of specific foods such as dairy products, wheat, laxatives, fruits. Other chronic disorders (diabetes).
   C. **Classification of Chronic Diarrhea:**
      1. **Secretory:** Diarrhea results from increased intestinal secretion secondary to toxin production or hormonal hypersecretion (thyrotoxicosis or carcinoid).
      2. **Osmotic:** Osmotically active solutes in the gut lumen result in loss of water. Magnesium or sulfate-containing substances (laxatives), or unabsorbed carbohydrates (lactase deficiency, fructose intolerance, celiac disease, or pancreatic insufficiency).
      3. **Exudative:** Mucus, blood, and proteins are discharged as a result of inflammatory bowel disease (ulcerative colitis, Crohn's disease, ischemic colitis).
      4. **Motor:** Systemic sclerosis, pseudo-obstruction, diabetes-associated neuropathic damage.
      5. **Functional:** No organic cause can be found, but psychological stress and sex hormones may play a role.

**IX.** **Laboratory Evaluation of Chronic Diarrhea**

A. The history can usually distinguish secretory from osmotic diarrhea.

B. Complete blood cell count (anemia or leukocytosis); serum electrolytes. Elevation of erythrocyte sedimentation rate suggests an inflammatory condition.

C. **Fecal Osmotic Gap:** Helpful in distinguishing between secretory and osmotic diarrhea.

Osmotic gap = plasma osmolality - [(fecal sodium + potassium) x 2]

In secretory diarrhea, the fecal osmotic gap is <40.

In osmotic diarrhea, fecal osmotic gap is >40.

D. **Secretory Diarrhea:**
1. Characterized by large stool volumes (>1 L per day), little or no decrease with fasting, and a fecal osmotic gap <40.
2. **Evaluation of Secretory Diarrhea:** Giardia antigen, Entamoeba histolytica antibody titers, Yersinia culture, fasting serum glucose, thyroid function tests, cholestyramine (Cholybar, Questran) trial.

E. **Osmotic Diarrhea:** Characterized by small stool volumes, a decrease with fasting, and a fecal osmotic gap >40. Postprandial diarrhea with bloating or flatus also suggests osmotic diarrhea. Osmotically active laxative use may be inadvertent (chewing sugarless gum containing sorbitol) or covert (with eating disorders).
1. **Evaluation of Osmotic Diarrhea:**
Trial of lactose withdrawal
Trial of antibiotic (metronidazole) for small-bowel bacterial overgrowth
Screening for celiac disease (anti-endomysial antibody, antigliadin antibody)
Fecal fat measurement (72 hr) for pancreatic insufficiency
Trial of fructose avoidance
Stool test for phenolphthalein and magnesium if laxative abuse suspected
Hydrogen breath analysis to help identify disaccharidase deficiency or bacterial overgrowth

F. **Exudative Diarrhea:**
1. Characterized by bloody stools, tenesmus (urge to defecate), urgency, cramping pain, nocturnal occurrence. Most often due to inflammatory bowel disease, which may be indicated by the presence of anemia, hypoalbuminemia, and an increased sedimentation rate.
2. **Evaluation of Exudative Diarrhea:** Complete blood cell count, serum albumin, total protein, erythrocyte sedimentation rate, electrolyte measurement, Entamoeba histolytica antibody titers, stool culture, Clostridium difficile antigen test, ova and parasite testing; flexible sigmoidoscopy and biopsies.

G. **Functional Diarrhea:** More common in women than men, and onset is usually before age 50. Patients usually give a long history of loose stools, typically exacerbated by stress. Episodes are often characterized by morning urgency and relief of abdominal pain after defecation.

H. **Small-Bowel Bacterial Overgrowth:** Common in patients with decreased motility (very elderly or diabetic patients), but can also occur in the absence of overt bowel disease.

I. **Diabetic Diarrhea:** The presence of neuropathy or gastroparesis suggests idiopathic diabetic diarrhea. In diabetic patients, withdrawal of foods that are high in fructose or sorbitol may dramatically improve diarrhea. An antibiotic (metronidazole, tetracycline) may be tried if bacterial overgrowth is suspected.

J. **Celiac Disease:** Supported by antiendomysial, antigiladin, or antireticulin antibodies; however, biopsy and improvement on a gluten-free diet are required for confirmation.

# Neurology

---

## Stroke

I. **Clinical Evaluation of the Stroke Patient**
   A. Determine when symptoms started and stopped, and whether symptoms came on abruptly or gradually. Hemorrhages and embolic strokes typically appear suddenly; thrombotic strokes may have a more stuttering course, with progressive neurologic symptoms such as a spreading numbness or weakness.
   B. A history of transient ischemic attacks (TIA), especially in a crescendo pattern, is a strong predictor of ischemic stroke. About 30% of patients with TIAs go on to have full-blown strokes, although less than half of patients have had a preceding TIA before a ischemic stroke.
   C. Markers of vascular disease such as diabetes, angina pectoris, and intermittent claudication point to cerebral infarction. A history of atrial fibrillation or MI suggests ischemic stroke from a cardiac embolus.
   D. Risk factors for stroke including smoking, hypertension, hyperlipidemia, diabetes mellitus, and heart disease.
   E. Sudden, explosive, headache pain, which is typically describes as "the worst headache of my life," are the classic signs of subarachnoid hemorrhage. Head pain is less common in ischemic strokes. Increased intracranial pressure from bleeding is also likely to trigger an emetic response or syncope. Other signs of subarachnoid hemorrhage include impaired consciousness, photophobia, and stiff neck.
   F. In younger people, about half of all strokes are hemorrhagic; in older people, 20-25% are hemorrhagic. Younger people are at greater risk for congenital aneurysms; older people have a higher risk of lacunar disease. Young people with sickle cell disease are at high risk for ischemic stroke. Hemophilia is a risk factor for hemorrhagic stroke.
   G. Migraine can cause pain severe enough to mimic subarachnoid hemorrhage, but migraines appear gradually (often with an aura), rather than suddenly. Hemiplegic migraine is more common in young women, who are unlikely to have atherosclerotic disease.
   H. Cocaine-related strokes are not common but should be considered in young adults; cocaine may be associated with either ischemia or hemorrhage.

II. **Neurologic Examination**
   A. Determine whether the patient's condition is acutely deteriorating or relatively stable. Key information includes level of consciousness, orientation; ability to speak and understand language; basic cranial nerve function, especially eye movements and pupil reflexes, facial paresis; neglect, gaze preference, arm and leg strength, sensation, reflexes, coordination in the arms and legs, and walking ability.
   B. Level of consciousness is the single most important predictor of short-term survival. A semiconscious or unconscious patient probably has a hemorrhage. A patient with an ischemic stroke may be drowsy but is unlikely to lose consciousness unless the infarcted area is large.
   C. All patients should be evaluated for the need for immediate surgery if there are signs of intracerebral, cerebellar, or subarachnoid hemorrhage. In an unconscious patient, consider the possibility of hydrocephalus from hemorrhage directly into the ventricles. This condition requires urgent surgery. Hydrocephalus after subarachnoid hemorrhage may be delayed, and may present with lethargy, stupor, gait difficulties, urinary incontinence, and cognitive dysfunction.
   D. Gaze deviations help localize a stroke. A stroke in the right hemisphere impairs motor actions (including the gaze centers) and perception on the left side of the body; consequently, the eyes will look toward the good side of the body and the bad side of the brain. Tell the patient to look to the left; with a right hemisphere lesion, the eyes will have trouble moving leftward across the midline because half the visual field is missing.

E. Left hemispheric syndromes are characterized by right-sided weakness with aphasia since the brain regions controlling motor function on the right half of the body are close to the regions controlling linguistic functions in the left frontal cortex.

F. Vertebrobasilar circulation syndromes are characterized by double vision, facial weakness, vertigo, and weakness or numbness on both sides of the body.

G. Impaired motor function in a large region of the body (such as paralysis of the face, arm, and leg on one side, or complete hemiparesis) points to a large area of cerebral infarction or to a smaller lesion in the white matter (internal capsule) or the upper brain stem.

H. The higher the initial BP, the more likely the stroke is a cerebral hemorrhage.

## III. CT Scanning and Other Diagnostic Studies

A. All patients with signs of stroke should undergo a noncontrast head CT to screen for bleeding and conditions that mimic stroke. A patient in acutely deteriorating condition should have an immediate CT to rule out expanding lesions such as subdural hematomas, epidural hematomas, or other indications for emergent surgery.

B. An initially negative CT scan is common early in ischemic strokes. CT is the most definitive modality for finding bleeds, but in infarction it does not detect the full extent of tissue damage until several days later. If the screening CT scan is equivocal or negative, consider MRI to localize a cerebral infarct; gadopentetate dimeglumine (Magnevist) contrast media may be used.

C. CT misses subarachnoid hemorrhage 5-10% of the time. If CT is negative, a lumbar puncture is mandatory when subarachnoid hemorrhage is suspected, such as when sudden onset of an excruciating headache has occurred.

D. **Laboratory Studies:** Blood glucose measurement, electrolytes, BUN, creatinine urinalysis; rapid plasma reagin (RPR) test to screen for syphilis.

E. **Complete Blood Count** may aid in detecting polycythemia or severe anemia. Platelet count, prothrombin time, and partial thromboplastin time may detect coagulopathies.

F. **Serum Thrombogenic Factors:** In younger patients with a history of miscarriages or deep vein thrombosis, anticardiolipoprotein, lupus anticoagulant, protein C, and protein S should be considered.

G. **12-lead ECG** should be assessed for signs of concomitant myocardial infarction (MI) or ischemia (ST segment elevations) or atrial fibrillation (a risk factor for stroke).

H. **Plain chest films** should exclude aspiration pneumonia. To evaluate swallowing ability, consider video fluoroscopic swallowing studies.

I. **Echocardiography and Holter monitoring** are recommended for evaluation of suspected cardiogenic embolism. Transesophageal echo should be obtained if transthoracic echo is negative, but a cardiogenic source if emboli is suspected.

J. **Carotid Ultrasonography with Doppler** in the subacute phase should be considered if the patient has sustained a non-disabling, anterior circulation stroke or TIA, and the patient is a candidate for endarterectomy.

K. **Electroencephalography** is indicated only if seizures have occurred. Up to 17% of patients with acute stroke have early seizures.

## IV. Differential Diagnosis of Stroke Syndromes

A. **Large Vessel Thrombotic Event:** Right hemiparesis associated with aphasia and right visual field cut is consistent with a large vessel thrombotic event causing a left hemispheric cortical infarction.

B. **Lacunar Stroke:**
  1. Characterized by focal hemiparesis without sensory loss, visual field cut, or a language disorder in an elderly patient, or pure sensory strokes, or dysarthria with clumsiness of one hand.
  2. Lacunar strokes are due to small hemorrhages or infarcts of deep cerebral white matter, usually in hypertensive patients but also in those with diabetes or carotid atherosclerosis.

C. **Cardiogenic Stroke** is characterized by sudden onset of a maximal deficit, presence of a potential cardioembolic source (atrial fibrillation, myocardial infarction, patent foramen ovale, or valvular disease), and presence of multiple, bilateral, conical infarctions by CT. Evidence of embolism to other organs may be apparent. Cardiac thrombi may be demonstrated by echocardiography. About 25% of all ischemic strokes are due to cardioemboli.

D. **Subacute Bacterial Endocarditis:** Fever and a new cardiac murmur is suggestive of embolism caused by endocarditis.

E. **Arterial Dissection:** Stroke following trauma to the head or neck raises the suspicion of a carotid or vertebral arterial dissection.

## V. Immediate Management of Stroke

A. **Airway and Breathing:** First secure the ABCs--airway, breathing, and circulation. Maintain normal oxygenation and near-normal $pCO_2$. Protect the upper airway from accumulated secretions. Labored or weak respirations are an indication for intubation and ventilation.

B. **Hypertension:**
1. May be either an initiating or a secondary event in patients with stroke. Diastolic blood pressure up to 110 mm Hg is not a concern unless there is end-organ compromise (heart failure) because pressure usually falls without treatment within days.
2. Blood pressure should not be aggressively reduced in ischemic stroke unless there is either severe hypertension (>220/120 mmHg), aortic dissection, heart failure or ischemia, hypertensive encephalopathy, or nephropathy. Overly aggressive blood pressure reduction reduces cerebral blood flow.
3. If treatment is needed, labetalol (Normodyne) is recommended. Reflex vasoconstriction and tachycardia are prevented by its alpha and beta blockade; 50 mg IV over 1 minute, repeated every 5 minutes if needed, maximum total dose of 200 mg. Nitrates are contraindicated because they increase intracerebral pressure.
4. Nitroprusside is a cerebral vasodilator and may increase intracerebral pressure, but it is readily titratable; start the dosage at 0.25 mcg/kg/min IV, and increase at increments of 0.25 mcg/kg/min to a maximum of 10 mcg/kg/min.

C. **Hypotension** should prompt a search for myocardial infarction, pulmonary embolism, internal hemorrhage, sepsis, or volume depletion.

D. **Hyperglycemia:** Existing diabetes can worsen after a stroke, and high blood glucose levels may increase tissue damage. Low doses of insulin should be administered if glucose levels rise above 160 mg/dL. Intravenous fluid routinely should be normal saline, not dextrose-saline.

E. **Hyperthermia** occurs in a third of stroke patients. An elevation of temperature by even one degree can increase brain damage. Acetaminophen is the first-line approach, and a cooling blanket should be used if necessary.

F. **Loss of Consciousness:** A unilateral stroke usually does not result in loss of consciousness or depressed mentation. Causes of depressed mentation and loss of consciousness include increased intracranial pressure (subarachnoid hemorrhage, hematoma), brainstem infarction, bihemispheric infarction. These complications should be rapidly evaluated and treated.

## VI. Emergency Interventions In Stroke

A. **Hemorrhagic Stroke:**
1. Immediate surgical evacuation may be required when a stroke is causing a shift within the brain, producing severe neurologic dysfunction. This is common with aneurysm-induced hematomas, intracerebral hematomas, or any cerebellar hematoma larger than 3 cm. Surgery should not be delayed until the patient is lethargic or comatose.
2. **Elevated Intracranial Pressure:**
   a. May result from hemorrhage or from cytotoxic edema (which complicates large infarcts), usually at about 24 to 48 hours. A common initial manifestation is reduced level of consciousness.
   b. Neurosurgical consultation for ventriculostomy should be obtained immediately, especially if the rise in pressure is due to a cerebellar infarct or hemorrhage.
   c. Management consists of raising the patient's head 30 degrees and minimizing

temperature elevations. Intubation and hyperventilation may be necessary temporarily to lower the $pCO_2$ level to 25 to 30 mm Hg.

    d. Mannitol may be given in a loading dose of 25-50 g over 30 minutes; 25-g doses can be repeated if necessary, as often as every 4 hours over 1 to 2 days. A rebound effect may occur when mannitol is discontinued.

    e. Furosemide (Lasix) is indicated for overhydrated patients, 20-40 mg IV.

  3. **Subarachnoid Hemorrhage:**

    a. Subarachnoid hemorrhage is the cause of 5% of strokes, and at least 8 of 10 are due to ruptured saccular aneurysms.

    b. Consider immediate neurosurgical consultation and angiographic evaluation. Emergent aneurysm clipping with clot removal will prevent rebleeding, lowering the rates of hydrocephalus and vasospasm.

    c. Nimodipine (Nimotop) should be considered to prevent vasospasm in subarachnoid hemorrhage; a semi-cerebroselective calcium channel blocker; two 30-mg capsules q4h, beginning no later than 48 hours from the hemorrhage and continuing for 21 days. Monitor BP carefully because hypotension is common.

B. **Ischemic Stroke**

  1. IV heparin is usually given only if (1) the stroke is actively evolving, and the patient's condition is worsening; (2) TIAs are increasing in frequency and severity (crescendo TIAs); (3) high-grade vertebrobasilar atherothrombotic disease places the patient at risk for basilar artery occlusion; (4) arterial dissection; or (5) the stroke was caused by a cardiac embolus and is not massive.

  2. Avoid heparin if the patient is at risk for intraparenchymal bleeding, uncontrolled hypertension, or bleeding at another site.

  3. Consider using thrombolytics only if hemorrhage has been definitively ruled out. Use of recombinant tissue plasminogen activator or urokinase has led to significant and sustained neurologic improvement when initiated within the first 6 hours.

VII. **Continuing Treatment**

A. **Ischemic Stroke**: When hemorrhage has been ruled out, consider long-term treatments that prevent recurrent clot formation: Aspirin 325 mg/d is used if heparin and warfarin are not indicated. Ticlopidine is appropriate for patients who cannot take aspirin or who were already on aspirin at the time of their stroke.

B. **Lacunar Infarction:** Should be treated with aspirin 325 mg PO qd and hypertension should be controlled.

C. **Cardiogenic Embolism:**

  1. In patients with cardiogenic stroke, anticoagulation reduces the recurrence rate and is indicated if (1) there are no contraindications, (2) bleeding is not seen on brain imaging studies, (3) the infarct is not large, and (4) bacterial endocarditis is not a cause.

  2. Heparin should be delayed for at least 48 hours after admission; later, it should be replaced by warfarin (Coumadin) titrated to a prothrombin time of 1.3-1.6 times control or an International Normalizing Ratio of 2-3.

  3. In patients with atrial fibrillation who cannot be given anticoagulants, aspirin reduces the risk of further stroke, but not by nearly as much as warfarin.

D. **General Care:** Deep vein thrombosis must be prevented by the use of low-dose heparin and elastic stockings in patients with an immobile limb. After the third day, small intracerebral hemorrhages do not contraindicate use of low doses of anticoagulants.

E. **Nutrition and Electrolyte Balance:**

  1. Nasogastric tube feeding is necessary if there is any compromise in swallowing (eg, if the patient coughs after drinking 100 mL of water). A soft diet with thickened liquids may be initiated later if tolerated.

  2. Electrolyte imbalances should be corrected. The syndrome of inappropriate antidiuretic hormone secretion may be manifest by hyponatremia, and it should be treated with fluid restriction.

# Transient Ischemic Attack

## Clinical Evaluation

A. **Transient Ischemic Attacks** are defined as a focal neurologic deficit due to a cerebrovascular event from which the patient recovers completely in less than 24 hours. Most TIAs last only 5 to 30 minutes, and little if any permanent brain damage results. When clinical manifestations persist beyond 24 hours, the event is considered a stroke.

B. TIAs develop rapidly, usually progressing from no symptoms to maximum symptoms in less than 5 minutes, and often in less than 1 minute. TIAs commonly last 2-20 minutes, but can last for as long as 24 hours.

C. TIAs are "ministrokes" that should prompt urgent evaluation, and hospitalization in an effort to prevent devastating consequences.

D. The most frequent mechanism of a TIA is embolization by a thrombus from an atherosclerotic plaque in a large vessel (stenotic carotid artery). TIAs may also occur as manifestations of intracranial atherosclerotic disease (lacunar TIAs) or large-vessel occlusion. In addition, they can be associated with (1) atrial fibrillation or mitral valve prolapse, (2) carotid or vertebral dissection, and (3) hypercoagulable states (antiphospholipid antibody syndrome).

E. **Uncommon Causes of TIAs:**
   1. Temporal arteritis; thrombotic diathesis (most commonly caused by lupus anticoagulant or anticardiolipin antibodies, often with smoking or birth control pills); classic migraine; blood dyscrasias (leukemia, thrombocytosis, sickle cell anemia); thrombotic thrombocytopenic purpura; chronic meningitis (syphilis); and drug abuse (cocaine, amphetamines, phenylpropanolamine, ephedrine, heroin).
   2. Unusual causes of TIA or stroke should be strongly considered in patients <45 years old, and in older patients without risk factors for vascular disease (hypertension, diabetes, coronary artery disease).

## II. Evaluation of TIA Symptoms

A. Determine the activity in which the patient was engaged, and the patient's physical position at the onset of the attack. Obtain a description of the specific symptoms of the attack, including the speed with which they developed, whether they were bilateral or unilateral, and their duration.

B. Ascertain history of hypertension, diabetes, cardiac disease, previous TIA or stroke, cigarette smoking, and use of street drugs.

C. TIAs are identified by their location in either the carotid or vertebrobasilar region.
   1. **Symptoms of Carotid TIAs:**
      a. Transient loss of vision in one eye (amaurosis fugax) resulting from retinal ischemia.
      b. Contralateral motor deficit in one or both extremities, which appears as weakness, paralysis, poor function, or clumsiness on one side.
      c. Contralateral sensory deficits (numbness) which present all at once and may be accompanied by a minor impairment of motor function.
      d. Aphasia or dysarthria can range from minor speech or language disturbances to global disturbances in reading, writing, or calculating.
   2. **Symptoms of Vertebrobasilar TIAs:** The manifestations of vertebrobasilar TIAs are more varied and complex than those associated with carotid TIAs. An episode should be considered a TIA only if two or more of the following symptoms occur in combination:
      a. Vertigo (with or without nausea and vomiting) is the most common symptom, occurring with other neurologic symptoms of brainstem or cerebellar ischemia (diplopia, dysphagia, or dysarthria).
      b. Binocular loss of vision, complete or partial.
      c. Motor deficit, appearing as weakness, clumsiness, or paralysis, in any combination of extremities.
      d. Sensory deficit appearing as numbness, loss of sensation, or paresthesia, in any combination of extremities or on both sides of the mouth or face.

      e. Ataxia, imbalance, unsteadiness, or disequilibrium.

D. **Differentiating TIAs From Other Entities:**
1. **Seizures:** Almost always involve a change in the level of consciousness or awareness, excessive motor activity and confusion, none of which characterizes a TIA.
2. **Syncope**Changes in cardiac output produce generalized, rather than focal, cerebral ischemia, characterized by loss of consciousness and a rapid heartbeat (often due to an arrhythmia).
3. **Benign Positional Vertigo:** Recurrent waves of dizziness which last 2-10 seconds, related to movement (standing up or sitting down)are likely to represent benign positional vertigo, an inner ear disorder.
4. **Meniere's Disease** causes episodic vertigo that does not involve impaired sensory or motor function, and vertigo is accompanied by tinnitus and hearing loss.
5. **Peripheral Neuropathy:** Transitory paresthesias involving one or both upper extremities, particularly when associated with neck or shoulder pain, are more likely to represent radicular compression related to cervical disk disease. Recurrent numbness of a hand occurring at night or while driving is most likely to represent carpal tunnel syndrome.
6. **Brain Tumors:** Tumors can cause symptoms similar to a TIA; however, patients with tumors show evidence of cranial nerve deficits, increased intracranial pressure, a progressive decline in intellectual capacity and awareness, and progressive disturbances in motor and sensory function.
7. **Migraine** can cause cerebral ischemia and TIA-like symptoms. Usually there is a history of unilateral headache with nausea and vomiting. The onset of migraine headaches occurs several decades before the typical onset of TIAs.

E. **Physical Exam:** Check heart rate, rhythm; blood pressure in both arms; peripheral pulses; skin lesions such as petechiae of embolic origin, or skin manifestations of connective tissue disease.

F. Auscultate for cervical bruits. Palpation of the carotid is not recommended because it can dislodge emboli. Ophthalmoscopic examination can detect arterial or venous occlusion and emboli.

G. The neurologic examination should be normal in TIA patients unless the patient has had a previous stroke or is currently experiencing a TIA or stroke.

III. **Laboratory Studies**

A. Urinalysis, complete blood count, erythrocyte sedimentation rate, blood chemistry, and fasting lipid panel.

B. ECG; Holter monitoring may be indicated in patients with suspected cardiac arrhythmias.

C. Chest x-ray may provide information about the cardiac, aortic and pulmonary diseases.

D. Cranial CT Scan or MRI is valuable in the differentiating hemorrhage from infarction. Either of these should be performed in any patient with suspected TIA or progressing stroke.

E. **Carotid Duplex Study:** Combination of a carotid Doppler study (measures degree of stenosis), and B-mode carotid ultrasound (defines plaque shape and structure) should be used for evaluation of carotid arteries if carotid endarterectomy is being considered.

F. **Transthoracic Echocardiography:** Indications include cardiac disease, age <45 years, patients >45 years without evidence of atheromatous disease. Transesophageal echocardiography should be considered if cardiogenic embolism is suspected despite a negative transthoracic echocardiography.

G. **Holter Monitoring:** Used to rule out suspected intermittent atrial fibrillation.

H. **Lumbar Puncture:** Indicated when there is suspicion of meningitis, or if serology is positive for syphilis.

I. **Electroencephalogram:** May help to exclude partial seizures if suspected.

IV. **Approach to Management**

A. Carotid Stenosis
1. **Aspirin** is an antiplatelet agent that irreversibly inhibits platelet cyclooxygenase.

Aspirin effectively reduces the incidence of nonfatal stroke by 22%; 325-500 mg PO qd.

2. **Ticlopidine** is an antiplatelet agent that reversibly inhibits platelet aggregation. A 30% reduction in ischemic stroke occurs with ticlopidine. Ticlopidine is indicated for patients who are intolerant to aspirin, or for patients who have had TIA's while taking aspirin. Superior to aspirin for stroke prevention, but has a greater number of side effects including rash, diarrhea, and potentially life-threatening neutropenia. White blood cell count should be monitored every 2 weeks for the first 3 months of therapy; 250 mg PO bid.

3. **Heparin** may be used only for crescendo TIAs or "stroke in evolution."

4. **Management of Symptomatic Carotid Stenosis:**
   a. Patients who have a carotid territory transient ischemic attack or minor stroke who are candidates for endarterectomy should undergo prompt carotid Doppler examination. Subsequent management and referral depend on the degree of stenosis and assessment of the patient's risk for angiography and endarterectomy. Carotid endarterectomy is not indicated if dementia, medical instability, or if no more TIAs occur after medical treatment.
   b. **Low-grade Stenosis:**
      (1) Patients with low-grade atherosclerosis (minor plaques or stenosis of up to 29% should be treated with aspirin and risk-factor reduction.
      (2) No benefit from carotid endarterectomy has been demonstrated in these patients.
   c. **Moderate Stenosis:**
      (1) Patients with moderate stenosis (30% to 69%) should be evaluated by carotid angiography to determine the precise degree of disease.
      (2) If moderate Stenosis is confirmed, the patient should be referred to a center participating in the North American Symptomatic Carotid Endarterectomy Trial (NASCET).
      (3) Patients with moderate degrees of stenosis and ulceration are also at higher risk for subsequent embolic events, and they should be considered for endarterectomy.
      (4) Patients with a prohibitive surgical risk factor (recent myocardial infarction, severe heart failure, inoperable coronary artery disease) should be treated with aspirin and risk-factor reduction.
   d. **High-grade Stenosis:**
      (1) Endarterectomy is the treatment of choice for symptomatic patients with severe (70% to 99%) ipsilateral stenosis of the internal carotid artery.
      (2) If patients are fit for surgery, they should first undergo arterial angiography.

B. **Cardioembolism:**
   1. TIAs may have an underlying source of cardiac emboli in up to 23% of patients. Heparin should be initiated if the TIA has a cardiogenic source of embolism.

C. **Vertebrobasilar Ischemia**
   1. **Mechanisms for Ischemia in the Posterior Circulation:** Large-vessel atherosclerosis affecting the vertebral or basilar arteries in 40% of cases, microvascular disease in 20%, cardioembolism in 20%, and artery-to-artery embolism in 20%.
   2. If an ongoing source of cardioembolism is present, then long-term warfarin therapy is indicated and aspirin is reserved for patients in the remaining categories.

# Dementia and Alzheimer's Disease

I. **Classification of Neurologic Syndromes**
   A. **Dementia** is characterized by a decline from a previous higher level of intellectual function of sufficient severity to interfere with social or occupational performance or both. Dementia is a syndrome produced by many disorders including Alzheimer's disease.
   B. **Age-Associated Memory Impairment (AAMI):** Consists of cognitive impairment without functional decline. This disorder is not dementia.
      1. Only memory is impaired
      2. Diminished timely retrieval of specific information
      3. Not disabling
      4. Awareness preserved
      5. Learning continues
   C. **Delirium** is a disorder of attention (abnormal consciousness), characterized by lethargy, stupor, coma.
   D. **Pseudodementia** is depression that mimics dementia. 10% of patients presenting with symptoms of dementia actually have primary depression.
      1. Dementia presents with a more global decline in cognitive function than does depression. Neuropsychiatric tests are often helpful in distinguishing depression from dementia.
      2. Patients with dementia often attempt to disguise their cognitive deficits with confabulation; dementia patients usually make a real effort to answer correctly. Social skills are preserved in dementia and patients become distressed when they make errors.
      3. Patients with primary depression often show diminished effort. They answer with "I don't know," and responses are characterized by low self esteem. Depression may be associated with altered appetite (usually decreased), weight change (usually weight loss), decreased energy, crying spells, anhedonia (loss of interest), and hypersomnia or insomnia.
      4. Patients with dementia, may exhibit depressive symptoms.

II. **Causes of Dementia**
   A. **Alzheimer's Disease**
      1. Most frequent cause of dementia; accounts for 50-80% of subjects with dementia
      2. Insidious onset with gradual progression over years
      3. Early difficulty with memory, then anomia, then more widespread cognitive impairment and behavioral alterations. Mental status changes, aphasia, memory loss, visuospatial deficits, neuropsychiatric changes (indifference, delusions) occur; motor function remains normal.
      4. The Neurologic exam is usually normal
      5. Risk Factors: Age, genetic influences, female gender, lack of education, head trauma, myocardial infarction
      6. **Neuroimaging:** CT and MRI may be normal or show atrophy
      7. **Diagnostic Criteria for Alzheimer's Disease:**
         a. Presence of dementia as established by clinical examination and mental status testing
         b. Deficits in two or more areas of cognition (affect, executive function, language, praxis, visual special relations, calculation, judgement orientation)
         c. Progressive worsening of memory and cognition
         d. Medical evaluation has excluded systemic disorders or other brain diseases that could account for the deficits in memory and cognition.
   B. **Other Causes of Dementia:**
      1. Frontal Lobe Degenerations
      2. Vascular Dementia (multi-infarct dementia)
      3. Normal pressure hydrocephalus
      4. Jakob-Creutzfeldt disease
      5. AIDS dementia complex (HIV encephalopathy)
      6. CNS infections (neurosyphilis)

7. Thyroid dysfunction, B12 deficiency
8. Hepatic encephalopathy, alcohol-related dementia
9. Iatrogenic (antihypertensives, psychotropics, anticonvulsants)

## III. Evaluation of the Dementia Patient

A. Assess the tempo of cognitive decline, the characteristics of deficits, family history, and exclude reversible causes of dementia.

B. **Mental Status Testing:** Orientation, recent and remote memory, language, praxis, visuospatial relations, calculations, judgment

C. **Neurologic Examination:** Usually normal in Alzheimer's disease. Focal abnormalities, extrapyramidal signs, movement disorders, abnormalities of gait should be sought to exclude other causes of dementia.

D. **Neuropsychological Testing:** Supports the diagnosis of dementia (multiple areas of dysfunction), and is useful for follow-up evaluation, but is not necessary to make a clinical diagnosis of Alzheimer's disease.

## IV. Laboratory Evaluation of Patients with Dementia

| Routine | When Indicated |
| --- | --- |
| CBC, ESR | CSF examination |
| Chemistry panel | EEG |
| Liver function panel | |
| syphilis serology | Neuropsychological testing |
| TSH | HIV testing |
| B12 level | |
| EKG | |

Neuroimaging: CT with and without contrast is adequate for exclusion of structural disorders. MRI is better for detecting ischemia.

## V. Tacrine (Cognex) Therapy for Alzheimer's Disease

A. **Cholinergic Hypothesis:** Proposes that the cognitive deficits of Alzheimer's disease are due to declining function of acetylcholine-mediated neuronal systems. Tacrine is a centrally acting cholinesterase inhibitor that increases levels of acetylcholine within synapses, thereby enhancing neurotransmitter activity.

B. **Efficacy:** Greater improvements are seen in memory and language deficits than in orientation deficits. Benefit occurs in patients' scores on functional ratings, and clinicians and caregivers subjectively report less decline in overall status. The degree of benefit is relatively small.

C. Tacrine is only indicated for the treatment of patients with mild to moderate Alzheimer's disease (MMSE score of 10 to 26) who are otherwise healthy. Tacrine is unlikely to benefit patients with severe Alzheimer's disease. Tacrine does not alter the underlying neurodegenerative process, and clinical deterioration can be expected to continue at the same rate.

D. Assessment of clinical response to tacrine relies largely on the subjective impressions of clinicians and caregivers.

E. **Drug Interactions:** Tacrine may increase theophylline concentrations two-fold. Tacrine plasma levels are significantly increased by cimetidine. Effects of anticholinergic medications may be diminished, and cholinomimetic drugs may produce a synergistic effect.

F. **Contraindications:** Asthma, atrioventricular conduction defects, hyperthyroidism, urinary tract obstruction (prostatic hyperplasia), peptic ulcer disease. Caution in seizure disorders, closed angle glaucoma, or history of liver disease.

G. **Management of Tacrine (Cognex) Therapy:**
1. Starting dosage 10 mg four times daily, given between meals on an empty stomach. Daily dosage may be increased at six-week intervals by increments of 40 mg per day if a clinical response is not initially observed. [10, 20, 30, and 40 mg capsules]

2. Dosage increases should be undertaken only if no evidence of significant hepatotoxicity by weekly transaminase monitoring.
3. Most patients who respond will require a dosage of at least 80 mg per day, but sustained benefit may be more likely at dosages of 120-160 mg per day. The maximum dosage is 160 mg/d.
4. Therapeutic effect may not be seen for 4 weeks. Evaluate for response after 6-12 weeks on the maximum dosage. Tacrine should be discontinued if clinical response does not occur. 30-50% have mild improvement, and there is an occasional dramatic response.
5. Wholesale cost to the pharmacist for a 30-day supply is $110.00. Laboratory monitoring substantially increases the total cost.

H. **Adverse Effects of Tacrine:**
1. Hepatotoxicity is the most common and most significant side effect. ALT elevations occur on 40% within eight weeks of initiation. When tacrine is discontinued, liver function values return to normal within 10 weeks in 95%.
2. **Routine Laboratory Monitoring:** Serum ALT levels should be monitored weekly for at least the first 18 weeks of treatment and weekly for an additional six weeks whenever the dose of tacrine is increased. ALT monitoring should be repeated every three months thereafter if values remain in the normal range.
3. **Other Adverse Effects:** Nausea, vomiting, diarrhea, anorexia, and abdominal pain occur in 9-35%. If gastrointestinal upset occurs, tacrine may be given with meals, but plasma levels will be reduced by 30-40%. Increased sweating, salivation, and frequency of micturition, myalgias, tremor, dizziness, skin flushing and rash may occur.

## VI. Alanine Aminotransferase Levels and Modification of Tacrine Dosage:

| ALT Value | Dosage Modification |
|---|---|
| Normal | Continue treatment, and increase dosage according to recommended titration |
| Above normal but <3x ULN | Maintain dosage but consider whether further dosage increases are likely to improve therapeutic effect. |
| >3x ULN but <5x ULN | Reduce daily dosage by 40 mg/day. Resume dosage titration when ALT level returns to normal. |
| >5 x ULN but <10x ULN | Discontinue immediately. Consider rechallenge when ALT level returns to normal. |
| >10x ULN | Discontinue immediately. |

ALT = alanine aminotransferase; ULN = upper limits of normal.

## VII. Treatment of Dementia with Depression

A. The selection of an antidepressant is based on the patient's clinical presentation. A withdrawn, lethargic patient may respond better to a strongly noradrenergic drug, such as bupropion HCL (Wellbutrin), 100 mg bid.

B. **Dosage Range for Antidepressants in the Elderly:**

| Drug | | Dosage Range (mg/day) |
|---|---|---|
| Amitriptyline | (Elavil, Endep) | 50-150 |
| Desipramine | (Norpramin) | 50-150 |
| Doxepin | (Sinequan) | 50-150 |
| Imipramine | (Tofranil) | 50-150 |
| Nortriptyline | (Pamelor) | 25-100 |
| Protriptyline | (Vivactil) | 15-30 |
| Trazodone | (Desyrel) | 50-300 |
| Maprotiline | (Ludiomil) | 50-150 |
| Amoxapine | (Asendin) | 50-150 |

| Fluoxetine | (Prozac) | 10-40 |
| Trimipramine | (Surmontil) | 50-150 |

## VIII. Treatment of Dementia with Anxiety and Agitation

A. Benzodiazepines may be useful when the main behavioral problems are agitation, restlessness, and insomnia related to anxiety.

B. Benzodiazepines can increase confusion and memory impairment in patients with dementia, and may cause oversedation and ataxia.

C. **Anxiolytics:**

Alprazolam (Xanax), 0.125 mg tid; useful if anxiety and agitation are accompanied by mild depressive symptoms.

Lorazepam (Ativan), 0.5 mg bid or tid; useful for anxiety.

Oxazepam (Serax), 5-30 mg PO tid-qid prn; useful for anxiety.

Temazepam (Restoril), 5-30 mg PO qhs prn; reserved for middle-of-the-night insomnia.

Zolpidem (Ambien), 5 mg PO qhs; useful for initial insomnia

## IX. Treatment of Dementia with Paranoia and Hallucinations

A. Paranoia and Hallucinations do not require treatment unless they are frightening to the patient.

B. Violent, threatening, or disruptive hallucinations should be treated with small doses of haloperidol (Haldol), 0.5 mg qd-bid. or thioridazine (Mellaril).

## X. Management of Physical Symptoms of Dementia

A. **Weight Loss:** Increase access to fingerfoods and allow frequent snacking; provide items that are easy-to-swallow, high in carbohydrates, and sweet-tasting, such as cake and ice cream.

B. **Urinary Incontinence:** Best handled with a 2-4 hour toileting regimen and "easy-on, easy-off" clothing such as jogging pants.

C. **Home Safety:** Doors should be equipped with safety locks, and grab bars by the toilet and in the shower.

D. Discuss "do not resuscitate" orders and health care proxy.

# Epilepsy

## I. Classification of Seizures
A. Seizures are classified into two broad categories, partial or generalized.
B. **Partial seizures** are characterized by signs and symptoms that depend on the focus of the seizure.
   1. Partial seizures produce either motor activity restricted to focal regions of the body (simple partial) or behavioral changes (complex partial). Partial seizures are subdivided into three types: Simple partial, complex partial, and secondarily generalized.
   2. **Simple partial seizures** are characterized by involuntary focal motor movements or abnormal sensations without any alteration in consciousness.
   3. **Complex Partial Seizures** are characterized by a change in consciousness during the seizure process, and are the most common form of seizures. Patients frequently experience postictal confusion, fatigue, and impaired or absent memory of the event.
   4. Complex partial seizures often secondarily generalize, culminating in a typical tonic-clonic seizure.
C. **Generalized Seizures:**
   1. Generalized tonic-clonic seizures are characterized by abrupt loss of consciousness and tonic extension of the extremities, followed by generalized clonic movements. The typical generalized seizure lasts less than 2 minutes, and is followed by a 5- to 10-minute postictal period of diminished responsiveness.
   2. Absence seizures are nonconvulsive, and are characterized by abrupt cessation of activity and a blank stare. Duration is generally less than 20 seconds.

## II. Clinical Evaluation of the Seizure Patient
A. **Characteristics of Seizure:** Obtain a complete description of the attack from a witness, including tonic-clonic movements, tongue biting, incontinence.
B. **Prodrome** symptoms occur hours or minutes before a seizure, and they include any warning or premonition of seizure, such as a dull headache, abdominal discomfort, fear, or unusual movements.
C. **Aura:** Emotional or experiential phenomenon perceived during the initial moments of a seizure; indicates the cortex location where the seizure originates.
D. **Seizure Beginning:** Seizures often begin with a motionless stare or extension of the arms (tonic activity).
E. **Convulsive Motor Movements** consist of movements at end of seizure (clonic activity).
F. **Precipitating Events:** Menstrual periods, lack of sleep, or stress may precipitate seizures.
G. **Neurologic Examination** can reveal focal neurologic abnormalities.
H. A first-time seizure may be the presenting clinical manifestation of a wide variety of conditions. Almost any central nervous system (CNS) insult and many systemic disorders can produce convulsions.
I. In adults, Illicit drug abuse and human immunodeficiency virus infection are becoming increasingly frequent causes of seizures. In older adults, cerebrovascular disease or metastatic malignancy may cause seizures. In patients older than 60 years of age seizures are caused by stroke in approximately one third of cases. In pregnant women, eclampsia is an important cause of generalized seizures.
J. Precipitating factors should be considered, including noncompliance with medications, photic stimulation, emotional stress, fatigue, and sleep deprivation.

**K. Common Causes of Generalized Seizures:**

Noncompliance with anticonvulsant meditations
Cerebrovascular accident
Central nervous system infection
Intracranial neoplasm
Primary
Metastatic
Head trauma
Alcohol abuse Intoxication
Withdrawal
Drug overdose
Cocaine
Amphetamines
Cyclic antidepressants

Theophylline
Isoniazid
Metabolic disorders
Hypoglycemia
Hyponatremia
Hypocalcemia
Hypoxia
Acidosis
Hyperosmolar states
Uremia
Eclampsia
Febrile illness
Idiopathic

## III. Laboratory Testing

A. **Electroencephalogram:**
  1. A routine study should include photic stimulation, hyperventilation, sleep deprivation, and awake and asleep tracings.
  2. If the clinical history indicates epilepsy but the EEG is normal, treatment should still be considered. Repeat EEG's or long-term EEG with video monitoring may be necessary.
  3. Many adults with epilepsy have a normal EEG between seizures. The diagnostic yield of EEG increases considerably with repeated studies.

B. **Magnetic Resonance Imaging (MRI):** All epileptic patients should undergo MRI because MRI has a higher diagnostic yield than CT scan.

C. Serum anticonvulsant levels should be measured if the patient has an established seizure disorder. If levels are low, loading doses of the appropriate medications should be administered.

D. **Initial Laboratory Evaluation for First-Time Seizure:** Serum electrolytes, glucose, calcium, magnesium BUN, creatinine; complete blood count, liver enzymes, toxicology screen, urinalysis, arterial blood gases. **As indicated:** Chest radiograph (to rule out aspiration), blood cultures.

E. **Lumbar Puncture** is unnecessary in the initial evaluation unless there is a specific reason to analyze cerebrospinal fluid.

## IV. Pharmacotherapy of Epileptic Seizures

A. Begin therapy with a single antiepileptic drug.

B. Initiate drug at a low dose, and slowly increase until serum level is in therapeutic range.

C. **Dosing Schedule:** Drug steady state is not reached until approximately five half-lives. With phenobarbital, a steady state is not reached for weeks. A loading dose is usually not necessary.

D. If seizures persist, increase dose until either toxic side effects occur or seizures are controlled. If toxic symptoms occur, reduce the dose. Many antiepileptic drugs cause sedation initially, but increasing the dosage slowly allows tolerance to develop.

E. Therapeutic serum levels are not absolute, and serum levels above the suggested therapeutic range may be necessary in some patients. Trough concentrations should be measured, preferably from serum samples drawn before the morning dose is taken. If seizures are controlled at a low drug level, the dose does not need to be increased.

F. If the initial agent fails to control seizures, switch to a second drug. Drug combinations should be tried only if monotherapy fails. Rarely are more than two anticonvulsants required

G. **Drug Choices for the Treatment of Epileptic Seizures:**

| Seizure Type | First-Line Therapy | Alternative Therapy |
|---|---|---|
| Partial (both simple and complex) | Carbamazepine (Tegretol)<br>Valproic acid (Depakote)<br>Phenytoin (Dilantin) | Phenobarbital<br>Primidone (Mysoline)<br>Felbamate (Felbatol)<br>Gabapentin (Neurontin)<br>Lamotrigine (Lamictal) |
| Generalized tonic-clonic | Carbamazepine<br>Valproic acid<br>Phenytoin | Phenobarbital<br>Primidone<br>Felbamate<br>Gabapentin<br>Lamotrigine |
| Absence | Ethosuximide (Zarontin)<br>Valproic acid | Clonazepam (Klonopin) |
| Atypical absence, myoclonic | Valproic acid | Clonazepam |

**Pharmacokinetics of Antiepileptic Drugs:**

| Drug | Reaction half-time (hours) | Time to steady state (days) | Time to peak (hours) |
|---|---|---|---|
| Carbamazepine (Tegretol) | 5-25 | 2- 4 | 4-8 |
| Phenytoin (Dilantin) | 9-40 | 7-28 | 4-8 |
| Valproic acid (Depakote) | 4-15 | 1-3 | 2-8 |
| Phenobarbital | 48-144 | 10-30 | 1-4 |
| Primidone (Mysoline) | 5-18 | 1-4 | 1-3 |
| Ethosuximide (Zarontin) | 30-60 | 6-12 | 1-7 |
| Felbamate (Felbatol) | 15 | 3-4 | 2-3 |
| Gabapentin (Neurontin) | 5-7 | 1-3 | 2-4 |
| Lamotrigine (Lamictal) | 24-59 | 5-12 | 2-4 |

**Pharmacologic Properties of Antiepileptic Drugs:**

| Drug | Starting Dose | Maintenance Dose | Dosage | Therapeutic Level |
|---|---|---|---|---|
| Carbamazepine (Tegretol) | 3 mg per kg per day (adults)<br>5 mg per kg per day (children) | 5 to 20 mg per kg per day (adults)<br>20 to 40 mg per kg per day (children) | Two to four times daily | 4 to 12 mcg per mL |
| Phenytoin (Dilantin) | 4 to 6 mg per kg per day (adults)<br>3 to 10 mg per kg per day (children) | Same<br><br>Same | One to three times daily | 10 to 20 mcg per mL |
| Valproic acid (Depakote) | 10 to 15 mg per kg per day | 15 to 30 mg per kg per day | Two to four times daily | 50 to 100 mcg per mL |
| Phenobarbital | 1to 3 mg per kg per day (adults)<br>3 to 5 mg per kg per day (children) | Same<br><br>Same | One to two times daily | 15 to 40 mcg per mL |
| Primidone (Mysoline) | 2to 4 mg per kg per day (adults) | 10 to 15 mg per kg per day (adults) | Two to three times daily | 4 to 12 mcg per mL |
| Ethosuximide (Zarontin) | 10 mg per kg per day | 10 to 20 mg per kg per day | Two times daily | 50 to 100 mcg per mL |

| | | | | |
|---|---|---|---|---|
| Felbamate (Felbatol) | 1,200 mg per day (adults) 15 mg per kg per day (children) | 3,600 mg per day (adults) 45 mg per kg per day (children) | Three times daily | N/A |
| Gabapentin (Neurontin) | 1,200 mg per day (adults) | 3,600 mg per day (adults) | Three times daily | N/A |
| Lamotrigine (Lamictal) | 50 to 100 mg per day (adults) | 100 to 400 mg per day (adults) | Two to three times daily | N/A |

H. **Carbamazepine:**
   1. Primary therapy for partial seizures because of its lack of cognitive and behavioral side effects. Carbamazepine has antiepileptic activity against partial and generalized (except absence) seizures.
   2. Adverse effects occur when serum concentrations rise above the accepted range. Dizziness, diplopia, agitation, and transient, benign leukopenia are common. Infrequently, a syndrome of inappropriate antidiuretic hormone secretion may occur. Aplastic anemia has been rarely reported.

I. **Phenytoin:**
   1. The antiepileptic activity of phenytoin is comparable to that of carbamazepine.
   2. Any condition that decreases albumin binding sites produces a greater proportion of free phenytoin because phenytoin is 90 percent protein-bound.
   3. Therapeutic serum concentration of phenytoin is 10-20 mcg per mL, some patients may require up to 30 mcg per mL.
   4. **Dose-related Adverse Effects:** Nausea, vomiting, nystagmus (> 20 mcg per mL), and ataxia (>30 mcg per mL). Non-dose-related adverse effects include gingival hyperplasia (20 percent), hirsutism, acneiform eruptions, and coarsening of facial features.

J. **Valproic Acid:**
   1. Valproic acid (Depakote) has the widest spectrum of activity of all drugs currently available for seizures, with efficacy against partial, generalized tonic-clonic and absence seizures; lacks negative cognitive effects.
   2. Initial dosage 10 to 15 mg per kg, increasing at one- to two-week intervals, to maximum of 60 mg/kg/day.
   3. Transient gastrointestinal symptoms and drowsiness occur at the onset of therapy. Tremor, thrombocytopenia, weight gain may occur. Rarely, fatal hepatotoxicity occurs in very young children. Periodic liver function tests may allow early detection.

K. **Phenobarbital:** Use of phenobarbital has declined in favor of other drugs; used for partial and generalized (except absence) seizures. The half-life of phenobarbital ranges from 3-4 days in adults; therefore, the full effects of dosage adjustment are not apparent for 2-3 weeks.

L. **Primidone:** Resembles phenobarbital in its spectrum of activity. The drug has active metabolites, phenobarbital and phenylethylmalonamide (PEMA); reserved for refractory patients.

M. **Ethosuximide (Zarontin)** is used exclusively for absence (petit mal) seizures.

N. **Felbamate (Felbatol):**
   1. Monotherapy or adjunctive therapy for partial seizures in adults.
   2. Broad spectrum of activity, similar to that of valproic acid. Principal advantage is its wide therapeutic index.
   3. **Adverse Effects:** Mild neurotoxicity, nausea and vomiting, insomnia and anorexia. Aplastic anemia rarely.

O. **Gabapentin (Neurontin):**
   1. Drug interactions are highly unlikely because it is not protein-bound, not metabolized, and does not induce liver enzymes.
   2. Adjunctive therapy for partial seizures with or without secondary generalization. It has a relatively short half-life (5-7 hours), necessitating multiple daily doses.

P. **Lamotrigine (Lamictal)** has demonstrated efficacy comparable to the other new agents, primarily in patients with partial seizures, especially with secondary generalization.

Q. **Indications for Surgical Treatment of Epilepsy:** Seizures continuing after a drug therapy may be amendable to surgical removal of the seizure focus.

V. **Status Epilepticus**
  A. Status epilepticus is defined as the occurrence of a seizure that is repeated or prolonged. If seizures are continuous or the patient does not awaken between repetitive seizures for longer than 10 minutes, treatment should be initiated immediately.
  B. The most common single cause of status epilepticus is noncompliance with anti-convulsant medications. Other common causes include metabolic disturbances (electrolyte imbalance, hypoglycemia, cerebral hypoxia), CNS infection, drug overdose, alcohol withdrawal, cerebrovascular disease, cerebral tumor, and trauma. In children febrile illness may produce status epilepticus.
  C. **Management of Status Epilepticus:**
    1. Maintain airway. The patient should be positioned laterally with the head down in order to promote drainage of secretions and prevent aspiration. The head and extremities should be cushioned to prevent injury.
    2. During the tonic portion of the seizure the teeth are tightly clenched. During the clonic phase that follows, however, a bite block or other soft object should be inserted into the mouth to prevent injury to the tongue.
    3. Secure IV access and draw blood for serum glucose analysis. Give **glucose, 50 mL of 50%** (1 amp) IV (in children, 4 mL/kg of 25% dextrose), and give **thiamine**, 50 mg IV.
    4. **Initial Control:**
       a. **Lorazepam (Ativan)** 4-8 mg (0.1 mg/kg; not to exceed 2 mg/min) IV at 1-2 mg/min. May repeat 4-8 mg q5-10min (max 80 mg/24h) **OR**
       b. **Diazepam** 5-20 mg slow IV at 1-2 mg/min. Repeat 5-10 mg q5-10 min prn (max 100 mg/24h).
    5. **Definitive Seizure Control:**
       a. **Phenytoin** 15-20 mg/kg loading dose in 100 mLs of normal saline at 50 mg/min. Repeat 100-150 mg IV q30min, max 1.5 gms. Hypotension may occur but should not preclude administration.
       b. **If Seizures Persist, Intubate Patient, and Administer Phenobarbital** 120-260 mg (10-20 mg/kg) IV at 50 mg/min, repeat 20 mg/kg q15min; additional phenobarbital may be given, up to max of 30-60 mg/kg.
    6. **Consider Intubation and General Anesthesia if necessary.**

# Headache

## I. Clinical Evaluation of Headache

A. **Age of Onset:** Migraines frequently have an onset in childhood, adolescence, or young adulthood. Suspect an organic cause if onset occurs later in life (temporal arteritis, cerebrovascular disease, tumor). Tension-type headaches may begin at any age.

B. **Location:** Migraine is suggested by unilateral pain that changes sides from episode to episode. Cluster headaches are strictly unilateral and orbital. Tension headaches are usually bilateral.

C. **Frequency:** Cluster headaches typically occur in brief attacks, lasting 30-90 minutes, 2-6 times a day. Migraines can also occur at sporadic intervals.

D. **Character and Severity of Headache:**
1. Subarachnoid hemorrhage causes an acute, rapid-onset, "thunderclap" headache that is often described as "the worst headache of my life."
2. Migraine is severe, throbbing.
3. Cluster headache pain is described as deep and boring.
4. Tension-type headaches are a dull, nagging, persistent, band-like tightening around the head.

E. **Clinical Course:** Progressively worsening or new headaches may indicate an organic cause such as an intracranial mass, and should be thoroughly evaluated.

F. **Prodrome and Aura:** Migraine is indicated by promontory sensations that occur before onset of headache.

G. **Precipitating Factors:** Migraine may be precipitated by bright lights, fatigue, lack of sleep, hypoglycemia, stress, alcohol, certain drugs and foods, and menstruation. Exercise or orgasm may trigger migraine or cause rupture of an aneurysm.

H. **Associated Signs and Symptoms:** Migraine commonly causes nausea and vomiting. Cluster is characterized by unilateral lacrimation and nasal congestion.

I. **Neurologic Dysfunction:** Weakness, paresthesia, aphasia, visual loss, diplopia, vertigo or loss of consciousness suggest a brain tumor or an intracranial aneurysm.

## II. Physical Examination

A. Evaluate for hypertension, fundoscopy (papilledema); temporal artery tenderness may indicate temporal arteritis. Percuss sinuses to detect sinusitis.

B. Tenderness in the hat-band area of the scalp and in the muscles of the neck is often a due to tension headache.

C. **Neurologic Examination:** Cranial nerve exam (especially pupil and eye movement); motor strength, sensation; meningeal irritation signs (neck stiffness).

## III. Differential Diagnosis

A. Life-threatening causes, such as subarachnoid hemorrhage or meningitis, are responsible for less than 1% of all headaches. If normal findings are found on general and neurologic examinations, abnormal results on CT scan are rarely present.

B. If the history is suggestive of intracranial bleeding, computed tomography (CT) scan without contrast should be performed. If the CT scan is normal, a lumbar puncture is mandatory to rule out intracranial bleeding.

## IV. Indications for CT or MRI Scan

A. An isolated, severe headache
B. Consistently localized head pain
C. Pain severe enough to disturb sleep
D. Abrupt onset, or onset during physical exertion (leaking aneurysm, elevated intracranial pressure, or arterial dissection)
E. Progressively worsening headaches
F. Abnormal neurologic findings, neck stiffness, or fever
G. The patient appears acutely ill and is confused or drowsy

## V. Characteristics of Migraine Headache
A. **Migraine Stages:**
1. **Prodrome Phase:**
   a. A prodrome is a sign of an impending headache that usually appears in the form of mood changes, irritability, thirst, fluid retention, lethargy, increased energy, euphoria, or food cravings.
   b. Appears several hours to 2 days before the onset of pain.
   c. 85% of migraine sufferers have prodrome.
2. **Aura:**
   a. Typically begins 10 minutes to 2 hours before the onset of headache.
   b. The aura may consist of visual phenomenon, paresthesias, weakness, or a peculiar odor.
   c. Visual auras are more common: Flashing or shimmering lights (scintillating scotoma), bright sparks or flashes (photopsia), or jagged, marching lines (fortification spectra).
   d. Only 15% of migraine patients experience an aura.
3. **Headache Phase:**
   a. The headache begins after the prodrome or aura.
   b. 60% of migraine patients have unilateral headaches, or unilateral pain that later becomes bilateral. Pain is typically throbbing, but may at times be steady.
   c. Migraine may be associated with nausea, photophobia, and phonophobia.
B. Hemiplegic migraine is accompanied by transient focal weakness. Basilar migraine is associated with transient aphasia, syncope, visual disturbances, and vertigo. Rarer forms are ophthalmoplegic migraine, with third cranial nerve palsy; and retinal migraine, with symptoms similar to amaurosis fugax.
C. Complicated migraine may consist of a migrainous infarction, marked by a neurologic deficit that persists after the headache resolves.
D. **Factors that May Trigger Migraine:**
1. **Dietary:**Alcohol, aspartame (NutraSweet), caffeine, cheese, chocolate, monosodium glutamate, nitrites (hot dogs, fast foods), nuts. Changes in diet (skipping meals, dieting).
2. **Sensorial:** Bright lights, flickering lights, odors
3. **Stress-Related:** Change of employment, crisis periods, intense activity (holidays, weddings), changes in sleeping pattern, menstruation.
4. **Drugs Associated with Migraine:** Oral contraceptives, estrogen, cimetidine, ranitidine, nifedipine, atenolol.

## VI. Characteristics of Tension-type Headache
A. Tension headaches are the most common type of headache; typically bilateral, constant, pressing, or band-like in quality; mild to moderate in intensity; occurs late in the day; precipitated by stress and poor sleep, and lasts from 1 hour to 3 days.
B. **Associated Symptoms:** No nausea or vomiting occurs; other associated symptoms are absent or mild (anorexia, photophobia, phonophobia).
C. Tension headaches are usually relieved by nonprescription analgesics, and patients usually do not seek medical attention.

## VII. Non-Pharmacologic Therapy of Migraine and Tension-type Headache
A. Avoiding known triggers, such as caffeine or too much or too little sleep. Stress reduction and biofeedback, application of local pressure, heat, or ice packs may ease the pain.
B. Patients with migraine (especially menstrual migraine) may improve after discontinuation of oral contraceptives.

## VIII. Abortive Drug Treatment for Migraine and Tension Headaches
A. **Abortive Therapy:** Aimed at stopping individual attacks after they have begun. Begin treatment as early as possible, at the first sign of impending headache.

## B. Drugs Used for Abortive Drug Treatment for Migraine and Tension Headaches

| Drug | Regimen |
|------|---------|
| **Analgesics** | |
| Acetaminophen | 650-1,000 mg q4h prn |
| Aspirin | 650 mg q4h prn |
| **Nonsteroidal Anti-inflammatory Drugs:** | |
| Ibuprofen (Motrin) | 400-600 mg at onset, then 300-800 mg PO qid [200, 300, 400, 600, 800 mg]. |
| Naproxen sodium (Aleve) | 825 mg followed 30 min later by 275-550 mg q30-60 min prn, max 1375 mg/d [275, 550 mg]. |
| Ketorolac (Toradol) | 30 or 60 mg IM initially followed by 30 mg every 6 hours as needed; or 10 mg PO q4-6h prn [10 mg]. |
| Ketoprofen (Orudis) | 50-75 mg PO tid [25, 50, 75 mg]. |
| Diclofenac (Voltaren) | 50 mg PO bid-tid [25, 50, 75 mg]. |
| Mefenamic acid (Ponstel) | 200-500 mg at onset then 250 mg PO qid [250 mg]. |
| **Combination** | |
| **Midrin** (isometheptene mucate 65 mg/ dichloralphenazone 100 mg/ acetaminophen 325 mg). | 2 capsules at headache onset, then take 1 q1h until relief; max 5 capsules in 12h. |
| **Esgic, Fiorinal** (aspirin 325 mg, caffeine 40 mg, butalbital 50 mg) | 1-2 tablets or capsules with onset of attack, then q4h; max 6 per attack. |
| **Fioricet** (acetaminophen 325 mg, caffeine 40 mg, butalbital 50 mg) | 1-2 tablets or capsules with onset of attack, then q4h; max 6 per attack. |
| **Fiorinal w/codeine** (aspirin 325 mg, caffeine 40 mg, butalbital 50 mg, codeine 30 mg) | 1-2 capsules with onset of attack, then q4h; max 6 per attack. |
| **Corticosteroid** | |
| Prednisone | 20 mg tid for 3 days, then bid for 3 days, then daily for 3 days. A short course may be stopped without further tapering in healthy patients. |
| **Ergot Preparations** | |
| Cafergot, Wigraine (ergotamine 1 mg/caffeine 100 mg) | 2 tablets at onset, then one q30min, max 6 per attack. Use for no more than 2 attacks/wk. Max: 10 tablets/wk. |
| Wigraine (ergotamine 2 mg/caffeine 100 mg suppositories) | 1 suppository at onset; may repeat once in 1 h; max 2 attacks/wk, 2 suppositories per attack. |
| Dihydroergotamine (DHE 45) | 1 mg self-injected SC q8-12h |
| **Narcotic Analgesics** | |
| Butorphanol nasal spray (Stadol NS) | 1 spray (1 mg) in one nostril at onset of headache; may repeat in 4 h prn. |
| **Serotonin Agonist** | |
| Sumatriptan injection (Imitrex) | 6 mg SC, max two injections in 24h; or 25-100 mg PO with fluids, repeat q2h prn, max 300 mg/d PO; or 6 mg SC and 200 mg PO in 24h |

## C. Sumatriptan (Imitrex):

1. In the emergency department, sumatriptan injection (Imitrex), the only specific agonist to serotonin (5-HT) receptors on intracranial vascular nerves, is the drug of choice. It is effective in 70-80% of patients, even when the headache has persisted for as long

as several days. Sumatriptan has minimal side effects compared to ergotamine and dihydroergotamine which cause significant nausea and vasoconstriction.

2. A 6-mg dose given subcutaneously (SC) often relieves headache and allows the patient to resume full activity in 1-2 hours. A second dose may be given in 1 hour.

3. **Oral Dose:** 25-100 mg PO with fluids, repeat q2h prn, max 300 mg/d PO; or start with 6 mg by subcutaneous injection, followed by 200 mg PO in 24h.

4. Sumatriptan is contraindicated in ischemic heart disease and pregnancy.

D. **Dihydroergotamine:**

1. Dihydroergotamine injection DHE. 45), a 5-HT receptor agonist, is highly effective in the emergency management of migraine. Relief occurs in 15-30 minutes following IM administration and persists for 3-4 hours.

2. Administer DHE, 1 mg IV over 2-3 minutes, and metoclopramide (Reglan), 10 mg mixed with 50 mL of 5% dextrose in water and given IV over 30 min IV q8h for 48 hours.

3. Discharge the patient with DHE to self-administer SC, 1 mg q8-12h, and propranolol HCL (Inderal), 40-80 mg po tid.

4. Contraindicated in ischemic heart disease and pregnancy.

E. **Ergotamine:**

1. Effective for treatment of migraine not relieved by simple analgesics, but often associated with rebound headaches; may cause peripheral vascular insufficiency and angina.

2. **Contraindications:** Coronary artery disease, peripheral vascular disease, hypertension, renal and hepatic disease, pregnancy.

3. **Side Effects:** Nausea, vomiting, and paresthesias; the occurrence of chest discomfort is a cause for concern.

F. **Narcotic Therapy for Migraine:**

1. Codeine combination analgesics such as Vicodin may occasionally be indicated for infrequent, severe attacks. When taken more than three times a week, codeine may cause rebound headache.

2. Butorphanol (Stadol) 1 spray in one nostril, may repeat in 60-90 minutes if needed. Repeat 1 dose sequence q3-4h prn [2.5 mL bottle].

IX. **Prophylactic Therapy for Migraine Headaches**

A. Prophylactic medications prevent headache from occurring, and should be used when attacks are more frequent than 2-3 per month, or if attacks are very severe.

B. **Drugs Used for Prophylactic Therapy of Migraine Headaches:**

| Drug | Regimen |
| --- | --- |
| **Valproic acid (Depakote)** | 250 mg bid for 3 days, then 500 mg bid |
| **beta-Blockers** | |
| Propranolol (Inderal) | 40-80 mg PO bid-tid [10, 20, 40, 60, 80 mg] |
| Propranolol timed-release (Inderal LA) | 80-160 mg PO qd [80, 120, 160 mg] |
| Atenolol (Tenormin) | 50-100 mg PO qd [25, 50, 100 mg] |
| Metoprolol (Lopressor) | 100 mg qd |
| Nadolol (Corgard) | 40-80 mg PO qd [20, 40, 80, 120, 160 mg] |
| **Tricyclic Antidepressants** | |
| Amitriptyline (Elavil) | 25-150 mg qhs |
| Desipramine (Norpramin) | 25-150 mg qd in AM |
| Doxepin (Sinequan) | 25-150 mg qhs |
| Nortriptyline (Pamelor) | 25-150 mg qhs |

C. **Valproic Acid (Depakote):** Highly effective for prophylactic therapy. Liver dysfunction and weight gain may occur.

D. **Beta Blockers:** Propranolol reduces the frequency of migraine in 51%. Contraindications: Congestive heart failure, diabetes, asthma. Side effects: depression, decreased exercise intolerance.

E. Amitriptyline HCl (Elavil) effectively reduces the frequency and severity of migraine.

F. Menstrual migraine responds to NSAIDs when given beginning 3-5 days before the expected onset of menses and continued through it. Naproxen sodium (Aleve, Anaprox) and meclofenamate sodium (Meclomen) are recommended.

**Cluster Headache**

A. Cluster headache has a rapid-onset; attacks are brief (30-90 minutes) and usually occur in clusters lasting weeks to months; predominantly affects men.

B. Strictly unilateral and excruciatingly severe. Ipsilateral nasal stuffiness, lacrimation, ocular redness and tearing are common.

C. No prodrome, aura, or gastrointestinal symptoms occur. Relief may be sought through activity such as pacing or head banging.

D. **Abortive Therapy for Cluster Headaches:**
   -Oxygen 100%, 8-10 L/min by mask for 10 min.
   -Ergotamine (same as in migraine).
   -Dihydroergotamine (same as in migraine).
   -Prednisone 40-120 mg PO qd x 2 weeks, followed by a tapering dose.
   -Lidocaine (Xylocaine) 4% applied to nasal mucosa in the area of the sphenopalatine ganglia.

E. **Prophylactic Therapy for Cluster Headaches:**
   -Verapamil (Calan) 80-120 mg PO tid-qid.
   -Lithium 300 mg PO bid-qid.

# Vertigo

I. **Differentiation of Central Causes of Vertigo from Peripheral Causes**
   A. Vertigo is a sensation of abnormal motion either of the surroundings or of the body; vertigo may be described as spinning, whirling, swaying, or "the room is moving."
   B. 85% of patients with vertigo have a peripheral vestibular disorder, 15% have a central nervous system disorder.
   C. Peripheral disorders may have associated hearing loss and tinnitus, without other neurologic deficits. Vertigo from peripheral lesions often develops acutely and is inter-mittent and shorter-lasting; peripheral lesions tend to cause more severe vertigo, with associated nausea and vomiting.
   D. Central lesions, such as cerebral tumors, are not associated with hearing loss, but may be accompanied by other neurologic signs reflecting brain-stem involvement. Symptoms of central lesions develop more insidiously and are longer-lasting and more continuous (except for vascular events); central lesions usually cause less severe vertigo and nausea.

II. **Peripheral Causes of Vertigo**
   A. **Benign Positional Vertigo:**
      1. Most common single cause of vertigo, occurring twice as frequently as any other vestibular disorder. Intense but brief episodes of vertigo are associated with changes in head position, usually when lying down. Resolves within 3-6 months, but may recur.
      2. **Neurologic Examination:** Normal, except for positional nystagmus (induced by rapid head movement).
      3. **Etiology:** May occur after trauma or viral infections; majority are idiopathic. Average age 51 years; increased incidence with advancing age. The mechanism may be sediment falling on the cupula of the semicircular canal.
      4. **Nylan-Barany Test** confirms the diagnosis of BPV. The patient's head is rotated to one side and then gradually lowered to 30° below the horizontal position. When the affected ear is in the downward position, nystagmus and vertigo is triggered after a few seconds. Vertigo fades within 30 seconds; nystagmus is usually rotatory and changes direction when the patient sits up.
   B. **Vestibular Neuronitis:**
      1. Sudden severe vertigo, lasting up to 10 days. Nausea and vomiting are common; no hearing loss or neurologic signs. Typically follows a viral upper respiratory infection.
      2. Residual unsteadiness may persist for several weeks after an attack.
   C. **Meniere's Disease:**
      1. Episodic vertigo, tinnitus, fullness in the ear, progressive sensorineural hearing loss; usually unilateral.
      2. Severe vertigo develops rapidly over a few minutes, and lasts for several hours.
      3. Caused by an abnormal accumulation of endolymphatic fluid in the inner ear.
   D. **Motion Sickness:**
      1. Nausea, dizziness, abdominal distress, increased salivation, and vomiting provoked by motion.
      2. Can be reduced by visually fixing eyes at the horizon.
   E. **Tumors of Cerebello-pontine (CP) Angle:**
      1. Acoustic neuroma or metastases of tumor to cerebropontine angle.
      2. Vertigo, deafness, nystagmus, ataxia; facial weakness, disturbance in taste
   F. **Other Disorders Associated with Vertigo:**
      1. Impacted cerumen or foreign bodies in the external auditory canal; otitis media, cholesteatoma, otosclerosis, mastoiditis, local ear trauma, and perilymphatic fistula.
      2. Ototoxic drugs: Aminoglycosides, loop diuretics, aspirin, quinine, caffeine, alcohol, phenytoin.

III. **Central Causes of Vertigo**
   A. Diseases affecting the brain stem and cerebellum may cause central vertigo; vertigo is

usually not the dominant manifestation of these disorders.

B. **Toxic:** Various medications/drugs, alcohol, narcotics, analgesics; dilantin nystagmus with excessive levels over 30

C. May be due to drug interaction, e.g., Darvon plus Tegretol--increased level of Tegretol

D. Volatile hydrocarbons/anesthetics/solvents

E. **Vascular:** Brain stem infarction--Wallenberg syndrome--lateral medullary syndrome
1. Ipsilateral ataxia, Horner's syndrome, palatal paralysis, loss of pain and temperature, nystagmus.
2. Contralateral loss of pain and temperature in extremities and trunk

F. **Tumors:** Cerebellar and other

G. **Infectious:** Brain stem encephalitis, basilar meningitis

H. **Traumatic:** Basilar skull fracture; brain stem/cerebellar contusion

I. **Other:** Multiple sclerosis and other demyelinating diseases

## V. Presyncope

A. Dizziness is associated with the feeling of an impending faint; no loss of consciousness; caused by a transient reduction in cerebral blood flow due to inadequate cardiac output, orthostatic hypotension, or noncardiac causes.

B. **Vasovagal Reflex Presyncope:** A common cause of presyncopy occurring after stressful, painful, or other noxious stimuli leads to peripheral vasodilatation with a drop in heart rate and cardiac output.

C. **Orthostatic Hypotension:**
1. Measurement of systolic blood pressure reveals a 20 mmHg or more BP drop within 3 minutes of assuming an upright posture.
2. **Factors Causing Orthostatic Hypotension:** Decreased intravascular volume from hemorrhage, dehydration, diarrhea, vomiting, or diuresis; antihypertensives, nitrates, phenothiazines, antidepressants, prolonged bedrest. Primary autonomic insufficiency due to diabetic multiple autonomic system atrophy (Shy-Drager's syndrome) is less common.

D. **Arrhythmias:** Bradycardia <40 beats per minute or tachyarrhythmias are a significant cause of dizziness and presyncope.

E. **Other Cardiac Causes of Presyncope:** Aortic stenosis, hypertrophic cardiomyopathy, ischemia, constrictive pericarditis, cardiac tamponade, carotid sinus hypersensitivity.

F. **Metabolic Causes of Presyncope:** Hypoglycemia and hypoxemia are rare causes of dizziness. True hypoglycemia is rare in nondiabetics and is usually a complication of insulin and oral hypoglycemics.

## V. Disequilibrium

A. Disequilibrium consists of unsteadiness most prominent with ambulation. Dizziness is absent when sitting or lying down, and is not associated with nystagmus.

B. **Syndrome of Multiple Sensory Deficits:** Most common cause of disequilibrium in the elderly. Multiple sensory defects are caused by peripheral neuropathies, vestibular abnormalities, visual impairment, and orthopedic problems.

C. Disequilibrium may frequently be a result of drug use, vestibular disease, cerebellar disease, Parkinsonism, anticonvulsants, psychotropics (lithium, haloperidol), and benzodiazepines.

## VI. Lightheadedness

A. Lightheadedness is described by the patient as a vague "giddy" or "woozy" sensation.

B. Anxiety disorder is commonly associated with lightheadedness secondary to hyperventilation, and reproduction of symptoms occurs with hyperventilation.

## VII. Clinical Evaluation of the Dizzy Patient

A. **Categorize the Form of Dizziness:** Differentiate vertigo (spinning or moving) from a nonvertiginous sensation (giddiness, unsteadiness, faintness).

B. Determine the onset and duration of the episodes, provoking factors, head position; associated nausea and vomiting, hearing loss or tinnitus.

C. **Differentiate Central Causes from Peripheral Causes:**
   1. **Central Causes** are indicated by neurological signs, dysphagia, diplopia, dysarthria or hemiparesis. Ataxia may suggest cerebellar disease.
   2. **Perform a Careful Neurologic Examination:**
   3. Ear, nose, throat exam should be done to rule out impacted cerumen, middle-ear disease, hearing loss.
   4. A history of hearing loss or tinnitus localizes the problem to the ear or the eighth nerve
   5. **Dizziness Simulation Tests:**

   | Type of Dizziness | Provoking Test |
   |---|---|
   | Vertigo | Nylan Barany Test |
   | Presyncope | Orthostatic blood pressure measurement |
   | Disequilibrium | Romberg test, tandem gait |
   | Lightheadedness | Hyperventilation |

D. **Additional Testing:** Electrolytes, glucose, complete blood count. Audiologic evaluation and electronystagmography may be indicated.
E. **If there are no neurologic abnormalities, hearing loss, or an ear abnormalities, the** most likely causes are BPV and vestibular neuronitis. Nylan-Barany test can establish the diagnosis of BPV. Assess blood pressure to exclude orthostatic hypotension.
F. **If the neurologic examination shows abnormal cranial nerve or cerebellar findings** an MRI should be used to rule out acoustic neuroma, tumor, or infarction.

VIII. **Management of Patients with Vertigo**
A. **Treatment of Acute Vertigo:**
   1. Stop vomiting with prochlorperazine (Compazine) suppository, 25 mg q4-6h prn
   2. Diazepam (Valium) 2 mg tid
   3. Meclizine (Antivert) 25-50 mg PO q6h prn [12.5, 25, 50 mg].
   4. Sodium restriction 4 gm. or less daily
   5. Correct sensory deficits if possible
B. **Benign Positional Vertigo:** Deliberate repetition of the head maneuvers that elicit the symptoms of vertigo may lessen the severity and duration.
C. **Vestibular Neuronitis:** Managed with bedrest and meclizine (Antivert) 25-50 mg PO q6h; diuretics and salt restriction.
D. **Lightheadedness:** Treat anxiety, depression, or panic attacks with anxiolytics or antidepressants. Hyperventilation is treated by deliberate slow breathing.
E. **Meniere's Disease:** Acute attacks are managed with meclizine and bed rest. For refractory cases, ablative surgery of the vestibular nerve or labyrinthectomy may relieve symptoms but sacrifice hearing on involved side.

# Chronic Fatigue Syndrome

. **Pathophysiology of Chronic Fatigue Syndrome**
   A. The etiology of CFS appears to be neurologic, and abnormalities in cerebral perfusion, hypothalamic function, and neurotransmitter regulation have been documented.
   B. Abnormalities of immune system activation or immune system dysfunction have also been associated with CFS.
   C. Most frequently occurs in working-age adults, both male and female, but has been described in all age groups. 70% of patients are female. Not associated with increased mortality.

. **Clinical Evaluation**
   A. CFS is characterized by profound fatigue worsened by exertion or exercise. Patients may also complain of headaches, sore throat, lymph node pain, abdominal pain, muscle and joint pain, temperature regulation symptoms, and cognitive difficulty.
   B. CFS is a diagnosis of exclusion. Clinical evaluation and laboratory tests should rule out treatable organic or mental disorders.
   C. Obtain a complete history of symptoms, including prior psychiatric illness. Abrupt onset of symptoms suggests an infectious or other organic etiology.
   D. Neurologic symptoms such as dizziness, balance disorder, paresthesias, and cognitive disturbances involving short-term memory and attention may also be present.
   E. Emotional symptoms of depression or panic disorder, sleep problems and fibromyalgia symptoms (muscle aches and tenderness), or allergies may be present.
   F. A protracted course is common, although the level of fatigue varies considerably from day-to-day. Physical or mental stress often exacerbates CFS.

. **Physical Examination**
   A. The patient characteristically looks healthy and has relatively minor abnormalities. Low-grade fever and pharyngitis may be present.
   B. Breast, pelvic, rectal, and neurologic examinations should be completed. Tender musculoskeletal points may indicate fibromyalgia.
   C. Examination may reveal minor lymphadenopathy; tenderness of the anterior, cervical, axillary, and inguinal lymph nodes is common.
   D. Check for hyperreflexia in the lower extremities, Romberg's sign, and impaired tandem gait.
   E. Psychological Evaluation: Psychiatric tests such as the General Health Questionnaire may reveal abnormalities.

/. **Diagnostic Criteria for Chronic Fatigue Syndrome**
   A. New onset of disabling fatigue for 6 mo with at least a 50% reduction in activity.
   B. Exclusion of other diagnostic possibilities
   C. **Six or More of the Following Symptoms:**

| | |
|---|---|
| Mild fever | Headaches |
| Sore throat | Migratory arthralgias |
| Painful lymph nodes | Neuropsychologic complaints |
| Muscle weakness | Sleep disturbance |
| Myalgia | Acute onset of symptom complex |
| Prolonged fatigue after exercise | |

   **PLUS Two or More of the Following Signs:**
   Low-grade fever
   Nonexudative pharyngitis
   Palpable or tender lymph nodes

. **Disorders that Exclude the Diagnosis of CFS**
   A. **Chronic Medical Conditions:** Malignancy, autoimmune disorders (rheumatoid arthritis, lupus erythematosus), inflammatory disease, endocrinopathy, neurologic disease; other

chronic organic diseases, postinfectious disease, HIV infection, tuberculosis; chronic active hepatitis B or C; Lyme disease, sarcoidosis.
   B. **Psychiatric and Behavioral Disorders:** Psychotic depression, bipolar disorder, schizophrenia, substance abuse.

VI.   **Disorders that may Coexist with CFS**
   A. **Medical Conditions:** Fibromyalgia (generalized muscle aches, fatigue), infectious mononucleosis.
   B. **Psychiatric and Behavioral Disorders:** Nonpsychotic depression, somatization, anxiety and panic disorders.

VII.  **Laboratory Evaluation**
   A. **All Patients:** Complete blood-cell count with differential, erythrocyte sedimentation rate, serum glucose, electrolytes, thyroid screening, urinalysis.
   B. **High-risk Patients:** Syphilis test, HIV, tuberculosis skin test, antinuclear antibody, rheumatoid factor, chest radiography, serum cortisol, immunoglobulin levels.
   C. **Geographic Risk Area:** Lyme titer
   D. **Angiotensin-converting enzyme (ACE) levels** may be increased in patients with chronic fatigue syndrome. This is a marker for sarcoidosis and for diseases involving the blood vessels. An increased ACE level is not in itself diagnostic of chronic fatigue syndrome. In patients with an elevated ACE level, sarcoidosis should be excluded by assessing for pulmonary symptoms, lymph nodes, eyes, and chest radiography.
   E. The hypothesis that Epstein-Barr virus is the cause has not been supported; antibody testing for this virus is of no value in clinical evaluation. Human herpesvirus 6 is unlikely to be causative.

VIII. **Treatment of Chronic Fatigue Syndrome**
   A. Treatment is largely supportive; the disorder may last months or years, but eventual improvement can be expected. Reassurance and education about the illness and the usually favorable prognosis may help reduce anxiety.
   B. Good nutrition and vitamin supplements may be useful. Adequate rest, and mild exercise to the point where fatigue occurs should be encouraged.
   C. Tricyclic antidepressants may help control pain, improve sleep, and alleviate depression. Initially give in low doses because many CFS patients are sensitive to side effects.
      -Fluoxetine (Prozac) 20 mg PO qAM; 20-40 mg/d [20 mg].
      -Bupropion (Wellbutrin) 100 mg PO bid-tid; 150-450 mg/d [75, 100 mg].
      -Sertraline (Zoloft) initial dose 50 mg PO qAM, max 200 mg PO qd [50, 100 mg].
   D. Nonsteroidal anti-inflammatory agents may relieve headaches, arthralgias, myalgias.
   E. Intramuscular gamma globulin (Gamastan) and intramuscular magnesium sulfate have been reported to relieve symptoms, but trials have yielded conflicting results.

# Dermatology

## Herpes Simplex Virus Infections

### Pathogenesis of Herpes Simplex

A. Any mucocutaneous surface or visceral site may be infected by HSV. Two strains of the virus, herpes simplex virus type 1 (HSV-1) and herpes simplex virus type 2 (HSV-2), cause clinically indistinguishable lesions.

B. Both HSV-1 and HSV-2 may cause genital and orofacial lesions. In genital infections, recurrences are more commonly caused by HSV-2 than HSV-1. The majority of genital herpes infections are asymptomatic.

C. Primary HSV infection occurs after first exposure, followed by a latency period while the virus remains dormant within a ganglionic nerve cell. The virus may reactivate in some patients, and recurrent disease results from migration of virus along axons to the skin and mucous membranes.

D. Antibody studies have shown that 60% of all US adults are positive, and 90% of inner city adults are positive.

E. Prevention of genital herpes through vaccination has not been effective.

### Clinical Features

A. **Diagnostic Features of HSV Infection:**
   1. Skin or mucous membrane location
   2. Grouped vesicles or a solitary vesicle with erythematous bases, progressing to ulceration
   3. Prodromal burning or itching (in recurrent disease)
   4. Reactivation along cutaneous nerves (in recurrent disease)
   5. Lesions are painful and persist for several days forming a honey-colored crust. Healing is usually complete within 3 weeks.

B. Immunosuppressed patients, especially HIV infected patients, have more frequent and more severe infections.

C. Contact with ulcerative lesions or with secretions may result in transmission. Asymptomatic viral shedding at a previously infected site may also cause infection.

D. The incubation period for primary HSV infections is 1-26 days, with a median of 6-8 days. Primary infections may be accompanied by flu-like symptoms. Primary HSV infections may involve both mucosal and extramucosal sites.

E. **Recurrent Disease:**
   1. Ninety percent of symptomatic HSV-2 infections and 60% of HSV-1 infections recur within 1 year. Patients usually experience 5-8 recurrences per year, but some may have outbreaks as frequently as every 2-3 weeks. The frequency and number of recurrences are highly variable. Median time to first recurrence is 50 days.
   2. Reported precipitating events for recurrent infection include menstruation, stress, sexual intercourse, sun exposure, cold, or local trauma.
   a potent sunscreen and sunscreen containing lip balm are recommended.
   3. Recurrent lesions usually arise at the site of the primary infection. Over time, the recurrences become less frequent; they peak during the early adult years.

F. HSV should be suspected as a cause of urethritis in men if dysuria is out of proportion to the urethral discharge. Perianal infections and proctitis are more common in homosexual men.

G. Sexual abuse should be suspected in children with anogenital HSV infections.

### . Differential Diagnosis of HSV Infections

A. Primary herpetic gingivostomatitis, erythema multiforme, Vincent's infection, streptococcal pharyngitis, genital herpes, primary syphilis (chancre), candidiasis, chancroid.

B. Fixed drug eruption, contact dermatitis, herpes zoster, aphthous stomatitis.

IV. **Clinical Variants of Herpes Simplex Infections**
  A. **HSV Infection and Erythema Multiforme:**
    1. HSV may trigger erythema multiforme and is the most common agent associated with this inflammatory skin condition. Erythema multiforme primarily affects healthy, young adults; more frequently men than women.
    2. Polymorphic skin lesions, including macules, papules, vesicles, bullae, wheals and target lesions, appear in a symmetric distribution. Tend to develop on the elbows, knees, palms and soles, and dorsal aspect of hands and feet.
    3. Erythema multiforme is characterized by recurrences and usually follows an HSV infection by 7-14 days. Not all episodes of erythema multiforme are preceded by definite herpetic lesions.
  B. **HSV Encephalitis:** HSV encephalitis must be considered in any case of nonbacterial encephalitis. Prompt treatment with IV acyclovir can be lifesaving.
  C. **Ophthalmic HSV Infection:** Primary and recurrent ocular infection may result in herpetic conjunctivitis, ulcerative herpetic keratitis, keratouveitis, or posterior segment disease.
    · Intravenous acyclovir and topical ophthalmic preparations are effective.

V. **Laboratory Tests**
  A. Diagnosis of genital herpes requires the characteristic history and physical appearance of lesions plus the selective use of viral culture. Viral culture is the gold standard for the diagnosis of genital herpes infection.
  B. Cytologic techniques such as the Tzanck and Papanicolaou smears may support a clinical diagnosis. Wright stained scrapings obtained from the base of a vesicle or ulcer reveal multinucleated giant cells. These tests do not distinguish between HSV infection and herpes zoster infection. Additionally, the sensitivities of these methods are so low that a negative smear cannot rule out infection.
  C. Viral culture requires 48-96 hours and has an accuracy rate of 85-90%.
  D. Immunofluorescent assays rapidly detect HSV in tissue samples or smears. Serologies have a minor role in the diagnosis of primary HSV infection since antibodies are absent at the onset of infection and become permanently positive after infection.

VI. **Therapy for HSV Infections**

| Type of infection | Dosage/regimen | Considerations |
|---|---|---|
| **Initial infection** | 200 mg PO five times per day for 10 days or until clinical resolution<br>or | Preferred route in the normal host |
| | 5 mg/kg IV q8h over one hour for 5-7 or until clinical resolution | Only for severe symptoms or complications |
| **Recurrent Infection** | | |
| **Episodic therapy** | 400 mg orally for tid for 5 days or 800 mg orally bid for 5 days | Treatment is most effective when initiated at the earliest sign of recurrence; it is of no benefit if initiated more than 48 hours after symptom onset |
| **Suppressive therapy** | 400 mg orally bid | Indicated for patients with frequent and/or severe recurrences (more than 6 outbreaks per year) |

  A. Acyclovir is the drug of choice for the treatment and suppression of genital herpes. Acyclovir does not cure genital herpes. Acyclovir is virtually nontoxic to normal cells because only HSV-infected cells preferentially take in acyclovir and convert it to the active form.

B. Acyclovir is eliminated primarily by the kidneys; therefore, the dosage should be individualized in patients with renal insufficiency.

C. To be effective, acyclovir must be started early. It acts only during active HSV replication, which occurs within approximately 48 hours of vesicle formation.

D. **Side Effects:** Usually well tolerated, but nausea, vomiting, rash, headache, lethargy, tremulousness, seizures, and delirium occur rarely.

E. Topical acyclovir has not shown significant efficacy in primary disease or recurrent infections.

F. **Oral analgesics:** Viscous lidocaine applied qid prn pain. Sitz baths. Keep area clean and dry--corn starch, baby powder, use a hair dryer. Pyridium may be useful for dysuria.

G. **Serious or Life-Threatening HSV Infections:** Intravenous acyclovir is indicated for serious or life-threatening episodes including herpes genitalis, oral herpes and herpetic whitlow. Dosage must be adjusted in impaired renal function.

H. **Immunocompromised Patients:**
   1. Treatment of genital herpes in the immunocompromised patient generally requires acyclovir therapy at higher doses and more frequent intervals.
   2. Acyclovir, 400 mg, PO three to five times daily until clinical resolution. Double dose if no response in 3-5 days. Intermittent or suppressive therapy may be needed

## VII. General Management Considerations

A. Patients should be informed that HSV autoinoculation from one body site to another is possible. Infected areas should be patted dry rather than wiped dry.

B. Patients are advised to abstain from sexual activity while lesions are present. Use of a latex condom is encouraged during all sexual exposures because of asymptomatic viral shedding.

C. The risk of neonatal transmission must be explained to male and female patients.

D. Recommended testing includes evaluation for gonorrhea, chlamydial infection, syphilis, trichomoniasis, genital warts, and human immunodeficiency virus (HIV).

## VIII. Treatment of Recurrences

A. **Episodic Acyclovir Therapy:**
   1. Early initiation of therapy has been shown to produce a statistically significant reduction in the duration of symptoms, but the degree of clinical improvement perceived by the patient is very limited.
   2. The patient should keep a supply of acyclovir and begin treatment at the earliest prodromal symptom in an attempt to abort an episode.

B. **Suppressive Acyclovir Therapy:**
   1. Suppressive acyclovir therapy has been shown to reduce the frequency of recurrence by 80% and to prevent recurrence in up to 30% of patients. Patients prefer suppressive over episodic therapy. Recommended for frequent recurrences ($\geq$6 per year)
   2. After one year of suppressive therapy, acyclovir should be discontinued to allow assessment of the patient's rate of recurrences. Daily suppressive therapy may be given for as long as five years.
   3. A patient maintained on episodic therapy could use a suppressive regimen during periods of increased stress or when optimal protection is desired, such as during a vacation or before a wedding.

# Herpes Zoster

I. **Clinical Evaluation**
   A. Zoster occurs in patients who have had chickenpox in the distant past. The disease occurs when the latent virus, within the nerve ganglion, reactivates and causes a new, localized rash of zoster.
   B. Zoster is usually heralded by dermatomal pain, sometimes accompanied by malaise and fever. Within a few days, the skin overlying the dermatome reddens and blisters. A few vesicles are usually grouped on one erythematous base, in contrast to the scattered, single vesicles of chickenpox. Several days later the vesicles become pustular and develop crusts, followed by scabs.
   C. Zoster may occur in any dermatome, but the thoracic dermatomes are most often affected. New lesions continue to appear for 2-3 days. Lesions usually develop crusts and scabs within 14 days. Elderly patients are at greater risk for postherpetic neuralgia. In more than 90% of immunocompetent patients, herpetic pain eventually disappears completely.
   D. The frequency of zoster increases markedly after age 55, but people of any age can be affected.
   E. Herpes simplex infections occasionally appear in a dermatomal pattern that mimics zoster, but frequent recurrences are a hallmark of herpes simplex infections.
   F. Less than 5% of immunocompetent patients who have one episode of herpes zoster will have another, and the episodes are usually separated by years. HIV-infected patients may be more likely to have recurrent herpes zoster and herpes simplex.

II. **Laboratory Evaluation**
   A. The diagnosis of herpes zoster can be made on clinical grounds without the need for laboratory tests in most patients.
   B. Viral isolation and culture assays are not useful for varicella-zoster. Herpes simplex and varicella-zoster cannot be differentiated by microscopic Tzanck smear.
   C. An isolated case of zoster in an apparently healthy young or middle-aged adult is probably not an indicator of an underlying immunodeficiency, and additional testing is unnecessary. Consider HIV testing when a patient who engages in high-risk behavior (sexual activities, drug use) develops herpes zoster. Testing for HIV is also indicated when herpes zoster is protracted, recurrent, or involves multiple dermatomes.

III. **Complications of Herpes Zoster**
   A. 15% of patients with zoster have involvement of the ophthalmic branch of the trigeminal nerve. Hutchinson's sign--a lesion on the tip of the nose--indicates corneal involvement and associated keratitis; however, ophthalmic involvement may occur even in the absence of Hutchinson's sign. Treatment with IV and topical antiviral agents is required to prevent blindness.
   B. Disseminated herpes zoster is present when 20 or more lesions occur outside of the primary contiguous dermatomes. These patients are at risk for visceral dissemination.

IV. **Symptomatic Therapy for Zoster**
   A. Wet dressings or compresses with aluminum acetate cream or Burow's solution (Domeboro) will protect sensitive areas.
   B. Topical agents include calamine-containing lotions and creams, and 10% salicylate (Aspercreme).
   C. Topical capsaicin cream is only indicated for postherpetic neuralgia, and is not appropriate in the acute stages of herpes zoster until the lesions have healed.
   D. **Systemic Analgesics:** Acetaminophen, nonsteroidal antiinflammatory drugs, or analgesics with codeine (Vicodin) may be needed.

V. **Antiviral Therapy for Zoster:**
   A. An antiviral can hasten the resolution of the rash by several days, although the benefit

is modest.

B. Relief of acute pain occurs relatively quickly, within two to three days after an antiviral is begun. The duration of pain associated with zoster has been reduced by about half.

C. Antiviral therapy is more likely to be of benefit if initiated within 48-72 hours following onset of the rash.

D. **Acyclovir (Zovirax):**
   1. The oral dose for zoster is 800 mg q4h five times a day (total of 4 g) for seven days. [400 mg and 800-mg tablet, 200 mg capsule].
   2. Oral acyclovir does not have significant adverse effects; nausea, vomiting, headaches, diarrhea, and constipation may sometimes occur. Dosage should be adjusted in renal failure.
   3. Oral acyclovir is sufficient for most patients. IV acyclovir is reserved for the severely immunosuppressed, such as bone marrow transplant patients with varicella, or disseminated zoster. IV acyclovir is also used for ophthalmic zoster.
   4. The IV dose for zoster is 10 mg/kg, administered over a one-hour, q8h. Reduce dosage in renal failure. Nephrotoxicity can usually be avoided if given over a period of one hour and the patient remains well-hydrated. Adverse effects of IV acyclovir include lethargy, confusion, and tremor.

E. **Famciclovir (Famvir)** for herpes zoster infections is equally effective to acyclovir; it offers increased bioavailability and a more convenient dosing interval; one 500-mg tablet tid for 7 days.

F. **Valacyclovir (Valtrex)** 1 g PO tid for 7 days [500 mg].

G. **Foscarnet sodium (Foscavir)** is helpful for acyclovir-resistant herpes zoster and herpes simplex infections.

H. Low-dose corticosteroids are not indicated because of the risk of potentiating the infection and because their benefits are not clear.

I. Ophthalmic distribution zoster is a medical emergency. IV Acyclovir will help to reduce ocular complications, but topical antivirals are also needed.

## VI. Postherpetic Neuralgia

A. The most common complication of herpes zoster is postherpetic neuralgia (PHN) defined as chronic pain persisting for at least one month after the skin lesions have healed.

B. The incidence of PHN is 5-50%. Those aged 60 and older have a 50% chance of developing PHN after herpes zoster. PHN resolves within two months in about half of those affected.

C. Antivirals are not effective for PHN. Aspirin and acetaminophen are usually ineffective.

D. **Topical Preparations:**
   1. Capsaicin cream 0.025% (Zostrix, Zostrix-HP), a derivative of hot peppers, reduces the pain. Apply the cream three to four times daily.
   2. Nonprescription, mentholated ointments such as Ben-Gay may offer similar relief at lower cost. Flex-all 454 and 10% salicylate (Aspercreme) may be useful.
   3. EMLA topical cream (lidocaine and prilocaine) may be useful.
   4. Amitriptyline (Elavil, Endep) is often effective; 10-25 mg qhs, increasing in weekly increments of 10-25 mg as needed.
   5. Transcutaneous electrical nerve stimulation (TENS) has been fairly successful in managing PHN that is resistant to drug therapy; 3-4 times daily or prn.
   6. Lidocaine (Xylocaine) injections, nerve block injections, permanent nerve blocks with alcohol nerve, and nerve resectioning have been used as a last resort.

# Acne Vulgaris

## I. Clinical Manifestations

A. Acne comedones are usually found on the forehead and upper cheeks of adolescents. Comedones may progress to inflammatory lesions on the lower cheeks, chin, chest, upper back, and shoulders.

B. In females, the possibility of androgenic disorders such as polycystic ovarian disease and Cushing's syndrome should be considered; the patient should be asked about menstrual irregularities and should be examined for hirsutism.

## II. Non-Pharmacologic Therapy for Acne

A. **Diet:** Patients should be advised to eat a well-balanced diet and to avoid foods which consistently result in acne flare-ups.

B. **Cleanliness:**
   1. Development of acne is not related to dirt. Excessive scrubbing, especially with abrasive cleaners and sponges, may worsen the condition.
   2. Patients who have oily skin should wash their faces using mild, unscented, antibacterial soap (Dial, Lever-2000) and water.

C. **Environment:** Very humid environments, heavy sweating, or exposure to pollution may aggravate acne.

D. **Mechanical Trauma:** Pressure, rubbing, and humidity from occlusive clothing can aggravate acne. Repeated picking of lesions can cause increased inflammation, scarring, and pigmentary changes.

E. **Cosmetics:** Heavy oils, greases or dyes in cosmetic creams and hair sprays can exacerbate acne. Water-based products should be used.

F. **Medications that Worsen Acne:** Corticosteroids, androgens, phenytoin, lithium, isoniazid, and cyclosporine. Some oral contraceptives with androgenic progesterones may promote acne eruptions.

## III. Pharmacologic Therapy

A. **Treatment of Comedonal Acne:**
   1. Mild noninflammatory acne can be treated with topical antibacterial agents such as benzoyl peroxide or comedolytic agents such as tretinoin (Retin-A). The combination of benzoyl peroxide in the morning and tretinoin at night is effective.
   2. Creams and lotions usually are less drying than gels and liquids.
   3. **Benzoyl Peroxide:**
      a. Potent antibacterial, mild comedolytic and exfoliant properties.
      b. Benzoyl peroxide is the first-line therapy for mild acne, and may be used with other agents. Available over-the-counter as 2.5%, 5%, and 10% gels, creams, lotions or soaps. The liquids and creams (Benoxyl, Oxy-10) are less irritating and may be useful for dry skin. The gel (Benzagel, Persa-Gel, Desquam-X) is more irritating but more effective for oily skin. Mild redness and scaling occurs during the first week.
      c. Start with 5% concentration. Apply qAM-bid after washing; increase strength as patient becomes tolerant of irritant effect [2.5, 5-10% gel, 5-10% cream or lotion].
   4. **Tretinoin (Retin A):**
      a. Most effective topical comedolytic agent. Retin-A cream (0.025, 0.05, 0.1%), Retin-A gel (0.01, 0.025%), and Retin-A liquid (0.05%).
      b. Start with 0.025% cream or gel. If no response occurs after a few weeks, use higher-concentration. The cream is best for dry skin; the gel is best for oily skin.
      c. Should be applied once a day at bedtime, 30 minutes after washing (to dry skin).
      d. Mild redness and peeling occurs; improvement may take 6-12 weeks; flare-ups of acne can occur during the first few weeks of therapy due to surfacing of the lesions; avoid excessive sun exposure, and use sunscreen.
   5. **Comedone Extraction** can accelerate resolution when used in addition to topical medications.

B. **Treatment of Papular Acne:**
1. Topical antibiotics are useful alone or in combination with benzoyl peroxide, tretinoin, or systemic antibiotics.
2. **Topical Antibiotics:**
   a. **Clindamycin:** Available in 1% solution, lotion or gel (Cleocin-T); apply to affected areas bid after cleansing.
   b. **Erythromycin:** 2% solution (EryDerm, A/T/S), gel (Erygel, Emgel), or pledgets (Erycette, T-stat); apply to affected areas bid; also available in a 3% gel combined with 5% benzoyl peroxide (Benzamycin) which is the most effective topical antibiotic.

C. **Treatment of Pustular Acne:**
1. Moderate or severe inflammatory acne requires oral antibiotics in addition to topical therapy. Side effects of oral antibiotics include gastrointestinal distress and vaginal candidiasis.
2. **Tetracycline:**
   a. Effective and low cost; first-choice oral antibiotic. Starting dosage is 250 mg qid or 500 mg bid, 1 hour before or 2 hours after meals; after 1-2 months reduce to maintenance dose of 250 mg PO qd.
   b. Antacids or dairy products can interfere with absorption; can cause dental discoloration; contraindicated in pregnancy or in children <12 years; photosensitizing.
   c. May reduce the efficacy of oral contraceptive pills. If tetracycline is used with OCP's, a backup birth control method should be advised. Erythromycin is a better choice in these patients.
3. **Minocycline (Minocin):** Highly effective because of its lipid solubility and ability to penetrate the sebaceous follicle; good absorption with food; high cost. The usual starting dose is 50 mg bid or 100 mg qd [50,100 mg].
4. **Doxycycline:** Less expensive than minocycline and is very effective. 100 mg once daily; photosensitivity, gastrointestinal distress may occur.
5. **Erythromycin:** Starting dosage is 250 mg qid or 500 mg bid. Propionibacterium acnes bacteria are more resistant to erythromycin than tetracycline; gastrointestinal side effects.
6. **Trimethoprim-Sulfamethoxazole (Bactrim DS):** Used for severe acne that is refractory to other antibiotics. One double-strength tablet qd-bid. Potential side effects include a severe eruptive reaction.

D. **Treatment of Nodulocystic Acne:**
1. **Isotretinoin (Accutane):**
   a. Vitamin A Derivative; decreases sebum production and reverses abnormal epithelial desquamation.
   b. **Initial Dose:** 0.5-1.0 mg/kg, or 40-80 mg/day [10,20,40 mg]. The usual duration of therapy is 4-5 months; response rate is 90%. Transient exacerbation of acne may occur during the initial month; only one course is usually needed.
   c. **Side Effects:** Cheilitis, dry skin, pruritus, epistaxis, photosensitivity. Decreased night vision, hypertriglyceridemia, abnormal liver function tests, electrolyte imbalance, elevated platelet count. Pseudotumor cerebri can occur if taken with tetracycline. Side effects are usually reversible once therapy is discontinued.
   d. **Teratogenic:** Exclude pregnancy with a serum test; contraception must be used.
2. **Corticosteroid Injection:** Intralesional injection of triamcinolone acetonide (Kenalog), 1.0-2.5 mg/mL solution, will lead to rapid resolution of most cystic lesions in 2-3 days. Stock solutions should be diluted in saline or 1% lidocaine (Xylocaine) to appropriate concentrations. Inject into cyst with 27-30 gauge needle.
3. **Systemic Hormones:** For female patients, low dose oral contraceptives can suppress ovarian androgen production. Oral contraceptives with norgestrel may exacerbate acne. Demulen is commonly used for acne-prone women.
4. **Less Commonly Used Treatments:**
   Spironolactone: 150-200 mg per day; reduces sebum production; brings significant improvement.

Isotretinoin Gel: Significantly reduces the number of both noninflamed and inflamed lesions.

IV. **Gram-negative Folliculitis**
   A. A form of severe acne caused by gram-negative organisms, characterized by a sudden increase in severity of acne **during** therapy with other antibiotics.
   B. The paranasal region is the most common site of involvement.
   C. **Trimethoprim-Sulfamethoxazole (Bactrim DS):** One double-strength tablet qd-bid.
   D. **Amoxicillin/clavulanate (Augmentin)** 500 mg PO tid for 7-10 days.
   E. For severe cases isotretinoin (Accutane) is the treatment of choice.

# Dermatitis and Verruca Vulgaris

. **Classification of Dermatitis (Eczema)**
A. **Contact dermatitis** is a nonallergic reaction caused by irritating substances.
   1. Any substance can act as an irritant, provided the concentration and duration of contact with the skin are sufficient.
   2. Irritants include water, soaps and detergents, aluminum salts in deodorants, urine, feces, acids, and alkalis.
B. **Delayed Type Hypersensitivity Reactions** are immunologic reactions to contact allergens of the delayed hypersensitivity type, occurring in sensitized individuals.
   1. Acutely, irritants produce erythema, microvesicles, and oozing, which may be indistinguishable from allergic contact dermatitis. If the agent is strong enough, blisters, erosions, and ulcerations can occur.
   2. The interval between introduction of the antigen and development of clinical symptoms varies from 3-12 days on the 1st exposure in a susceptible patient.
   3. An already sensitized individual will react to the substance within 12-48 hours.
   4. **Common Topical Sensitizers:**
      a. Toxicodendrons (poison ivy, oak, and sumac, ragweed pollen)
      b. Ethylenediamine (a stabilizer in many topical creams)
      c. Nickel (10% of females are allergic to nickel found in jewelry)
      d. Benzocaine
C. **Atopic Dermatitis:**
   1. A constitutional and inherited ability to react with pruritus and inflammation of the skin; pathogenesis is unknown.
   2. Associated with asthma, hay fever, urticaria, and high levels of IgE.
   3. **Clinical Presentation:**
      a. Commonly begins as infantile eczema that presents as dermatitis of the cheeks, face, and upper extremities. This remits or may change to a flexural dermatitis of the antecubital fossae and neck.
      b. Flexural involvement usually lasts from ages 4-10 years old, but may go on longer.
      c. Most atopic childhood eczema fades in adult life, but sometimes recurs at times of stress or for unknown reasons. In adults it may appear as recalcitrant hand eczema or as a localized or generalized dermatitis.
   4. Atopic skin is particularly susceptible to bacterial and viral infections that may become widespread. These patients may develop widespread herpes infections of the skin, and they should be protected from people with active herpetic lesions.

I. **Treatment of Dermatitis/Eczema**
A. Identify and avoid offending agents. Remove the antigen as soon as possible with warm, soapy water.
B. **Acute Dermatitis That Is Wet, Vesicular, or Weeping:** Use wet compresses with either tap water or an antibacterial solution to cleanse the area and soothe itching.
C. Oral antihistamines such as diphenhydramine or trazodone are useful for pruritus.
D. **Topical Corticosteroids:** In the intertriginous and facial areas, use only low-potency steroids, such as 1% hydrocortisone cream, as there is risk of causing atrophy in these areas. Stronger steroids should be reserved for other areas of the skin.
E. **Low-Potency Topical Corticosteroids:**
   Hydrocortisone apply tid-qid [cream 1, 2.5%; ointment 1, 2.5%; lotion 1, 2, 2.5%].
   Triamcinolone acetonide (Aristocort, Kenalog) apply to affected area tid-qid [ointment 0.1, 0.5%; cream 0.1, 0.5%; lotion 0.1%].
F. **High-Potency Topical Corticosteroids:**
   Betamethasone dipropionate Augmented (Diprolene) apply to affected areas bid [oint, lotion 0.05%]
   Clobetasol propionate (Temovate) apply to affected areas bid [cream, oint 0.05%]
   Diflorasone diacetate (Florone) apply to affected areas qd-qid [cream, oint 0.05%]

Halobetasol propionate (Ultravate) apply to affected area bid [cream, oint 0.05%]

G. **Systemic Corticosteroids** are reserved for severe, widespread reactions, or for severe involvement of the hands, face, or genitals.
  1. Prednisone 1-2 mg/kg PO, tapering over 10-18 days.
  2. For patients who are at risk for complications of fluid retention due to the mineralocorticoid effects of prednisone, substitute dexamethasone (Decadron), 0.75 mg/kg PO; particularly effective in older patients with cardiac problems or if taking diuretics.

H. Antibiotic therapy should be initiated prophylactically if there is a risk for secondary infection.
  -Erythromycin 250 mg PO bid-tid with meals.
  -Dicloxacillin (if staphylococci resistance is possible) 250 mg PO qid [250, 500 mg].

I. All patients with chronic forms of dermatitis should only use mild soap for cleaning, and they should lubricate the skin with lotion or petroleum jelly on a regular basis to keep the skin well hydrated.

## III. Verruca Vulgaris (Common Skin Warts)

A. Verruca vulgaris warts are benign, usually self-regressing papilloma of the skin and adjacent mucous membranes caused by the human papilloma virus (HPV).

B. The peak incidence of warts occurs during the second decade of life with about 10% of teenagers having them.

C. Warts can occur at every location on the skin, but warts in different locations often assume different appearances:
  1. Plantar or mosaic warts on the soles are hyperkeratotic.
  2. Common warts on the hands have a dome shape and velvety surface.
  3. Flat warts occur over the face, arms, or around the knees.
  4. Anogenital warts, called condylomata acuminata, occur on the genitalia or anorectal area.
  5. Buschke-Lowenstein tumor or verrucous carcinoma appears as a persistent, large wart of the foot or anogenital region that can become malignant.

D. **Differential Diagnosis:**
  1. **Molluscum contagiosum:** Shiny, dome-shaped, papilla like a wart, but has an umbilicated center.
  2. **Calluses:** Can look like warts, but lack the thrombosed punctate capillaries of warts.

E. **Treatment of Verruca Vulgaris:**
  1. **Cryotherapy and Chemical Agents:**
    a. Chemicals such as cantharidin or liquid nitrogen are favored over electrodesiccation which can scar. Cryosurgery with liquid nitrogen should freeze wart and about 1 mm of surrounding tissue.
    b. **Over-the-counter Wart Preparations:** Mediplast (for plantar use) salicylic acid plaster for home use.
    c. **Prescription Wart Preparation:** Duofilm, Occlusal, Occlusal-HP, Podofilox (Condylox), Viranol (gel), cantharidin alone or in combination (Cantharone, Cantharone Plus, Verrusol).
    d. Unresponsive or diffuse warts can be treated with topical 5-fluorouracil or dinitrochlorobenzene (DNCB).
  2. **Surgery:** Anesthetize area, and use a dermal curet to bluntly dissect the wart and completely remove. Potential for scarring, and recurrent warts may form in the scar.
  3. Vaccines prepared from wart tissue are not advisable because of the oncogenicity of HPV.

# Common Skin Diseases

**I. Alopecia Areata**

A. Characterized by asymptomatic, noninflammatory, non-scarring areas of complete hair loss most commonly involving the scalp, but may involve any area of hair-bearing skin.

B. Probably caused by auto-antibodies to hair follicles. Emotional stress is sometimes a precipitating factor. The younger the patient and the more widespread the disease, and the poorer the prognosis.

C. Regrowth of hair after the first attack takes place in 6 months in 30% of cases, with 50% regrowing within 1 year and approximately 80% growing within 5 years. 10-30% of patients will not regrow hair; 5% progress to total hair loss. In active lesions, "exclamation point" hairs (loose hairs 3-10 mm in size with a tapered, less pigmented proximal shaft) are seen at the margins.

D. Lesions are well defined, single or multiple, round or oval areas of total hair loss. In active lesions, "exclamation point" hairs (loose hairs 3-10 mm in size with a tapered, less pigmented proximal shaft) are seen at the margins.

E. **Differential Diagnosis:** Tinea capitis, trichotillomania, secondary syphilis, and lupus erythematosus.

F. A VDRL or RPR test for syphilis should always be obtained. A CBC, SMAC, sedimentary rate, thyroid function tests, antinuclear antibody should be done to screen for pernicious anemia, chronic active hepatitis, thyroid disease, lupus erythematosus, and Addison's disease.

G. **Therapy:** Topical steroids, intralesional steroids, and topical minoxidil may be somewhat effective. Hair regrowth will usually occur in 1 year without therapy.

**II. Scabies**

A. Characterized by an extremely pruritic eruption usually accentuated in the groin, axillae, navel, breasts, and finger webs, with sparing the head.

B. Scabies is spread by skin to skin contact. The diagnosis is established by finding the mite, ova, or feces in scrapings of the skin, usually of the finger webs or genitalia.

C. Treatment of choice for nonpregnant adults and children is gamma benzene hexachloride (Kwell), applied for 8-12 hours, then washed off. CNS toxicity has been reported in infants in whom it was used too frequently.

D. Elimite, a 5% permethrin cream, is more effective but more expensive than lindane (Kwell). With the availability of Elimite, crotamiton (Eurax) has little use in the management of scabies.

E. Treatment should be given to all members of an infected household simultaneously. Clothing and sheets must be washed on the day of treatment. Treatment failures usually result from incomplete treatment or failure to treat all members of the household simultaneously.

**III. Head Lice**

A. Look for crabs in the axillae, abdominal hair, and eyelashes.

B. RID, NIX, or A-200 are now the treatment of choice. Kwell is not very effective.

C. Pubic lice (crabs) are still usually Kwell sensitive, but repeated treatments may be required.

**IV. Seborrheic Dermatitis**

A. Seborrheic dermatitis is often called cradle cap, dandruff, or seborrhea. It has a high prevalence in infancy, and then is not common until after puberty. Predilection is for the face, retroauricular region, and upper trunk.

B. **Clinical Findings:**

1. Infants present with an adherent, waxy, even asbestos-like, laminated, scaly lesions on the scalp vertex also known as "cradle cap."

2. In adults, the eruption is bilaterally symmetrical, affecting the scalp with patchy or diffuse, dull, yellow-like erythema, and waxy yellow, greasy scaling on the forehead, retroauricular region, auditory meatus, eyebrows, cheeks and nasolabial folds.

3. Trunk areas affected include the presternal, interscapular regions, the umbilicus, intertriginous surfaces of the axilla, inframammary regions, groin, and anogenital

crease.

4. Pruritus is mild. Bacterial infection is indicated by vesiculation and oozing.

C. **Differential Diagnosis:**
   1. Lupus erythematosus - has telangiectasias almost always.
   2. Psoriasis - thick, micaceous white scale.
   3. Tinea versicolor - fine scale, usually tan or pink; positive KOH.

D. **Treatment:**
   1. **Scalp:** Selenium sulfide or tar shampoos; sulfur and salicylic acid lotions as keratolytics; topical corticosteroid lotions.
   2. **Face, neck, and intertriginous regions:** Hydrocortisone 1 or 2 ½%.
   3. **Trunk:** Fluorinated steroids can be used if severe.

## V. Drug Eruptions

A. Drug eruptions, may be type I, type II, type III, or type IV immunologic reactions.

B. Cutaneous drug reactions may start within 7 days of initiation of the drug or within 4-7 days after the offending drug has been stopped.

C. The cutaneous lesions usually become more severe and widespread over the following several days to 1 week and then clear over the next 7-14 days.

D. Lesions most often start first and clear first from the head and upper extremities to the trunk and lower legs. Palms, soles, and mucous membranes may be involved.

E. Most drug reactions appear as the typical maculopapular drug reaction. Tetracycline is associated with a fixed drug eruption; phenytoin (Dilantin) and sulfonamides have a tendency to erythema multiforme-like drug eruptions; thiazide diuretics have a tendency for photosensitivity eruptions.

F. Specifically question the patient concerning medications, eye drops, nasal sprays, suppositories, immunizations, vitamins, laxatives, analgesics, and aspirin. These drugs are capable of causing cutaneous reactions.

G. **Treatment of Drug Eruptions:**
   1. Oral antihistamines are very useful. Diphenhydramine (Benadryl), 25-50 mg q4-6h.
   2. Soothing, tepid water baths in Aveeno or corn starch or cool compresses are useful.
   3. Drying antipruritic lotions such as Caladryl and calamine with menthol and/or phenol are sometimes helpful.
   4. **Severe Signs and Symptoms:** A 2-week course of systemic steroids (prednisone starting at 60 mg per day and then tapering) will usually stop the symptoms and prevent further progression of the eruption within about 48 hours of the onset of therapy.

## VI. Groin Rashes

A. In adults groin rashes may be due to Candida or tinea.

B. Candida lesions are often moist, red and confluent with peeling borders that are surrounded by satellite lesions. Candida tends to involve intertriginous areas and scrotum.

C. Tinea clears centrally, has a sharp border with a scale, and spares the scrotum.

D. **Treatment:** Imidazoles are effective for both tinea and Candida, but nystatin only treats Candida.
   - Miconazole (Micatin), apply to affected area bid; cream: 2% [15, 30 gm]
   - Clotrimazole (Lotrimin), apply to affected area bid; cream: 1% [15, 30, 45, 90 gm], lotion: 1% [30 mL]
   - Econazole (Spectazole), apply to affected area once daily; cream: 1% [15, 30, 85 g]
   - Ketoconazole (Nizoral), apply to affected area qd-bid; cream: 2% [15, 30, 60 gm]
   - Oxiconazole (Oxistat), apply to affected area qd; cream: 1% [15, 30, 60 gm], lotion: 1% [30 mL]
   - Nystatin (Mycostatin), apply to affected area bid; cream, oint: 100,000 U/gm [15, 30 gm]

E. Allylamines (naftifine and terbinafine) are more effective against tinea, but have little activity against Candida.
   - Naftifine (Naftin) 1%, apply to affected area qd-bid; [cream 15, 30, 60 gm]; [gel 20, 40, 60 gm]; minimal Candida coverage.

-Terbinafine HCL (Lamisil), apply to affected area bid; cream: 1% [15, 30 g]; minimal Candida coverage.

## VII. Lesions of the Nail Fold

A. Acute paronychia presents as tender, red, swollen areas of the nail fold, but not the nail itself. Pus may be seen through the nail plate or at the paronychial fold.

B. In acute cases, the most common causative bacteria are staphylococci, beta-hemolytic streptococci, and gram-negative enteric bacteria.

C. Chronic paronychia infections of the nail fold are due almost universally to Candida albicans.

D. Predisposing factors include minor trauma, foreign bodies or splinters under the nail. Moisture predispose to Candida.

E. **Diagnosis of Paronychial Lesions:** Acute lesions are usually bacterial and may be cultured for bacteria. Chronic lesions are usually caused by Candida and may be diagnosed by KOH prep or by fungal culture (DTM culture).

F. **Treatment of Acute Bacterial Paronychia:**
   1. Wet compresses made with Burow's solution (Bluboro Powder, Domeboro Powder and Tablets) or hot, bland soaks.
   2. **Oral Antibiotics:**
      -Dicloxacillin 500 mg PO qid.
      -Cephalexin (Keflex) 500 mg PO qid.
      -Cefadroxil (Duricef) 500 mg PO bid.
      -Erythromycin 500 mg PO qid.
   3. If redness and swelling do not resolve, and a pocket of pus remains, surgical drainage is indicated.

G. **Treatment of Chronic Candida Paronychia:**
   1. Stop all wet work and apply clotrimazole (Lotrimin) 1% solution or nystatin (Mycostatin) cream to the nail folds tid.
   2. Resistant cases can be treated with a 3-6 week oral course:
      Fluconazole (Diflucan), 100 mg PO daily
      Itraconazole (Sporanox) 200 mg-400 mg PO daily.
      Ketoconazole (Nizoral), 200 mg PO daily

## VIII. Tinea Versicolor

A. Caused by Malassezia furfur, a normal skin resident.

B. **Predisposing Factors:** Pregnancy, serious underlying diseases, genetic predisposition, corticosteroid therapy.

C. Lesions may be spotty, hyper- or hypopigmentated with slightly hyperkeratotic papules; the upper two-thirds of the horny layer has splits and mild scaling. Lesions favor scalp margins, upper trunk, neck and shoulders. Rarely it may involve the flexures, distal parts of the extremities, and the face.

D. A glass slide can be used to scrape the lesion, and prepare a KOH prep. Gnarled, angulated, short hyphae and clusters of spores will be visible. A negative KOH examination virtually excludes the diagnosis, unlike dermatophyte infections, where a positive KOH may be difficult to obtain.

E. **Treatment:**
   1. Selenium sulfide shampoo or lotion 2.5% qhs for 15 minutes for 7 days or
   2. Topical imidazole bid for 4 weeks.
      -Miconazole Nitrate (Micatin); apply to affected areas bid; cream: 2% [15, 30 gm]
      -Clotrimazole (Lotrimin), apply to affected area bid for up to 4 wk; cream: 1% [15, 30, 45, 90 gm], lotion: 1% [30 mL]
      -Ketoconazole (Nizoral) apply to affected area(s) qd-bid; cream: 2% [15, 30, 60 gm]
   3. Oral ketoconazole (Nizoral) in a single dose or for several days, 200 mg PO qd, may be useful for resistant disease. 200 mg PO daily for 2-4 weeks is advised if recurrences occur.
   4. Relapses are very common. Prophylactic therapy, once weekly to monthly, with topical or oral agents should be encouraged if relapses occur.

IX. **Dermatophytosis**
A. Dermatophytosis is a superficial fungal infection caused by fungi belonging to the genera Microsporum, Trichophyton, or Epidermophyton. May be anthropophilic (transmitted from person to person) or zoophilic (transmitted by animals, especially cats).
B. **Pathophysiology:** Dermatophyte fungi grow only within the keratin layers of the skin, and within the hair. Hydration and occlusion of the skin (by shoes) facilitate infection.
C. **Clinical Findings:**
1. **Tinea Capitis:** Most often noninflammatory, presenting with scalp patches of scaling and alopecia.
2. **Tinea Pedis:** Most commonly presents with scaling, maceration, and fissuring in the toe webs and soles.
3. **Tinea Manuum:** Usually presents with diffuse scaling of one or, less commonly, both palms. Frequently there is fine scaling in the skin creases.
4. **Tinea Corporis and Tinea Cruris:** Erythematous, scaly plaques occur on the trunk or other non-hairy areas or groin. The border of the lesion is exceedingly well demarcated (without satellite lesions as in Candida) with increased scaling or erythema, papules, or vesicles. There may be central clearing.
5. **Tinea Unguium:** Affects the toenails more commonly than the fingernails. Subungual hyperkeratosis and a whitish or yellowish discoloration of the nail.
6. Candida does not invade the nail plate.
D. **Diagnostic Tests:**
1. **Potassium Hydroxide Exam:** Scales are scraped from the lesion and digested with 10% KOH with gentle heating, fungal hyphae and spores may be visible. If negative, the scales may be cultured on a fungal medium.
2. Wood's lamp examination is of limited value, since the most commonly found pathogenic agents for tinea do not fluoresce.
E. **Differential Diagnosis:** Noninflammatory tinea capitis may be confused with seborrheic dermatitis, or secondary syphilis. Tinea cruris may be confused with intertriginous dermatitis that usually spares the crease. Tinea unguium may be confused with nail psoriasis.
F. **Treatment:**
1. **Tinea of the Scalp:**
   -Ketoconazole (Nizoral) 200 mg PO daily for 6-8 weeks or topical imidazole solution bid for 6-8 weeks.
   -Griseofulvin, 500 mg PO day in single or divided doses for 6-8 weeks [250, 500 mg]
2. **Skin Folds, Palms, and Soles:**
   -Miconazole (Micatin); apply to affected areas bid; cream: 2% [15, 30 gm]
   -Ketoconazole (Nizoral) apply to affected area qd-bid; cream: 2% [15, 30, 60 gm]
   -Econazole Nitrate (Spectazole) apply to affected area bid; cream: 1% [15, 30, 85 g]
   -Clotrimazole (Lotrimin), apply to affected area bid for up to 4 wk; cream: 1% [15, 30, 45, 90 gm], lotion: 1% [30 mL]
   -Naftifine (Naftin), apply to affected area qd-bid; cream: 1% [15, 30, 60 gm]; not effective for Candida.
   -Itraconazole (Sporanox) 200 mg-400 mg PO daily for 1 week
3. **Nail Infections:**
   -Naftifine (Naftin),1% apply to affected area qd-bid; gel: 1% [20, 40, 60 gm]
   -Terbinafine (Lamisil), 125 mg PO bid for 6 months.
   - Itraconazole (Sporanox) PO 100 mg bid for the first 7 days of each month for 3 months.
   -Griseofulvin 500 mg PO daily in a single or divided dose; for fingernails 6-8 months, or for toenails 9-12 months. Patients should be followed by CBC and SMAC every 3 months due to hematologic, hepatic and renal toxicity.

X. **Pityriasis Rosea**
A. An acute inflammatory dermatitis characterized by self-limited, lesions distributed on the trunk and extremities. A viral cause is hypothesized. Most common between the ages

of 10 and 35.

B. **Clinical Manifestations:**
1. The initial lesion, called the "herald patch", can appear anywhere on the body, and is 2-6 cm in size, and begins a few days to several weeks before the generalized eruption. The hands, face, and feet are usually spared.
2. The lesions are oval, and the long axes follow the lines of cleavage. Lesions are 2 cm or less, pink, tan, or light brown. The borders of the lesions have a loose rim of scales, peeling peripherally, called the "collarette."
3. Pruritus is usually minimal. Fever and malaise are occasionally associated.

C. **Differential Diagnosis:** Secondary syphilis (always check VDRL for atypical rashes), drug eruptions, viral exanthems, acute papular psoriasis, tinea corporis.

D. **Treatment:**
1. Topical antipruritic emollients (Caladryl) relieve itching. Ultraviolet therapy may be used within the first week.
2. The disease resolves in 2-14 weeks and recurrences are unusual.

# Bacterial Infections of the Skin

## I. Furuncles and Carbuncles

A. A furuncle, or boil, is an acute perifollicular staphylococcal abscess of the skin and subcutaneous tissue. Lesions appear as an indurated, dull, red nodule with a central purulent core, usually beginning around a hair follicle or a sebaceous gland. Furuncles occur most commonly on the nape, face, buttocks, thighs, perineum, breast, and axillae.

B. A carbuncle is a coalescence of interconnected furuncles that drain through number of points on the skin surface.

C. The most common cause of furuncles and carbuncles is coagulase-positive S aureus. Cultures should be obtained from all suppurative lesions.

D. **Treatment of Furuncles and Carbuncles:**

1. Warm compresses and cleansing.
2. Dicloxacillin (Pathocil) 500 mg PO qid for 2 weeks or other penicillinase-resistant antibiotic.
3. Manipulation and surgical incision of early lesions should be avoided, because these maneuvers may cause local or systemic extension. However, when the lesions begin to suppurate and become fluctuant, drainage may be performed by "nicking" the lesion with a No. 11 blade.
4. Draining lesions should be covered with topical antibiotics and loose dressings. Placement of rubber drains or wicks may prevent healing and lead to scarring and should be avoided. A lesion typically resolves within 2 weeks.

## II. Superficial Folliculitis

A. Superficial folliculitis is characterized by small dome-shaped pustules at the ostium of hair follicles; caused by coagulase-positive S aureus.

B. Multiple or single lesions appear on the scalp, back, and extremities. In children, the scalp is the most common site.

C. Gram stain and bacterial culture supports the diagnosis.

D. **Treatment:** Local cleansing and erythromycin 2% solution applied topically bid to affected areas.

## III. Hot Tub Folliculitis

A. Caused by Pseudomonas aeruginosa that flourish in pools that have low chlorine levels and high water temperatures.

B. Characterized by small erythematous papules topped by pustules on areas of the body that were submerged in the hot tub; the head, neck, and mucous membranes are spared. Very pruritic and usually begins 6 hours to 5 days after exposure.

C. Diagnosis is supported by gram stain and bacterial culture of a pustule.

D. **Treatment:** Erythromycin 2% solution bid for 2-3 wk or until 1 wk after lesion has healed. Bacitracin neomycin polymyxin B ointment bid-tid for 2-3 wk or until 1 wk after lesion has healed. Immunosuppressed patients should avoid recreational use of hot tubs.

## IV. Impetigo

A. Small superficial vesicles appear that eventually form pustules and develop a stuck-on honey-colored crust. A halo of erythema often surrounds the lesions.

B. Impetigo contagiosa occurs most commonly on exposed surfaces such as the extremities and face, where minor trauma, insect bites, contact dermatitis, or abrasions may have occurred.

C. Gram stain of an early lesion or the base of a crust often reveals gram-positive cocci. Bacterial culture yields S aureus, group A beta-hemolytic streptococci, or both.

D. **Treatment of Impetigo:**

1. A combination of systemic and topical therapy is recommended for moderate to severe cases of impetigo for a 7- to 10-day course:
   a. Dicloxacillin 250-500 mg PO qid; should be the initial treatment because of erythromycin-resistant strains of S aureus.
   b. Erythromycin 250-500 mg PO qid

    c. Cephalexin (Keflex) 500 mg PO bid
2. Mupirocin (Bactroban): Highly effective against all staphylococci, including methicillin-resistant S aureus and Streptococcus pyogenes. Applied bid-tid for 2-3 weeks or until 1 week after lesions heal. Bacitracin (neomycin, polymyxin B) ointment tid may also be used.

E. **Complications:**
  1. Acute glomerulonephritis is a serious complication of impetigo, with an incidence of 2-5%; most commonly seen in children under the age of 6. Treatment of impetigo does not alter the risk of acute glomerulonephritis.
  2. Rheumatic fever has not been reported after impetigo.

. **Cellulitis**
A. Cellulitis is a diffuse suppurative bacterial inflammation of the subcutaneous tissue.
B. Localized erythema, warmth, and tenderness are characteristic. Cutaneous erythema is poorly demarcated from uninvolved skin; may be accompanied by malaise, fever, and chills.
C. The most common causes are beta-hemolytic streptococcal and S aureus. Complications include gangrene, metastatic abscesses, and sepsis.
D. **Treatment:**
  1. Dicloxacillin or cephalexin provide adequate coverage for either streptococci and staphylococci. Penicillin may be added to increase activity against streptococci.
  2. The affected body part should be kept elevated.
  3. **Antibiotic Therapy:**
    a. Dicloxacillin (Dycill, Pathocil) 15 mg/kg per day in 4 divided doses for 7-12 days; adults: 500 mg qid
    b. Cephalexin (Keflex) 50 mg/kg per day PO in 2 divided doses for 7-10 days; adults: 500 mg PO bid
    c. Azithromycin (Zithromax) 500 mg on day 1, then 250 mg PO qd for 4 days
    d. Erythromycin ethylsuccinate 30-40 mg/kg per day in 3 divided doses for 7-10 days; adults: 250-500 mg qid
    e. Amoxicillin/clavulanate (Augmentin) 500 mg PO tid for 7-10 days
    f. Mupirocin (Bactroban) ointment apply topically to affected areas bid-tid.

# Psoriasis

I. **Clinical Presentation**
   A. Psoriasis is a chronic skin disease characterized by epidermal hyperplasia and a accelerated rate of epidermal turnover. Psoriasis is a lifelong disorder that may consist of only a few patches on the scalp, elbows or knees, or it may be extensive with total skin involvement.
   B. It has an unpredictable course with improvement or exacerbation of lesions. Onset occurs at any age with equal frequency in males and females. The mean onset of age is 27.8 with 35% having an onset before 20 years.
   C. The lesion is elevated and erythematous with thick, micaceous, silver, loosely adherent scales cover the lesion.
      1. Scraping off the scale and leaves a bleeding point (Auspitz sign).
      2. Lesion predilection is in the sacral region, and over extensor surfaces (elbows, knees, lumbosacral), and scalp. The appearance of disease is often associated with superficial cutaneous trauma (Koebner phenomenon).
      3. Mucosal psoriasis consist of circinate, ring-shaped, whitish lesions on the tongue, palate, or buccal mucosa.
   D. Onycholysis, or separation of the nail plate from the underlying nail bed is frequently seen, as well as a yellow-brown discoloration underneath the nail, known as an "oil spot."
   E. **Aggravating Factors:** Stress, infection, certain drugs (lithium and some beta-blockers).
   F. 5-10% of the patients have an associated arthritis characterized by asymmetrical distal oligoarthritis involving small joints; a smaller number of patients have a rheumatoid arthritis-like picture involving symmetrical larger joints or a spondyloarthropathy. The arthritis may be mutilating and very destructive.

II. **Treatment of Psoriasis**
   A. **Topical corticosteroids:**
      1. Hydrocortisone 1 to 2½% on face, neck, axilla, groin, intertriginous regions.
      2. Fluorinated corticosteroids in plaque regions.
      3. Occlusive dressings can be used to flatten out psoriatic lesions. Intralesional steroid are also useful.
      4. **Scalp psoriasis:** Remove scales with warm oil before shampooing with tar. Topical corticosteroid lotion can be massaged into the scalp.
      5. **Nail psoriasis:** Apply topical corticosteroids to the nail under occlusion 2-3 times weekly.
   B. **Low Potency Agents:**
      -Hydrocortisone apply tid-qid [cream 1, 2.5%; ointment 1, 2.5%; lotion 1, 2, 2.5%; gel 0.5%; solution 1%].
      -Triamcinolone acetonide (Aristocort, Kenalog) apply to affected area tid-qid [ointment 0.1, 0.5%; cream 0.5%].
   C. **Medium Potency Agents:**
      -Betamethasone valerate (Valisone) apply qd-bid [cream, oint, 0.1%].
      -Fluocinolone acetonide (Synalar) apply bid-qid [cream 0.025, 0.2%; oint 0.025%].
   D. **High Potency Agents:**
      -Betamethasone dipropionate augmented (Diprolene) apply to affected areas qd-bid [gel, oint, 0.05%]
      -Clobetasol propionate (Temovate) apply to affected areas bid [cream, oint 0.05%]
      -Flurandrenolide (Cordran) apply bid-tid [oint, cream 0.05%].
      -Halcinonide (Halog) apply bid-tid [cream 0.025, 0.1%; oint 0.1%].
      -Betamethasone dipropionate apply qd-bid [oint, cream, 0.05%].
      -Amcinonide (Cyclocort) apply bid-tid [cream, oint 0.1%].
   E. **Vitamin D Analog:**
      -Calcipotriene (Dovonex) 0.005% ointment, apply a thin layer to affected skin bid [30, 60, 100g]

F. **Crude Coal Tar:**
   1. Used to reduce the thickness of psoriatic plaques.  Effect is potentiated when combined with UV light in the B range (UVB).
   2. Topical 5% coal tar solution, cream or 1-2% crude coal tar ointment applied qd. Adding salicylic acid enhances penetration of tars, dissolves scales.
G. **Systemic Agents:**  Indicated for severe, extensive psoriasis.
   Etretinate (Tegison) 0.75 mg/kg/day in divided doses PO [caps: 10, 25 mg].
   Methotrexate 2.5 mg PO at 12 hour intervals for 3 doses or 10-25 mg/week; liver toxicity is a major problem.
H. **UV Light:** Effective for widespread psoriatic lesions; however, overexposure can exacerbate the disease.
   1. **Goeckerman Regime:** Tars and UVL twice daily, tar is removed, followed by bathing. The procedure continues for 4-6 weeks; remission lasts weeks to months.
   2. **Modified Goeckerman Regimen:** Uses tar at night with a.m. ultraviolet light in the B range (UVB), corticosteroids in the daytime.
   3. **PUVA Regimen:** Combination of UV light in the A range (UVA) and psoralen. Four treatments a week for 4 weeks causes 93% clearing, but maintenance therapy must be continued weekly to prevent recurrences.

# Nephrology

## Renal Failure

I. **Clinical Presentation of Acute Renal Failure**
   A. Acute renal failure is defined as a sudden decrease in renal function sufficient to increase the concentration of nitrogenous wastes in the blood, manifest by an increasing BUN or creatinine. Creatinine is a more reliable indicator of renal failure than BUN, because BUN can be elevated by a high protein diet, endogenous protein degradation, dehydration, heart failure, or obstructive uropathy.
   B. Significant renal failure (loss of 25-50% of total function) can occur before any increase in creatinine is detectable.
   C. **Oliguria** is a common indicator of acute renal failure, and is marked by a decrease in urine output to less than 30 mL/h. Acute renal failure may be oliguric or nonoliguric (>30 mL/h). Anuria (<100 mL/day) is unusual, and its presence suggests obstruction or a vascular cause.
   D. Acute renal failure may less commonly be manifest by encephalopathy, volume overload, pericarditis, bleeding, anemia, hyperkalemia, hyperphosphatemia, hypocalcemia, and metabolic acidemia.

II. **Clinical Causes of Renal Failure:**
   A. **Prerenal Insult:**
      1. Prerenal insult is the most common cause of acute renal failure, accounting for 70%. Prerenal failure is usually caused by reduced renal perfusion pressure secondary to extracellular fluid volume loss (diarrhea, diuresis, GI hemorrhage), or secondary to extracellular fluid sequestration (pancreatitis, sepsis), inadequate cardiac output, renal vasoconstriction (sepsis, liver disease, drugs), or inadequate fluid intake or replacement.
      2. Most patients with prerenal azotemia have oliguria, a history of large fluid losses (vomiting, diarrhea, burns), and evidence of intravascular volume depletion (thirst, weight loss, orthostatic hypotension, tachycardia, flat neck veins, dry mucous membranes). Patients with congestive heart failure may have total body volume excess (distended neck veins, pulmonary and pedal edema, cardiac gallops) but still have compromised renal perfusion and prerenal azotemia due to diminished cardiac output.
      3. The causes of prerenal failure are usually reversible if recognized and treated early; otherwise, prolonged renal hypoperfusion can lead to acute tubular necrosis and permanent renal insufficiency
      4. Nonsteroidal anti-inflammatory drugs and angiotensin converting enzyme inhibitors can cause prerenal failure through their effects on hemodynamics; this type of renal failure is generally mild and reversible.
   B. **Intrarenal Insult:**
      1. Insult to the renal parenchyma (tubular necrosis) causes 20% of acute renal failure. Acute tubular necrosis is characterized by an abrupt decline in renal function caused by ischemic or toxic injury to the renal tubules.
      2. Prolonged hypoperfusion is the most common cause of tubular necrosis.
      3. Nephrotoxins (aminoglycosides, radiographic contrast) are the second most common cause of tubular necrosis. Less common nephrotoxins include cisplatin, amphotericin, pentamidine, and tetracycline.
      4. Pigmenturia induced renal injury can be caused by intravascular hemolysis or rhabdomyolysis. Traumatic rhabdomyolysis and non-traumatic rhabdomyolysis (from cocaine use, seizures, heatstroke, alcoholism, strenuous exercise, infections, drug overdose) are causes of renal injury.
      5. Other causes of tubular necrosis include pyelonephritis, thrombosis, emboli, malignant hypertension, thrombotic thrombocytopenic purpura, hemolytic-uremic syndrome, and

vasculitis.

6. Acute glomerulonephritis or acute inflammation of renal interstitium (acute interstitial nephritis) (usually from allergic reactions to beta-lactam antibiotics, sulfonamides, rifampin, NSAIDs, cimetidine, phenytoin, allopurinol, thiazides, furosemide, analgesics) are occasional causes of intrarenal kidney failure.

7. The presence of a disease known to cause chronic renal insufficiency (diabetes mellitus) may suggest chronic renal failure. The presence of normochromic normocytic anemia, hypercalcemia, and hyperphosphatemia also suggests chronic renal insufficiency.

C. **Postrenal Insult:**

1. Postrenal damage results from obstruction of urine flow. Postrenal insult is the least common of the three causes of acute renal failure, accounting for 10%.

2. Postrenal insult may be caused by Extrarenal obstructive uropathy due to prostate cancer, benign prostatic hypertrophy, or renal calculi occlusion of the bladder outlet.

3. Postrenal insult may be caused by intrarenal obstruction of the distal tubules by amyloidosis, uric acid crystals, or multiple myeloma, or by drugs such as methotrexate and acyclovir.

## III. Clinical Evaluation of Acute Renal Failure

A. **Initial evaluation** of renal failure should determine whether the cause is decreased renal perfusion, obstructed urine flow, or disorders involving the renal parenchyma. Review recent clinical events and drug therapy, including volume status (orthostatic pulse, blood pressure, fluid intake and output, daily weights, hemodynamic parameters), nephrotoxic medications, and pattern of urine output.

B. **Prerenal azotemia** is likely when there is a history of heart failure or extracellular fluid volume loss or depletion.

C. **Postrenal azotemia** is suggested by a history of decreased size or force of the urine stream, anuria, flank pain, hematuria or pyuria, or cancer of the bladder, prostate, or pelvis. Anuria (complete absence of urine) usually results from obstructive uropathy; occasionally anuria indicates cessation of renal blood flow and rapidly progressive glomerulonephritis.

D. **Acute tubular necrosis** is suggested by a history of prolonged volume depletion (often post-surgical), pigmenturia, hemolysis, rhabdomyolysis, or nephrotoxins.

E. **Intrarenal insult** is suggested by recent radiocontrast, aminoglycoside use, or vascular catheterization. Glomerulonephritis may be implicated by a history of medication rash, fever, or arthralgias. Transient eosinophilia occurs in 80% of cases. Urinary studies may reveal hematuria, sterile pyuria, eosinophiluria, mild proteinuria (<2 g/24 h) and, rarely, white blood cell casts. NSAID-induced acute interstitial nephritis occurs most often with the use of ibuprofen, fenoprofen, and naproxen. This complication usually presents after several months of drug use and without systemic symptoms.

## IV. Physical Examination

A. Assess cardiac output, volume status, bladder size, and systemic disease manifestations.

B. Prerenal azotemia is suggested by impaired cardiac output (neck vein distention, pulmonary rales, pedal edema). Volume depletion is suggested by orthostatic changes, weight loss or negative intake and output.

C. Examine for flank, suprapubic, or abdominal masses that may indicate an obstructive cause.

D. Skin rash may suggests drug-induced interstitial nephritis; palpable purpura suggests vasculitis; nonpalpable purpura suggests thrombotic thrombocytopenic purpura, hemolytic-uremic syndrome, or livido reticularis--all of which are compatible with intrarenal kidney failure.

E. **Bladder Catheterization:** Useful to rule out suspected bladder outlet obstruction; a residual volume of more than 100 mL suggests bladder outlet obstruction.

F. **Central Venous Monitoring:** Measure cardiac output and left ventricular filling pressure if prerenal failure is suspected.

**V. Laboratory Evaluation**

A. **Spot Urine Sodium Concentration:**
1. Spot urine sodium can help distinguish between prerenal azotemia and acute tubular necrosis.
2. Prerenal failure causes increased reabsorption of salt and water, and will manifest as a low spot urine sodium concentration <30 mEq/L and a low fractional sodium excretion <1%.

   Fractional Excretion of Sodium (%) = [Urine Sodium/Plasma Sodium] + [Urine creatinine/Plasma creatinine] x 100)
3. If tubular necrosis is the cause, the spot urine concentration should be >50 mEq/L, and fractional excretion of sodium >1% because necrosed tubules do not efficiently reabsorb sodium.

B. **Urinalysis:**
1. Normal urine sediment is a strong indicator of prerenal azotemia or may be a possible indicator of obstructive uropathy.
2. Hematuria, pyuria, or crystals may be associated with postrenal obstructive azotemia.
3. Urine sediment containing abundant cells, casts, or proteins suggests an intrarenal disorders.
4. Red cells alone may indicate vascular disorders; RBC casts and abundant protein suggest glomerular disease (glomerulonephritis).
5. White cell casts and eosinophilic casts indicate interstitial nephritis.
6. Renal epithelial cell casts and pigmented granular casts are associated acute tubular necrosis.

C. **Laboratory Findings in Prerenal Failure:** Hemoconcentration (increased albumin and hematocrit), elevated BUN and creatinine, and a BUN to creatinine ratio >20. Urinalysis may reveal a specific gravity greater than 1.015 but is otherwise unremarkable.

D. **Ultrasound:** Useful for evaluation of suspected postrenal obstruction (nephrolithiasis) after bladder outlet obstruction has been ruled out by catheterization. Ultrasonography can be used to look above the bladder for dilated ureters. The presence of small (<10 cm in length), scarred kidneys is diagnostic of chronic renal insufficiency.

**VI. Management of Acute Renal Failure**

A. Rule out reversible disorders such as obstruction, correct hypovolemia with adequate volume replacement, and maintain adequate cardiac output to ensure adequate renal perfusion.

B. **Extracellular Fluid Volume Expansion:** Infusion of a crystalloid fluid bolus may confirm suspected volume-depleted, prerenal azotemia.

C. In the critically ill patient with respiratory failure, sepsis, pulmonary edema, or coma; physical examination and chest film are often inadequate guides to hemodynamic status. A pulmonary artery catheter should be used for monitoring.

D. If the patient remains oliguric despite euvolemia, consider measures to restore urine output with IV diuretics or renal vasodilators. Nonoliguric tubular necrosis is easier to manage than oliguric renal failure, and metabolic complications are less likely.
1. A large single dose of furosemide (200 to 300 mg) may be administered intravenously to promote diuresis. If urine flow is not improved, a second dose of furosemide alone or in combination with metolazone (Zaroxolyn) may be given. Additional large doses of loop diuretics are not beneficial and can result in ototoxicity.
2. Mannitol 12.5-25 gm IV can also be effective, but it may worsen pulmonary edema if oliguria persists.
3. Urine flow may also be improved with low dose dopamine, 1-3 mcg/kg/min IV.

E. Modify either dosage or dosing intervals of renally excreted drugs, and monitor drug levels. Monitor blood count, electrolytes, creatinine, calcium, and phosphorus.

F. Remove potassium from IV solutions; hyperkalemia is among the most dangerous complications of renal failure.

G. **Fluids:** After normal volume has been restarted, fluid intake should be reduced to an amount equal to urinary and other losses plus insensible losses of 300-500 mL/day. In oliguric patients, daily fluid intake may need to be restricted to less than 1 L.

H. **Nutritional Therapy:** Enteral nutrition is preferable to parenteral nutrition. Daily dietary high biologic value protein of 0.6 to 0.8 g/kg, sodium 2 g, potassium 1 mEq/kg, and at least 35 kcal/kg of nonprotein calories can reduce hyperkalemia and azotemia without excessive catabolism.

I. **Hyperkalemia** is the most immediately life-threatening complication. Serum potassium values greater than 6.5 mEq/L may lead to arrhythmias and cardiac arrest. Potassium binding resins (Kayexalate), orally or by enema, or urgent dialysis may be required. Hyperkalemia may be treated with sodium polystyrene sulfonate (Kayexalate), 15-30 gm orally every 4-6 hours.

J. **Hyperphosphatemia** can be controlled with antacids containing calcium carbonate, calcium acetate, or aluminum compounds given with meals to bind dietary phosphorus. Antacids that contain magnesium are contraindicated.

K. **Metabolic Acidosis** can further aggravate hyperkalemia, alter cardiac function, and decrease pulmonary reserve. Treated with sodium bicarbonate to maintain the serum pH >7.2 and the bicarbonate level >20 mEq/L.

L. **Dialysis:** Indications for dialysis include uremic pericarditis, severe hyperkalemia, pulmonary edema, severe metabolic acidosis (pH less than 7.2), and symptomatic uremia. Institute hemodialysis to keep the BUN below 100 and to keep the serum creatinine below 10 mg/dL.

## VII. Complications of Renal Failure

A. Uremic pericarditis is life-threatening and requires emergency dialysis.
B. Gastrointestinal complications include anorexia, nausea, and vomiting. Bleeding from gastritis and peptic ulcers can occur because of impaired platelet function.
C. Hematologic complications include anemia and coagulation disorders. The presence of anemia suggests gastrointestinal bleeding or hemolysis.
D. Infectious complications are the most common cause of death in hospitalized patients with acute renal failure; the respiratory and urinary tracts are frequent sources of infection.
E. Neurologic complications include asterixis, neuromuscular irritability, mental status changes, seizures, coma.

## VIII. Prevention of Renal Failure:

A. Prompt replacement of lost extracellular fluids prevents ischemic tubular damage associated with trauma, burns, surgery, and GI hemorrhage. Aggressive treatment of septic and cardiogenic shock will also prevent tubular damage.
B. Nephrotoxic medications and radiographic contrast agents should be used sparingly and closely monitored. Volume repletion and administration of furosemide before the diagnostic test is important for patients at high risk.

## IX. Chronic Renal Insufficiency

A. Chronic renal failure is an end-result of damage to the kidney arising from many different causes. The onset is frequently insidious and gradual; overt symptoms may not appear until renal failure is far advanced.
B. **Common Etiologies:** Tubular necrosis, glomerulonephritis, interstitial nephritis (including pyelonephritis), nephrosclerosis, diabetic nephropathy, and polycystic kidney disease. The etiology of the renal failure may be unidentifiable.
C. **Stages of Progressive Renal Insufficiency:**
   1. **Renal Insufficiency:**
      a. Glomerular filtration rate is 30-50% of normal.
      b. Mild azotemia, anemia, and the inability to concentrate the urine become manifest.
      c. Challenges such as fluid and salt restriction, vomiting, diarrhea or blood loss may lead to severe azotemia and acidosis.
   2. **Renal Failure:**
      a. GFR is 10-25% of normal.
      b. Widespread excretory and endocrine failure results in anemia, alterations in calcium and phosphorus metabolism, acidosis, and other electrolyte abnormalities.
   3. **Uremia:**
      a. Cardiovascular: Hypertension, atherosclerosis, cardiovascular events, and

      pericarditis.
    b. Pulmonary: Uremic pneumonitis, pulmonary edema, pleural effusions.
    c. Hematologic: Anemia due to decreased erythropoietin production; shortened red cell survival, and inhibitors of erythropoiesis.
    d. Osteodystrophy due to hypocalcemia.

D. **Indications for Renal Biopsy:**
    1. Oligoanuria persisting longer than 3 weeks.
    2. Clinical signs and symptoms suggestive of glomerular, vascular, or systemic disease.
    3. Renal failure with no obvious cause.
    4. Suspected drug-induced renal failure.

E. **Management of Chronic Renal Failure:**
    1. **Specific therapy for the underlying disorder:** Immunosuppressives, corticosteroids, plasmapheresis, antibiotics.
    2. **Avoidance of factors that are known to accelerate renal insufficiency** such as control of hypertension, prevention of volume contraction, control of congestive heart failure, and avoidance of nephrotoxins (radiocontrast media, nephrotoxic antibiotics).
    3. **Manage metabolic abnormalities:** Hyperphosphatemia, hyperuricemia, hypercalcemia, hyperkalemia.
    4. Dialysis and/or transplantation is appropriate for uremic patients.
    5. Anemia may be treated with recombinant erythropoietin, 50 units/kg 3 times/week IV or SC; maintenance, 25-100 units/kg 3 times/week.
    6. When serum creatinine reaches 2.5 mg%, protein should be restricted to 0.6-0.7 gm/day of high quality protein rich in essential amino acids.

# Hematuria

## I. Pathophysiology of Hematuria

A. Hematuria may be a sign of urinary tract malignancy or renal parenchymal disease. Up to 18% of normal persons excrete red blood cells into the urine, averaging 2 million RBC's per 24 hours or 2 RBC's per high-power field (HPF).

B. Improper collection and improper analysis can yield false-positive or false-negative results. Exercise or jogging can cause an increase in RBC excretion, and hematuria may be intermittent.

C. The dipstick detects hemoglobin and myoglobin; microscopic examination of the urinary sediment is required before diagnosing hematuria.

## II. Clinical Evaluation of Hematuria

A. The patient should be asked about frequency, dysuria, pain, colic, fever, fatigue, anorexia abdominal, flank, or perineal pain. Exercise, jogging, menstruation. History kidney stones.

B. Examine for hypertension, edema, rash, heart murmurs, or abdominal masses (renal tumor, hydronephrosis from obstruction). Costovertebral-angle tenderness may be a sign of renal calculus or pyelonephritis.

C. Genitourinary examination may show a foreign body in the penile urethra or cervical carcinoma invading the urinary tract. Prostatitis, carcinoma, or benign prostatic hyperplasia may be found.

## III. Laboratory Evaluation

A. At least one of the following criteria should be met before initiating a workup for hematuria.
   1. More than 3 RBC's/HPF on two of three properly collected clean-catch specimens (abstain from exercise for 48 hours before sampling; not during menses).
   2. One episode of gross hematuria.
   3. One episode of high-grade microhematuria (>100 RBC's HPF)

B. Obtain a properly collected, freshly voided specimen for red blood cell morphology, evaluate character of the sediment, and check for proteinuria.

C. RBC casts are pathognomonic of glomerulonephritis; WBC casts and granular casts are indicative of pyelonephritis. Cytodiagnostic urinalysis by Pap smear technique on urinary sediment often aids in visualizing casts.

D. Culture urine to rule out urinary tract infection that may cause hematuria.

E. Evaluate serum blood urea nitrogen and creatinine levels to rule out renal failure. Impaired renal function is seen more commonly with medical hematuria.

F. Fasting blood glucose levels should be obtained to rule out diabetes; obtain a complete blood count to assess severity of blood loss and to evaluate for the presence of infection.

G. Serum coagulation parameters should be measured to screen for coagulopathy. Skin tests for tuberculosis should be completed if risk factors are present. Sickle cell prep should be completed for all black patients with hematuria.

## IV. Classification of Hematuria

A. Hematuria is Divided into Two Broad Groups:
   1. **Medical Hematuria** is due to a glomerular lesion; plasma proteins filter into urine out of proportion to the amount of hematuria. Characterized by glomerular RBC's distorted with crenated membranes and an uneven hemoglobin distribution casts. Microscopic hematuria and a urine dipstick test of 2+ protein is more likely to have a medical cause.
   2. **Urologic Hematuria** is due to a urologic lesion such as a urinary stone or carcinoma, characterized by minimal proteinuria with plasma protein in urine proportional to the amount of whole blood added. Non-glomerular RBC's (disk shaped with an even hemoglobin distribution) and absence of casts are characteristic.

V. **Diagnostic Evaluation of Medical Hematuria**
   A. **Renal Ultrasound:** Evaluate kidney size and rule out hydronephrosis or cystic disease.
   B. **24-hour Urine:** Creatinine, creatinine clearance and protein to assess renal failure.
   C. **Immunologic Studies:** Third and fourth complement components, antinuclear antibodies, cryoglobulins, anti-basement membrane antibodies; serum and urine protein electrophoresis (to rule out IgA nephropathy).
   D. **Audiogram:** If a family history of Alport syndrome is present.
   E. **Skin Biopsy:** Can reveal dermal capillary deposits of IgA in 80% of patients with Berger's disease (IgA nephropathy); the most common cause of microhematuria in young adults.

VI. **Diagnostic Evaluation of Urologic Hematuria**
   A. **Intravenous Pyelography** is the best screening test for upper tract lesions if serum creatinine is normal. Usually contraindicated if renal insufficiency. If renal insufficiency is present, renal ultrasound and cystoscopy with retrograde pyelogram should be used to search for etiologic causes of hematuria such as stones or malignancy.
   B. **If the IVP Is Normal:** Cystoscopy with washings for cytology may reveal the cause of bleeding.
   C. **Other Tests:**
      1. Lesions in the kidney visualized on IVP can be evaluated by renal ultrasound to asses cystic or solid character; CT-guided aspiration of cysts may be considered.
      2. Filling defects in the ureter may be evaluated by retrograde pyelogram and ureteral washings; ureteroscopic brushings or biopsy is useful to rule out tumors, stones, or strictures.
      3. Renal arteriogram to rule out arteriovenous fistula.

VII. **Idiopathic Hematuria**
   A. Idiopathic hematuria is a diagnosis of exclusion; 5-10% of significant hematuria will have no diagnosis.
   B. Suspected urologic hematuria with a negative initial workup should be followed every 6-12 months with urinalysis and urine cytology. An IVP should be done every 2-3 years.
   C. Monitor renal function and proteinuria. If renal function declines or if proteinuria is >1 gm/day, renal biopsy is indicated.

# Hyperkalemia

I. **Pathophysiology of Potassium Homeostasis**
   A. 98% of body K is intracellular. Only 2% of total body potassium, about 70 mEq, is in the extracellular fluid, where it is measured in serum at a normal concentration of 3.5-5 mEq/L.
   A. The normal upper limit of plasma K is 5-5.5 mEq/L, with a mean K level of 4.3
   B. **External Potassium Balance:** Normal dietary K intake is 1-1.5 mEq/kg in the form of vegetables and meats. The kidney is the primary organ for preserving external K balance, excreting 90% of the daily K burden.
   C. **Internal potassium balance** is defined as potassium transfer to and from tissues.
   D. **Factors Affecting the External and Internal Balance of Potassium:**
      1. **External:** Potassium intake, stool losses, renal potassium excretion
      2. **Internal:** Insulin, acid-base status, catecholamines, aldosterone, plasma osmolality, cellular necrosis, glucagon, drugs

II. **Clinical Disorders of External Potassium Balance**
   A. **Chronic Renal Failure:** The kidney is able to excrete the normal dietary intake of potassium until the glomerular filtration rate falls below 10 cc/minute, or until urine output falls below 1 L/day. Renal failure is advanced before hyperkalemia occurs.
   B. **Impaired Renal Tubular Function:** Renal diseases may cause hyperkalemia. The renal tubular acidosis caused by these conditions may worsen hyperkalemia.
   C. **Primary Adrenal Insufficiency (Addison's disease):**
      1. Now a rare cause of hyperkalemia.
      2. **Diagnosis** is indicated by the combination of hyperkalemia and hyponatremia, and is confirmed by a low aldosterone and a low plasma cortisol level that does not respond to adrenocorticotropic hormone treatment.
      3. **Treatment** requires glucocorticoid and mineralocorticoid agents and volume replacement with normal saline.
   D. **Drugs** are among the most common causes of hyperkalemia including nonsteroidal anti-inflammatory drugs, angiotensin-converting enzyme inhibitors, cyclosporine, potassium-sparing diuretics. Hyperkalemia is especially common when these drugs are given to patients at risk for hyperkalemia (diabetics, renal failure, hyporeninemic hypoaldosteronism, advanced age).
   E. **Excessive Potassium Intake:**
      1. Long-term potassium supplementation results in hyperkalemia most often when an underlying impairment in renal excretion already exists.
      2. Oral ingestion of 1 mEq/kg may increase the serum K level by 1 mEq/L, an hour afterward, in normal individuals. A frank hyperkalemia results when 2.5 mEq/kg is ingested. A single intravenous administration of 0.5 mEq/kg over 1 hour increases serum levels by a peak of 0.6 mEq/L. Hyperkalemia results when infusions of greater than 40 mEq/hour are given.
      3. **Acute K Overload** may result from infusion from the dependent portion of an unmixed potassium mixture, and ingestion of salt substitutes.

III. **Clinical Disorders of Internal Potassium Balance**
   A. **Diabetic patients** are at particular risk for severe hyperkalemia because of renal insufficiency and hyporeninemic hypoaldosteronism.
   B. **Acidosis:** Systemic acidosis reduces the excretion of potassium.
   C. **Drugs:** Hyperkalemia caused by drugs that alter internal potassium balance by extrarenal mechanisms is uncommon. Beta-blockers may occasionally cause hyperkalemia, especially in diabetics or renal failure. A minimal increase in serum K occurs with succinylcholine or digoxin (in toxic amounts).
   D. **Endogenous potassium release** from muscle injury, tumor lysis, chemotherapy may elevate serum potassium.

## IV. Manifestations of Hyperkalemia

A. Hyperkalemia, unless severe, is usually asymptomatic. The effect of hyperkalemia on the heart becomes significant above 6 mEq/L. As levels increase, the initial ECG change is tall peaked T waves, especially in the precordial leads. QT interval is normal or diminished.

B. As K levels rise further, the PR interval becomes prolonged, then the P wave amplitude decreases. QRS complexes widen into a sine wave pattern, representing a form of ventricular flutter, with subsequent cardiac standstill.

C. The electrocardiogram occasionally may display Q waves or ST elevation similar to myocardial infarction. Cardiac contractility is not impaired.

D. At serum K levels of 7 mEq/L, an ascending muscle weakness may lead to a flaccid paralysis that spares cranial nerve function and cerebration. Sensory abnormalities lead to impaired speech and respiratory arrest.

## V. Pseudohyperkalemia

A. Potassium may be falsely elevated by hemolysis during phlebotomy, when K is released from ischemic muscle distal to a tourniquet, and because of erythrocyte fragility disorders.

B. Falsely high laboratory measurement of serum potassium may occur in normokalemic subjects who have markedly elevated platelet (>$10^6$ platelet/mm$^3$) or white blood cell (>50,000/mm$^3$) counts.

## VI. Diagnostic Approach

A. The serum K level should be repeat tested to rule out laboratory error, poor phlebotomy technique, or pseudohyperkalemia. If significant thrombocytosis or leukocytosis is present, a plasma potassium level should be determined.

B. Renal and extrarenal causes of hyperkalemia should be distinguished as follows:
1. Measure urine output, urinary K concentration, blood urea nitrogen, and serum creatinine.
2. Renal K retention is diagnosed when urinary K excretion is less than about 20 mEq/day while the serum K level is increased.
3. High urinary K and K excretion >20 mEq/day is indicative of excessive intake of K as the cause.

## VII. Renal Hyperkalemia

A. If urinary K is low and urine output is in the oliguric range and creatinine clearance is lower than about 20 cc/minute, renal failure is the probable cause. Prerenal azotemia resulting from volume depletion must be ruled out because the hyperkalemia will respond to volume restoration.

B. When urinary K is low, yet blood urea nitrogen and creatinine levels are not elevated and urine volume is at least 1 L daily, and renal sodium excretion is adequate (about 20 mEq/day), then either a defect in the secretion of renin or aldosterone or a tubular resistance to aldosterone is likely. Low plasma renin and aldosterone levels, will confirm the diagnosis of hyporeninemic hypoaldosteronism. A specific cause of this entity should then be sought. If plasma aldosterone is low despite high renin values, the use of heparin should be suspected. Addison's disease and isolated hypoaldosteronism should be considered.

C. When inadequate K excretion is not caused by hypoaldosteronism, a tubular defect in K clearance is suggested. Consider urinary tract obstruction, renal transplant, lupus, or a medication.

## VIII. Extrarenal Hyperkalemia

A. When hyperkalemia occurs along with high urinary K, and K excretion is >20 mEq/day, excessive intake of K is the cause. Potassium excess in IV fluids, diet, or medication should be sought. A concomitant underlying renal defect in K excretion is also likely to also be present.

B. Measure blood sugar to rule out insulin deficiency; check blood pH and serum bicarbonate to rule out acidosis.

C. Medications causing internal K imbalance, such as beta-blockers, should be ruled out.

D. Rule out endogenous sources of K, such as tissue necrosis, hypercatabolism, hematoma gastrointestinal bleeding, or intravascular hemolysis.

IX. **Management of Hyperkalemia**

A. The degree of elevation of serum K and severity of electrocardiographic changes determines the proper management of hyperkalemia.

B. **Acute Treatment of Hyperkalemia**

1. **Calcium Chloride:**

a. Calcium chloride should be given IV if the electrocardiogram shows loss of P waves or widening of QRS complexes; calcium reduces the membrane threshold potential, but will not lower the potassium level.

b. 10% calcium gluconate should be given as 2-3 ampules over 5 minutes. In patients with circulatory compromise, give 1 ampule of calcium chloride IV over 3 minutes.

c. If the serum level of K is greater than 7 mEq/L (even if normal ECG), calcium should be given because of imminent cardiac toxicity. If digitalis intoxication is suspected, calcium must be given cautiously. Coexisting hyponatremia should be treated with hypertonic saline.

2. **Insulin:**

a. If only peaked T waves are present on the electrocardiogram, and the serum level is under 7 mEq/L, begin treatment with insulin (regular insulin, 5-10 U by IV push) with an infusion of 10% glucose to avoid hypoglycemia (unless the blood sugar is already substantially elevated).

b. Repeated insulin doses of 10 U can be given every 15 minutes for maximal effect, combined with glucose infusion as needed.

3. **Sodium Bicarbonate:**

a. Promotes cellular uptake of K. Should be given as two 50-mEq ampules IV over 5 minutes. Bicarbonate is most effective when acidosis is present; however, alkalinization may be used even in the absence of low pH.

b. Avoid bicarbonate if severe heart failure or hypernatremia. If the serum calcium is low (as in uremic acidosis), calcium should also be given to avoid hypocalcemic tetany during alkali therapy.

4. **Potassium Elimination Measures:**

a. Furosemide (Lasix)100 mg IV should be given immediately to promote kaliuresis; normal saline may be added to avoid volume depletion.

b. Sodium polystyrene sulfonate (Kayexalate) is a cation exchange resin that binds stool K. Give 30 g with 50 cc of 20% sorbitol orally. A retention enema of 50 g in 200 cc of 20% sorbitol has a more rapid effect.

c. Emergent dialysis specifically for hyperkalemia is not usually necessary, even in renal failure. Hemodialysis is more efficient at K elimination than peritoneal dialysis.

# Hypokalemia

### Pathophysiology of Hypokalemia

A. Hypokalemia is indicated by a serum K concentration of less than 3.5 mEq/L. Because 98% of K is intracellular; serum potassium concentration is not an accurate reflection of total body potassium content.

B. **Cellular Redistribution of Potassium:** Hypokalemia may result from the intracellular shift of potassium by insulin (exogenous or glucose load), beta2 agonist drugs, stress induced catecholamine release, thyrotoxic periodic paralysis, alkalosis-induced shift (metabolic or respiratory), familial periodic paralysis, cellular proliferation (vitamin B12 treatment), hypothermia, acute myeloid leukemia.

C. **Nonrenal Potassium Loss:**
   1. Gastrointestinal loss caused by diarrhea, laxative abuse, villous adenoma, biliary drainage, enteric fistula, clay ingestion, potassium binding resin ingestion
   2. Sweating, prolonged low potassium ingestion, hemodialysis and peritoneal dialysis may also account for nonrenal potassium loss.

D. **Renal Potassium Loss:**
   1. **Hypertensive High Renin States:** Malignant hypertension, renal artery stenosis, renin-producing tumors.
   2. **Hypertensive Low Renin, High Aldosterone States:** Primary hyperaldosteronism (adenoma or hyperplasia).
   3. **Hypertensive Low Renin, Low Aldosterone States:** Congenital adrenal hyperplasia (11 or 17 hydroxylase deficiency), Cushing's syndrome or disease, exogenous mineralocorticoids (Florinef, licorice, chewing tobacco), Liddle's syndrome
   4. **Normotensive:**
      a. Metabolic acidosis--renal tubular acidosis (type I or II)
      b. Metabolic alkalosis (urine chloride <10 mEq/day)--vomiting
      c. Metabolic alkalosis (urine chloride >10 mEq/day): Bartter's syndrome, diuretics, magnesium depletion, normotensive hyperaldosteronism

### Clinical Effects of Hypokalemia

A. **Cardiac Effects:**
   1. The most lethal consequence of hypokalemia is cardiac arrhythmias.
   2. **Electrocardiographic Effects:** U waves >1 mm in height, T waves in the same lead; ST segment depression; T wave flattening, followed by inversion.
   3. Atrial and ventricular ectopy, including ectopic atrial tachycardia, atrioventricular blocks, premature ventricular contractions, ventricular tachycardia and fibrillation. Arrhythmias of digitalis intoxication are worsened by hypokalemia and hypercalcemia.

B. **Musculoskeletal Effects:** Initial manifestation of K depletion is muscle weakness that can lead to paralysis. In severe cases, respiratory muscle paralysis may occur. Crampy pain, swelling, and paresthesias occur early.

C. **Gastrointestinal Effects:** Nausea, vomiting, constipation occurs, and paralytic ileus may develop.

### Diagnostic Evaluation

A. Determine 24-hour urinary potassium excretion.

B. If >20 mEq/day, excessive urinary K loss is the cause. If <20 mEq/d, low K intake or excess, or nonurinary K loss is the cause.

C. In patients with excessive renal K loss and hypertension, determine plasma renin and aldosterone to differentiate adrenal from non-adrenal causes of hyperaldosteronism.

D. If hypertension is absent and patient is acidotic, renal tubular acidosis should be considered.

E. If hypertension is absent and serum pH is normal to alkalotic, a high urine chloride (>10 mEq/d) suggests hypokalemia secondary to diuretics or Bartter's syndrome. A low urine chloride (<10 mEq/d) suggests vomiting as a probable cause.

IV. **Emergency Treatment of Hypokalemia**
   A. **Estimated Potassium Deficit:**
      At a serum K <3 mEq/L there is a K deficit of more than 300 mEq
      At a serum K <2 mEq/L there is a K deficit of more than 700 mEq
   B. **Indications for Urgent Replacement:** Electrocardiographic abnormalities consisted with severe K depletion, myocardial infarction, hypoxia, digitalis intoxication, or marked muscle weakness or respiratory muscle paralysis.
   C. **Intravenous Potassium Therapy:**
      1. Intravenous KCL is usually used unless concomitant hypophosphatemia is present (diabetic ketoacidosis), where potassium phosphate is indicated. Intravenous should be administered via a large peripheral or central vein. When infusing K via central vein verify that the catheter is in the superior vena cava, and not the right atrium or ventricle, to avoid intracardiac injection of potassium.
      2. Intravenous K infusions should be mixed in dextrose-free solutions because dextrose will stimulate endogenous insulin release with subsequent K shift intracellularly.
      3. The maximal rate of intravenous K replacement is 20 mEq/hour. Keep the concentration of IV fluids at 40 mEq/L or less if given via peripheral vein.
      4. Frequent monitoring of serum K and constant electrocardiographic monitoring a required.
   D. If large doses of K fail to correct hypokalemia, or if diuretic-induced hypokalemia present, determination of the serum magnesium level is indicated. Magnesium levels le than 2 mg/dL will impair normalization of K.

V. **Non-Emergent Therapy of Hypokalemia**
   A. Attempts should be made to normalize K levels if <3.5 mEq/L.
   B. Oral supplementation is significantly safer than IV. Upper and lower gastrointestin irritation, bleeding, and poor palatability are common. Micro-encapsulated and sustained release forms of KCL are less likely to induce gastrointestinal disturbances than are wal matrix tablets or liquid preparations.
      -KCL elixir, 1-3 tablespoon qd-tid PO after meals (20 mEq/Tbsp 10% sln).
      -Micro-K, 10 mEq tabs, 2-3 tabs tid PO after meals (40-100 mEq/d).

# Hypermagnesemia

### Clinical Evaluation of Hypermagnesemia

A. Serum magnesium has a normal range of 0.8-1.2 mMol/L. Magnesium homeostasis is regulated by renal and gastrointestinal mechanisms. Hypercalcemia inhibits tubular magnesium reabsorption.

B. Hypermagnesemia is usually iatrogenic and is frequently seen in conjunction with renal insufficiency.

C. **Causes of Hypermagnesemia:**
1. **Renal:** Creatinine clearance <30 mL/minute.
2. **Nonrenal:** Excessive use of magnesium cathartics, especially with renal failure; iatrogenic overtreatment with magnesium sulfate.
3. **Combined Renal and Nonrenal:** Excessive magnesium in dialysates, iatrogenic overdosage of magnesium in patients with renal insufficiency.
4. **Less Common Causes of Mild Hypermagnesemia:** Hyperparathyroidism, Addison's disease, hypocalciuric hypercalcemia, lithium therapy.

D. Hypermagnesemia is commonly due to overzealous replacement of presumed magnesium losses, inadequate adjustment of Mg dosage for renal insufficiency, and overuse of magnesium-containing cathartics.

E. **Manifestations of Hypermagnesemia** may include stupor and obtundation, respiratory failure, and cardiac arrhythmias, and it should always be considered in patients with renal failure, in those receiving therapeutic magnesium, and in laxative abuse.
1. **Cardiovascular:**
   a. **Lower levels of hypermagnesemia <10 mEq/L or 5 mMol/L:** Delayed interventricular conduction, first-degree heart block, prolongation of the Q-T interval.
   b. **Levels greater than 10 mEq/L or 5 mMol/L:** Heart block progresses to complete heart block and asystole occurs at levels greater than 12.5 mMol/L (>6.25 mMol/L).
   c. Hypotension may occur but is usually only transient. Contractility is not affected.
2. **Neuromuscular Effects:**
   a. Hyporeflexia occurs at a Mg level >4 mEq/L (>2 mMol/L); an early sign of magnesium toxicity is diminution of deep tendon reflexes due to neuromuscular blockade.
   b. Respiratory depression due to respiratory muscle paralysis occurs at levels >13 mEq/L (>6.5 mMol/L).
   c. Somnolence and coma occur at very elevated levels.

### Treatment of Hypermagnesemia

A. **Asymptomatic, Hemodynamically Stable Patients:**
1. Moderate hypermagnesemia can be managed by elimination of intake and maintenance of renal magnesium clearance.
2. Saline diuresis and loop diuretics increase renal clearance of magnesium. Diuresis is adequate treatment if cardiovascular or respiratory compromise are absent.

B. **Severe Hypermagnesemia:**
1. Severe hypermagnesemia requires loop diuretics, saline diuresis, and correction of acute cardiovascular or respiratory symptoms. Furosemide 20-40 mg IV q3-4h as needed. Frequently monitor input, output, and patient weight. Initiate saline diuresis with 0.9% or 0.45% saline infused at 150 cc/h to replace urine loss.
2. Calcium gluconate (10% sln; 1 gm per 10 mL amp) 1-3 ampules may be added to saline infusate to reverse acute cardiovascular toxicity and ameliorate respiratory failure. Calcium administration can be continued and given over a longer period of time (15 mg/kg, given as calcium gluconate over a 4-hour period) to increase renal excretion of magnesium.

C. **If Renal Failure or Massive Overdose:** Dialysis with magnesium-free dialysate is life-saving.

# Hypomagnesemia

I. **Pathophysiology**
   A. Hypomagnesemia is rare in healthy subjects due to the abundance of Mg in the food and water supply. Absorption of ingested Mg occurs in the small intestine; the kidney regulate Mg balance.
   B. **Causes of Hypomagnesemia:**
      1. Decreased Mg intake
      2. Increased Mg losses
      3. Alterations in the distribution of Mg
   C. **Decreased Magnesium Intake:** Protein-calorie malnutrition is a common cause hypomagnesemia. Inadequate caloric intake, prolonged parenteral (Mg-free) flu administration, and catabolic illness also cause hypomagnesemia.
   D. **Gastrointestinal Losses of Magnesium:**
      1. Gastrointestinal losses of Mg may result from prolonged nasogastric suction, laxativ abuse, pancreatitis, extensive small bowel resection, short bowel syndromes, biliar and bowel fistulas, enteropathies, cholestatic liver disease, and malabsorptic syndromes.
   E. **Renal Losses of Magnesium:**
      1. Renal loss of Mg may occur secondary to renal tubular acidosis, glomerulonephriti interstitial nephritis, or acute tubular necrosis.
      2. Hyperthyroidism, hypercalcemia, and hypophosphatemia may cause Mg loss.
      3. **Drugs Causing Mg loss:** Diuretic agents (furosemide, thiazides) induc hypomagnesemia by increasing Mg excretion. Digitalis, aminoglycoside antibiotic cyclosporine, terbutaline, methotrexate, amphotericin, pentamidine, ethanol, an calcium are associated with hypomagnesemia.
   F. **Alterations in Magnesium Distribution:**
      1. Redistribution of circulating Mg occurs by extracellular to intracellular shifts, chelatio sequestration, hungry bone syndrome, or by acute administration of glucose, insuli or amino acids.
      2. Hypomagnesemia noted after cardiopulmonary bypass may be related to the shift Mg into cells.
      3. Mg depletion occurs during severe pancreatitis due to decreased intestinal absorptic of Mg, prolonged nasogastric suction, administration of large quantities of parenter fluids, and pancreatitis-induced sequestration of Mg.

II. **Clinical Manifestations of Hypomagnesemia**
   A. **Cardiovascular:** Ventricular tachycardia, ventricular fibrillation, atrial fibrillatio multifocal atrial tachycardia, ventricular ectopic beats, hypertension, enhancement digoxin-induced dysrhythmias, cardiomyopathies, coronary artery spasm.
   B. **Neuromuscular and Behavioral:** Convulsions, confusion, psychosis, weakness, ataxi spasticity, tremors, tetany, agitation, delirium, depression.
   C. **ECG changes:** Prolonged PR and, QT intervals; ST segment depression, T wav inversions, wide QRS complexes, tall T waves.
   D. **Concomitant Electrolyte Abnormalities:** Na, K, Ca, PO4

III. **Clinical Evaluation**
   A. Hypomagnesemia is diagnosed when the serum Mg concentration is less than 0.7-0 mMol/L, and symptomatic Mg deficiency occurs when the serum Mg concentration is les than 0.5 mMol/L.
   B. **Urinary Magnesium Determinations:**
      1. 24-hour urine collection for Mg determination should be completed.
      2. In hypomagnesemic states due to renal Mg loss, Mg excretion exceeds 1.5-2 mMol/day.
      3. Low urinary Mg excretion (<1 mMol/day) with concomitant serum hypomagnesemi

suggests Mg deficiency due to decreased intake, nonrenal losses, or redistribution of Mg.

## IV. Treatment of Hypomagnesemia

### A. Asymptomatic Magnesium Deficiency:

1. The daily recommended dietary allowance of Mg in healthy young, non-pregnant subjects is 4.5-5 mg/kg/day. In hospitalized patients, the daily Mg requirements can be provided through either a balanced diet, as oral Mg supplements (0.18-0.23 mMol/kg/day), or 8-15 mMol/day in a parenteral nutrition formulation.

2. Magnesium oxide tablets contain 111 mg (4.5 mMol, or 9 mEq) of elemental Mg. Magnesium oxide is better absorbed and less likely to cause diarrhea.

### B. Symptomatic Magnesium Deficiency

1. Serum Mg 0.5 mMol/L or less, requires IV Mg repletion with electrocardiographic and respiratory monitoring.

2. 600 mg of elemental Mg should be infused IV over 3 hours with a maximum rate of 15 mg/minute. An additional 600-900 mg of Mg should be provided as intermittent bolus therapy or by continuous infusion over the next 24 hours. Parenteral Mg preparations use the sulfate (4 mMol/g) or the chloride (4.5 mMol/g) salt. $MgSO_4$ is more frequently used than $MgCl_2$.

3. States of severe Mg deficiency may require additional therapy over a number of days due to slow repletion of cellular Mg stores.

# Disorders of Water and Sodium Balance

## I. Pathophysiology of Water and Sodium Balance

A. Volitional intake of water is regulated by thirst.

B. Maintenance intake of water is the amount of water sufficient to offset obligatory losses.
   **Maintenance Water Needs:**
   - = 100 mL/kg for first 10 kg of body weight
   - + 50 mL/kg for next 10 kg
   - + 20 mL/kg for weight greater than 20 kg

C. **Clinical Signs of Hyponatremia:** Confusion, agitation, lethargy, seizures, and coma. The rate of change during onset of hyponatremia is more important in causing symptoms than is the absolute concentration of sodium.

D. **Pseudohyponatremia**
   1. A marked elevation of the blood glucose creates an osmotic gradient that pulls water from cells into the extracellular fluid, diluting the extracellular sodium. The contribution of hyperglycemia to hyponatremia can be estimated using the following formula:
      Expected change in serum sodium = (Serum glucose - 100) x 0.016
   2. With normalization of the serum glucose level, the serum sodium level rises as a result of redistribution of body water.
   3. Marked elevation of plasma solids (lipids or protein) can also result in erroneous hyponatremia due to laboratory inaccuracy. The percentage of plasma water can be estimated with the following formula:
      % plasma water = 100 - [0.01 x lipids (mg/dL)] - [0.73 x protein (g/dL)]

## II. Diagnostic Evaluation of Hyponatremia

A. Exclude pseudohyponatremia, then determine the cause of the hyponatremia based on history, physical exam, urine osmolality, and urine sodium level. Determine if the patient is volume contracted, normal volume, or volume expanded.

B. **Classify Hyponatremic Patients Based on Urine Osmolality:**
   1. **Low Urine Osmolality (50-180 mOsm/L):** Indicates primary excessive water intake (psychogenic water drinking).
   2. **High Urine Osmolality (urine osmolality > serum osmolality):**
      a. **High Urine Sodium (>40 mEq/L) and Volume Contracted:** Indicates a renal source of sodium and fluid loss (excessive diuretic use, salt-wasting nephropathy, Addison's disease, osmotic diuresis).
      b. **High Urine Sodium (>40 mEq/L) and Normal Volume:** Most likely due to water retention caused by a drug effect, hypothyroidism, or the syndrome of inappropriate antidiuretic hormone secretion (SIADH). Drugs that can cause water retention: Chlorpropamide (Diabinese), carbamazepine, amitriptyline, cyclophosphamide. In SIADH, the urine sodium level is usually high, but may be low if the patient is on a salt-restricted diet. SIADH is found in the presence of a malignant tumor or a disorder of the pulmonary or central nervous system.
      c. **Low Urine Sodium (<20 mEq/L) and Volume Contraction:** Dry mucous membranes, decreased skin turgor, and orthostatic hypotension indicate an extrarenal source of fluid loss (gastrointestinal disease, burns).
      d. **Low Urine Sodium (<20 mEq/L) and Volume-expanded, Edematous:** Caused by congestive heart failure, cirrhosis with ascites, and nephrotic syndrome; effective arterial blood volume is decreased. Decreased renal perfusion causes increased reabsorption of water.

## III. Treatment of Water Excess Hyponatremia

A. Determine the volume of water excess:
   Water excess = total body water x [(140/measured sodium) -1]

B. **Treatment of Asymptomatic Hyponatremia:** Restrict water intake to 1,000 mL/day. Food alone in the diet contains this much water, so no liquids should be consumed. If an intravenous solution is needed, an isotonic solution of 0.9% sodium chloride (normal saline) should be used. Dextrose should not be used in the infusion because the dextrose is metabolized into water.

C. **Treatment of Symptomatic Hyponatremia:**
1. If neurologic symptoms of hyponatremia are present, the serum sodium level should be corrected with hypertonic saline. Excessively rapid correction of sodium may result in a syndrome of central pontine demyelination.
2. Raise the serum sodium at a rate of 1 mEq/L per hour. If chronic hyponatremia, limit the rate to 0.5 mEq/L per hour. Aim for a serum sodium of 125-130 mEq/L, then continue water restriction until the level normalizes.
3. The amount of hypertonic saline needed is estimated using the following formula:
   Sodium needed (mEq) = 0.6 x wt in kg x (desired sodium - measured sodium)
4. 3% sodium chloride contains 513 mEq/L of sodium. The calculated volume required should be administered over the period required to raise the serum sodium level at a rate of 0.5-1 mEq/L per hour.
5. Concomitant administration a furosemide may be required to lessen the risk of fluid overload, especially in the elderly.

## IV. Hypernatremia

A. **Clinical Manifestations of Hypernatremia:**
1. Signs of volume overload or volume depletion may be prominent. Clinical manifestations include tremulousness, irritability, ataxia, spasticity, mental confusion, seizures, and coma. Symptoms are more likely to occur with acute increases in plasma sodium.

B. **Causes of Hypernatremia:**
1. Net sodium gain, net water loss
2. Failure to replace obligate water losses, as in the case of patients unable to obtain water due to an altered mental status or severe debilitating disease.
3. Diabetes Insipidus: If urine volume is high but $U_{osm}$ is low, diabetes insipidus is the most likely cause.

## V. Management of Hypernatremia

A. Acute treatment of hypovolemic hypernatremia depends on the degree of volume depletion.
1. If there is evidence of hemodynamic compromise (e.g., orthostatic hypotension, marked oliguria), fluid deficits should be corrected initially with isotonic saline.
2. Once hemodynamic stability is achieved, the remaining free water deficit should be corrected with 5% dextrose water or 0.45% NaCl.
3. The water deficit can be estimated using the following formula :
   Water deficit = 0.6 x wt in kg x [1 - (140/measured sodium)]

B. The change in sodium concentration should not exceed 1 mEq/liter/hour. Roughly one half of the calculated water deficit can be administered in the first 24 hours, followed by correction of the remaining deficit over the next 1-2 days. The serum sodium concentration and ECF volume status should be evaluated every 6 hours.

C. Excessively rapid correction is dangerous as it may lead to lethargy and seizures secondary to cerebral edema.

D. Maintenance fluid needs from ongoing renal and insensible losses must also be provided. If the patient is conscious and able to drink, water should be given orally.

## VI. Mixed Disorders

A. **Water Excess and Saline Deficit:** Occurs when severe vomiting and diarrhea occur in a patient who is given only water; clinical signs of volume contraction and a low serum sodium are present. Replace saline deficit and restrict free water intake until the serum sodium level has normalized.

B. **Water and Saline Excess:** Often occurs with heart failure with edema and a low serum sodium. An increase in the extracellular fluid volume, as evidenced by edema, is a saline excess. A marked excess of free water expands the extracellular fluid volume, causing apparent hyponatremia. However, the important derangement in edema is an excess of sodium. Sodium restriction and use of diuretics (furosemide) are usually indicated, in addition to treatment of the underlying disorder. Requires restriction of both sodium and water, plus an increase in diuretic dosage.

C. **Water and Saline Deficit:** Frequently caused by vomiting and high fever, and is characterized by signs of volume contraction and an elevated serum sodium. Replace saline and free water in addition to maintenance amounts of water.

D. **Water Deficit and Saline Excess:** Characterized by edema with cirrhosis, fever, and stupor and an elevated serum sodium. Restrict sodium, replace free water, and administer diuretics.

# Endocrinology

## Diabetic Ketoacidosis

### Clinical Presentation

A. Diabetes is newly diagnosed in 20% of cases of diabetic ketoacidosis. The remainder of cases occur in known diabetics in whom ketosis develops after a precipitating factor, such as infection.

B. **Symptoms of DKA:** Polyuria, polydypsia, fatigue, nausea, and vomiting developing over 1 to 2 days. Abdominal pain is prominent in 25%.

C. **Physical Exam:**
1. Patients are typically flushed (despite hypotension) and tachycardiac. Tachypnea is common; Kussmaul's respiration, with deep breathing and air hunger, occurs when serum pH is between 7.0 and 7.24.
2. A fruity odor on the breath indicates the presence of acetone, a by-product of diabetic ketoacidosis.
3. Fever is seldom present even though infection is common. Hypothermia may occur.
4. 80% of patients with diabetic ketoacidosis have altered mental status. Most are awake but confused; 10% are comatose.

D. **Laboratory Findings:**
1. Serum glucose level >250 mg/dL
2. pH <7.35
3. Bicarbonate level below normal with an elevated anion gap,
4. Presence of ketones in the serum

### Differential Diagnosis

A. Diabetic ketoacidosis must be differentiated from other causes of ketosis, acidosis, and hyperglycemia.

B. **Differential Diagnosis of Ketosis-Causing Conditions:**
1. Ketosis may result from alcoholic ketoacidosis or starvation. The majority of patients with alcoholic ketoacidosis do not have diabetes, and the serum glucose level is not elevated. Alcoholic ketoacidosis occurs with heavy drinking and vomiting.
2. Starvation ketosis occurs after 24 hours without food and is not usually confused with diabetic ketoacidosis because glucose and serum pH are normal.

C. **Differential Diagnosis of Acidosis-Causing Conditions:**
1. Metabolic acidoses are divided into increased anion gap (>14 mEq/L) and normal anion gap (anion gap is determined by subtracting the sum of chloride plus bicarbonate from sodium).
2. All ketoacidoses increase the anion gap (DKA, lactic acidosis, uremia, poisoning from salicylates or methanol).
3. Acidoses without an increased anion gap are associated with a normal glucose level and absent serum ketones. Acidoses that do not increase the anion gap are caused by renal or gastrointestinal electrolyte losses.

D. **Hyperglycemia Caused by Hyperosmolar Nonketotic Coma:**
1. Causes severe hyperglycemia that must be distinguished from DKA. Patients are usually elderly and have type II diabetes and a precipitating illness.
2. Serum glucose level is markedly elevated (>600 mg/dL), and osmolarity is increased. In hyperosmolar coma, ketosis is minimal. Patients may be acidotic from lactic acidosis and renal failure resulting from dehydration.
3. Treatment of hyperosmolar, nonketotic coma consists of hydration and potassium replacement. Administration of insulin is less important and should be begun after fluid resuscitation is under way.

### III. Treatment of Diabetic Ketoacidosis

  A. **Fluids**

    1. Fluid deficits average 5 L (50 to 100 mL/kg).

    2. Give 1 liter of normal saline solution in the first hour and the second liter over the second and third hours. Thereafter, ½ normal saline solution should be infused at 250-500 mL/h. These rates are lower than recommended in the past, because lower rates cause fewer electrolyte abnormalities.

    3. Higher rates of fluid administration may be required in patients who are extremely dehydrated.

    4. Lower rates are indicated for patients with chronic renal failure because they have not had major fluid losses.

    5. When the glucose level reaches 250 mg/dL, 5% dextrose should be added to the replacement fluids to prevent hypoglycemia. If the glucose level declines rapidly, 10% dextrose should be used.

  B. **Insulin**

    1. Insulin 0.1 U/kg IV bolus, followed by an infusion of 0.1 U/kg per hour. The biologic half life of IV insulin is less than 20 minutes, so an IV bolus without a follow-up infusion has a very short-lived effect, and serum glucose will rise rapidly if the insulin infusion is discontinued.

### IV. Monitoring of Therapy

  A. The serum bicarbonate level and anion gap should be monitored to determine the effectiveness of insulin therapy.

  B. Follow-up evaluation of acidosis, not just of glucose level, is very important because in some patients glucose levels may normalize early in therapy, but the acidosis takes longer to resolve. Continued insulin infusion is needed to resolve the acidosis.

  C. **Glucose Levels**: Check glucose level at 1-2 hour intervals during IV insulin administration

  D. **Electrolyte Levels:** Assess q2h for first 6-8 h and then q4h

  E. Use a flow sheet to record of intravenous fluid administration, insulin infusion rate, urine output, glucose and electrolyte levels, and anion gap.

  F. Phosphorus and magnesium levels should be checked after about 4 hours of treatment and replacement therapy should be started if they are significantly below normal.

  G. Testing for plasma and urine ketones is helpful in diagnosing diabetic ketoacidosis, but is not necessary during therapy.

  H. When the bicarbonate level is greater than 16 mEq/L and the anion gap is less than 16 mEq/L, the insulin infusion rate should be decreased by half. However, if the bicarbonate level is not rising and the anion gap is not falling after 2 hours of treatment, the insulin infusion rate should be doubled.

### V. Potassium

  A. The most common preventable cause of death in patients with DKA is hypokalemia. Deficits are caused by osmotic diuresis and cellular shifts. The typical deficit is between 300 and 600 mEq.

  B. Replacement therapy with potassium chloride should be started when fluid therapy is started. In most patients, the initial rate of potassium replacement is 20 mEq/h, but those with hypokalemia need more aggressive replacement (40 mEq/h) and monitoring.

  C. All patients should receive potassium replacement, except for those with known chronic renal failure, no urine output, or an initial serum potassium level greater than 6.0 mEq/L.

### VI. Determination of Underlying Cause

  A. Infection is the underlying cause of diabetic ketoacidosis in about 50% of cases. Infection of the urinary tract, skin, sinuses, or teeth should be sought. Fever is unusual in diabetic ketoacidosis and indicates infection when present; an elevated white blood cell count is usually present whether or not there is infection.

  B. Physical examination, chest film, and urinalysis should be completed to exclude infection. If infection is suspected, antibiotics should be started empirically.

C. Omission of insulin doses (common in adolescents) is often a precipitating factor.

D. Patients using a subcutaneous insulin pump can become ketotic within hours if the pump becomes disconnected.

E. Myocardial infarction, cerebrovascular accident, and abdominal catastrophes may precipitate DKA.

## II. Sodium

A. Patients with diabetic ketoacidosis often have a low serum sodium level, because the high level of glucose has a dilutional effect. For every 100 mg/dL that glucose is elevated, the sodium level should be corrected upward by 1.6 mEq/L.

B. Rarely, patients have an initial serum sodium greater than 150 mEq/L, indicating severe dehydration. Initial rehydration fluid should consist of 50% normal saline.

## III. Phosphate

A. Diabetic ketoacidosis depletes phosphate stores.

B. Serum phosphate level should be checked after 4 hours of treatment. If it is below 1.5 mg/dL, potassium or sodium phosphate should be added to the IV solution.

## X. Bicarbonate

A. Administration of bicarbonate is ineffective in diabetic ketoacidosis, even in severely acidotic patients.

B. Bicarbonate administration may exacerbate hypokalemia and cause a paradoxic intracellular acidosis, a negative shift in the oxygen dissociation curve, and late alkalemia.

## . Additional Therapies

A. A nasogastric tube should be inserted in semiconscious patients to protect against aspiration.

B. Deep vein thrombosis prophylaxis should be provided for patients who are elderly, unconscious, or severely hyperosmolar; subcutaneous heparin, 5,000 U every 8 hours.

## I. Initiation of Subcutaneous Insulin

A. When the serum bicarbonate level is normal and the patient is ready to eat, subcutaneous insulin can be started.

B. It is critical to overlap intravenous and subcutaneous administration of insulin to avoid redevelopment of ketoacidosis. The intravenous infusion may be stopped 1 hour after the first subcutaneous injection of regular insulin.

C. Estimation of Subcutaneous Insulin Requirements:

1. Multiply the final insulin infusion rate times 24 hours and divide the total into morning and evening doses.

2. Two thirds of the total dose is given in the morning, as two thirds NPH and one third regular insulin. The remaining one third of the total dose is given before supper as one half NPH and one half regular insulin.

3. Adjust subsequent doses according to the patient's blood glucose response.

## II. Complications

A. Death from diabetic ketoacidosis can be caused by hypokalemia, untreated infection, aspiration, thromboembolism, cerebral edema, and myocardial infarction.

B. The glucose level should be carefully monitored as it declines to avoid hypoglycemia.

C. Excessive use of normal saline solution can result in fluid overload and hypernatremia.

D. Cerebral edema occurs in 1 of 200 patients with diabetic ketoacidosis, usually in those younger than age 20. It is manifested by abrupt worsening of the mental status. Patients should be treated aggressively with dexamethasone and mannitol.

# Insulin-Dependent (Type I) Diabetes Mellitus

### I. Pathophysiology of Type I Diabetes
A. Peak incidence occurs at age 15. Most patients have developed hyperglycemia by age 30, but a few patients may present at an older age.
B. Chronic hyperglycemia is associated with the chronic microvascular complications of diabetes including retinopathy, nephropathy, and neuropathy.

### II. Diagnosis
A. Insulin-dependent (type I) diabetes mellitus typically presents with severe dehydration, diminished mental status, coma (ketoacidosis), elevated blood glucose, elevated blood acetone, and low blood pH.
B. Patients may experience polyuria, polydipsia, polyphagia, weight loss; frequent bacterial or fungal mucocutaneous infections, or blurred vision.
C. **Physical Findings:** Dehydration (orthostatic hypotension), coexisting infection, acetone odor on breath.
D. **Diagnostic Tests:**
1. Generally the diagnosis of type I diabetes may be confirmed immediately in the outpatient setting by fingerstick blood glucose and urine dipstick ketone testing.
2. Blood glucose is usually greater than 250 mg/dL.
3. Evidence of acidemia (low blood pH and bicarbonate level) confirms the diagnosis.
4. Oral glucose tolerance testing is not indicated in the diagnosis of type I diabetes.
5. Glycohemoglobin may be elevated, but the short duration of hyperglycemia in many type I diabetics prior to diagnosis, precludes this test from being helpful.

### III. Differential Diagnosis
A. The only two common causes of chronic hyperglycemia are type I and type II diabetes mellitus. They are generally distinguished by the presence or absence of ketosis.
B. Age of onset is a less reliable indicator, as a subset of type II diabetics present as teenagers, and type I diabetes may present at any age.
C. Measurement of anti-islet cell antibodies is not necessary.

### IV. Treatment Strategy
A. All type I diabetics should immediately be started on insulin injections when the diagnosis is made. Dietary modification or oral hypoglycemic agents should not be used in place of insulin in type I diabetics.
B. At the initial diagnosis, the goals of therapy can be defined more loosely. Commonly a "honeymoon" phase occurs within the first months after the diagnosis, and exogenous insulin requirements are decreased for a period of weeks or even months.
C. Human insulin is recommended. A minimum of 2 injections per day is generally needed to achieve adequate control, although three or four smaller injections per day are preferable. Single-dose insulin therapy is never adequate
D. **Diet:**
1. 60% of calories should be in the form of carbohydrates, 20% as protein, and no more than 20% as fat. Cholesterol intake should be less than 300 mg/day.
2. High-fiber foods and artifical sweeteners should be encouraged.
3. Diet should be consistent from day to day, and meals should not be skipped.

### V. Intensive Insulin Therapy
A. The Diabetes Control and Complications Trial Study has demonstrated that improved glycemic control is extremely important for preventing diabetic complications (retinopathy, nephropathy, neuropathy) and for reversing many complications secondary to diabetes.
B. Intensive insulin therapy aimed at tight glucose control is recommended in all patients except patients with recurrent severe hypoglycemia or hypoglycemic unawareness, or patients with far advanced complications, such as renal failure, or patients with coronary artery disease or cerebral vascular disease, or children younger than age 13.
C. The general goal of insulin therapy is to control the blood glucose at a level as close to

normal as is possible without incurring a significant risk of dangerous hypoglycemia.
D. Severe acute hypoglycemia can result in seizures, coma, irreversible brain damage, myocardial infarction, and death.

## VI. Therapeutic Goals

A. **Target Blood Glucose Levels for Patients with IDDM:**

|  | Ideal | Acceptable |
|---|---|---|
| Pre-meal | 70 to 105 | 70 to 130 |
| 1 hour after meal | 100 to 160 | 100 to 180 |
| 2 hours after meal | 80 to 120 | 80 to 150 |
| 2 AM to 4 AM | 70 to 100 | 70 to 120 |

Glycosylated Hemoglobin 4%-6% above the upper range of normal

B. **In older individuals or those with severe chronic diabetic complications, major medical problems, or a past history of severe hypoglycemia "Loose" control consists of the following goals:**

| Preprandial Glucoses | 130-180 mg/dL |
|---|---|
| Postprandial Peaks | <240 mg/dL. |
| Glycosylated Hemoglobin | 6% above the upper range of normal |

C. Goals should be tempered for individual patients; less stringent goals should be set for patents with hypoglycemic unawareness.

## VII. Monitoring

A. **Home Blood Glucose Monitoring:** Diabetics should check their blood sugar levels prior to each meal, at bedtime, and at least once a week at 3 AM to detect asymptomatic hypoglycemia. Patients should also periodically monitor their blood sugar 1-2 hours after eating to make certain that the preprandial dose of regular insulin was appropriate for that meal.

B. **Glycosylated hemoglobin:**
   1. The percentage of hemoglobin A1 molecules which are glycosylated is dependent on mean blood glucose level, and is a reliable marker of the mean blood glucose concentration during the previous 60-120 days.
   2. The Hb A1c level should be tested routinely in stable patients every 3 to 4 months.

## VIII. Insulin Regimens

A. An insulin regimen must provide (1) basal insulin to suppress background glucose production by the liver, and (2) bolus insulin (given before meals) to limit postprandial glucose elevation.

B. Doses of regular insulin are either added to or deleted from the basic insulin regimen to bring the next blood glucose value into target range.

C. **Action Times of Commonly Used Human Insulins:**

| Insulin type | Onset (hr) | Peak (hr) | Duration (hr) | Maximum duration (hr) |
|---|---|---|---|---|
| Regular | ½-1 | 2-3 | 3-6 | 4-6 |
| NPH | 2-4 | 4-10 | 10-16 | 14-18 |

D. **Estimation of Total Daily Insulin Dose:**
   Prior to designing an insulin regimen, the estimated total daily insulin dose should be calculated.
   Total Daily Dose of Insulin = Weight in kg (0.5 - 0.7 U/kg)

E. **Regular Insulin** is given to control postprandial glucose levels and should be injected 15-30 minutes before meals. Blood testing 1 hour postprandially and just before the next meal helps determine the appropriate dose. Regular insulin has a peak onset within 1 hour and a duration of action of 4-6 hours.

F. **NPH Insulin:** The intermediate-acting insulins are used to provide basal insulin. The effect of intermediate insulins can best be monitored by determining predinner and fasting blood glucose levels. Onset of action occurs at 2 hours and peak occurs at 8 to 10 hours after injection; duration of action is 16-24 hours. NPH insulin given at dinner may peak at 2 to 3 AM and cause hypoglycemia. This problem can be avoided by moving the NPH insulin to 9-10 PM.

G. **Premixed Insulin Preparations:** The 70/30 preparation is 70% NPH and 30% regular insulin, and the 50/50 preparation is 50% NPH and 50% regular insulin. Premixed preparations can be helpful in treating children and older individuals who have difficulty mixing insulin.

H. Subcutaneous insulin remains standard therapy. Available methods for insulin delivery include syringes, pen injectors, jet injectors, and continuous subcutaneous infusion pumps.

IX. **NPH/Regular Insulin Regimens**

A. **Regimen 1:** Consists of NPH and regular insulin twice a day, and is the most frequently used regimen. Its main advantage is simplicity. Its disadvantages are that nighttime hypoglycemia is common, and the noon meal is not always well covered. Two-thirds of the daily insulin dose is given before the breakfast, and one-third is administered before dinner. Give 2/3 of total insulin requirement as NPH and ⅓ as regular.

B. **Regimen 2:** Moves NPH insulin to bedtime to avoid nighttime hypoglycemia and to control the fasting blood glucose level better. However, this regimen may not always give control after the noon meal.

C. **Regimen 3:** Adds regular insulin at noon to the basic two-injection regimen. It provides better control after the noon meal, but it does not always control nighttime hypoglycemia and fasting blood glucose levels.

D. **Most Common NPH/Regular Insulin Regimens:**

|  | Morning | Noon | Evening | Bedtime |
|---|---|---|---|---|
| Regimen 1 | NPH/regular |  | NPH/regular |  |
| Regimen 2 | NPH/regular |  | Regular | NPH |
| Regimen 3 | NPH/regular | Regular | NPH/regular |  |

E. **Control of High Fasting Glucose Levels:**

1. Causes of high fasting blood glucose level in a patient on a regimen of two injections a day:
   a. Insufficient basal insulin overnight.
   b. Excessive basal insulin, resulting in hypoglycemia at 2 AM, and leading to a rebound increase of the fasting glucose level (Somogyi effect).
   c. The dawn phenomenon (increased early morning glucose secondary to cortisol secretion).
2. In patients with high fasting blood glucose, before a change is made in the insulin schedule, blood glucose determinations at 2 to 3 AM for several nights may be needed. If the glucose level is low at this time, the amount of NPH insulin should be decreased or the injection moved to bedtime. If the glucose value is elevated, the amount of NPH insulin should be increased. Doses should be adjusted 1 or 2 units at a time.

X. **Supplementation of Insulin Dosage**

A. Once the basic insulin regimen has been established, supplements can be used with the goal of bringing the next scheduled glucose determination into target range.

B. If supplements are consistently needed at a particular time of day the basic insulin dose should be increased.

C. **Insulin Sliding Scale for Supplementation:**

| Post Prandial Blood glucose level | Preprandial Action needed |
|---|---|
| <70 | Reduce regular insulin by 1-2 units |
| 71-120 | Take prescribed amount of regular insulin |
| 121-150 | Increase regular insulin by 1 unit |
| 151-200 | Increase regular insulin by 2 units |
| 201-250 | Increase regular insulin by 3 units |
| >250 | Increase regular insulin by 4 units |

D. If the planned meal is larger than usual, increase preprandial regular insulin by 1 to 2 units. If the planned meal is smaller than usual, decrease preprandial regular insulin by 1 to 2 units.

E. **Exercise:**
1. Glucose levels drop after exercise, and hypoglycemia may occur either shortly after exercise or hours later as the exercised muscles take up glucose.
2. If the planned activity after eating is unusually vigorous, the patient should eat extra carbohydrates and decrease regular insulin dose by 1 to 2 units.

## XI. Treatment of Hypoglycemia

A. Hypoglycemia is most frequently precipitated by inadequate or missed meals, excessive and unexpected exercise, or over-insulinization.

B. Symptoms of hypoglycemia include sweating, palpitations, hunger, nausea, blurred vision, headache, weakness, irritability, and confusion.

C. Diabetic sugar cubes will raise the blood sugar 20 points per tablet.

D. A half-can of regular Coke will raise the blood sugar approximately 80 points.

E. For severe hypoglycemia, Glucagon (1 mg) IM may be administered.

## XII. Chronic Complications of Diabetes

A. **Retinopathy:** Ophthalmologic evaluation should be performed annually for patients who have had diabetes for at least 5 years, and on every patient who is older than 30. Unexplained changes in vision or fundoscopy should be referred to an ophthalmologist.

B. **Renal Disease:**
1. 10-20% of patients with type I diabetes develop end-stage renal failure and require dialysis. The complete syndrome includes proteinuria, hypertension, edema, and renal insufficiency.
2. As the renal clearance of insulin diminishes with the rising creatinine level, insulin doses typically must be reduced.
3. At the microalbuminuria stage, the renal disease can probably be reversed. Once there is clinically detectable proteinuria (dipstick-positive for protein), the long-term prognosis is guarded.
4. **Microalbuminuria Screening:** Screening for microalbuminuria in patients with either type I or type II diabetes is recommended. Microalbuminuria is a sensitive index of early nephropathy.
   a. Microalbuminuria should be checked annually on all diabetic patients, and is accomplished by checking urine albumin/creatinine ratio.
   b. If albumin is high--exceeding 30 mg/g on at least two occasions--the adequacy of blood sugar and hemoglobin A1c levels should be reevaluated.
   c. If glycemic control is the best that can be achieved and microalbuminuria persists, an angiotensin-converting enzyme inhibitor or calcium channel blocker should be strongly considered, even if the patient's blood pressure is normal.

C. **Peripheral Neuropathy:**
1. Neuropathies have an insidious onset, are usually progressive, and generally progress from the most distal to the more proximal areas of the body.
2. Persistent painful neuropathies may be treated with low doses of antidepressants, such as amitriptyline (Elavil) 25-75 mg po hs, and nonsteroidal anti-inflammatory drugs.
3. Pentoxifylline (Trental), 400 mg four times a day, and capsaicin (Zostrix) applied topically prn may provide some relief.
4. Peripheral neuropathy can cause a misalignment of the joints of the feet, and Charcot's fractures can occur and the foot becomes grossly distorted. Heavy calluses and plantar ulcers can develop.
5. Orthotics and other special footwear may be required. Any evidence of tissue breakdown or infection should be treated aggressively and requires early podiatric consultation.

D. **Autonomic Neuropathy:**
1. Signs of cardiovascular autonomic neuropathy include resting tachycardias, exercise intolerance, painless myocardial infarction, and orthostatic hypotension.
2. Signs of GI autonomic neuropathy include upper GI discomfort (reflux), autonomic

gastropathy with delayed gastric emptying, diabetic diarrhea, severe constipation, fecal incontinence. GI autonomic neuropathy can be assessed by liquid- and solid-phase radionucleotide gastric emptying studies.

3. Signs of genitourinary autonomic neuropathy include erectile impotence, retrograde ejaculation, and bladder dysfunction with recurrent infections.

4. Hypoglycemic unawareness results from autonomic neuropathy, wherein the hyperadrenergic manifestations of hypoglycemia (sweating, tachycardia, tremulousness) are absent.

## XIII. Cardiac Risk Factors

A. Hyperlipidemia should be screened for, and more aggressively treated, in diabetics: Screening should include measurements of HDL, LDL cholesterol, and triglycerides. Levels should be checked after the patient is in good diabetic control, because hyperglycemia alone can raise LDL cholesterol.

B. Signs of coronary ischemia are often absent in patients with diabetes because of autonomic neuropathy. Therefore, exercise stress test screening is indicated for asymptomatic patients with diabetes for more than 10 years, or if other risk factors for coronary disease are present.

# Non-Insulin Dependent (Type II) Diabetes

I. **Pathophysiology**
   A. 80% diabetics have type II (non-insulin-dependent) diabetes. In type II diabetes, impaired insulin secretion and peripheral insulin resistance cause hyperglycemia.
   B. Most patients are over age 50, overweight, and have a strong family history of type II diabetes.
   C. The Diabetes Control and Complications Trial (DCCT) conclusively showed that tight glycemic control reduces the risk of microvascular complications by 50-75% in patients with type I diabetes. Complications of type II diabetes also respond to tight control.

II. **Diagnosis of Type II Diabetes**
   A. The diagnosis of diabetes is readily made when patients exhibit the classic clinical picture of polydipsia, polyuria, weight loss, and blurred vision. Also typical are fatigue and a vague sense of "not feeling well." Female patients may present with vulvovaginitis or fungal infections of the intertriginous areas.
   B. A complete lack of symptoms is a very common presentation in most patients. Many patients are hyperglycemic several years prior to diagnosis. Type II diabetics rarely develop ketosis except under conditions of extreme stress.
   C. Two fasting serum glucose values in excess of 140 mg/dl, or random serum glucose values in excess of 200 mg/dl establish the diagnosis of Type II diabetes.
   D. A glycosylated hemoglobin more than 3 SD above the mean of normal will also establish the diagnosis of diabetes.
   E. The diagnosis of type II diabetes can be established without oral glucose tolerance testing in most patients.
   F. Type I diabetes is distinguished from type II by the young age of onset and by the production of ketones. Type II diabetes may occur in adults and young patients, and ketones are not present.

III. **Initial Evaluation of Type II Diabetes Patients**
   A. A history and physical examination should be completed with emphasis on the eye (visual acuity, cataracts, macular edema, retinopathy), the feet (neuropathy and vasculopathy), and blood pressure.
   B. **Initial Laboratory Evaluation of Patients with Diabetes:**
   Fasting plasma glucose
   Glycated hemoglobin
   Fasting lipid profile: Total cholesterol, HDL, triglycerides, LDL cholesterol
   Electrolytes, BUN, creatinine, liver function tests,
   Urinalysis (glucose, ketones, protein, sediment)
   Measurement of microalbuminuria by 24 hour or overnight urine collection
   ECG

V. **Dietary Management of Type II Diabetes**
   A. Dietary modification is usually the first step in controlling hyperglycemia. Caloric intake should be uniformly spread throughout the day, usually among breakfast, lunch, supper, and a bedtime snack.
   B. Weight Reduction: For most type II diabetics a weight reduction diet is indicated. Weight loss will ameliorate insulin resistance and may prevent the need for hypoglycemic drugs.
   C. Complex carbohydrates are preferred to simple concentrated sugars.
   D. Saturated fats (animal, dairy) should be avoided, and cholesterol intake should be reduced.
   E. If diet and exercise fail to control hyperglycemia, diet medications such as phentiramine (Fastin) and fenfluramine (Pondimin) should be considered to enhance weight loss.

V. **Hypoglycemic Drug Treatment of Type II Diabetes:**
   A. **Sulfonylureas:**
      1. Sulfonylureas are used in monotherapy and in combination with insulin, and they lower

blood glucose levels by stimulation of beta cells to produce more insulin and by lowering both peripheral and hepatic insulin resistance.

2. The principal side effect is hypoglycemia, which is mainly related to an increase in insulin production. Most cases are mild and caused by increased exercise or delayed meals. These episodes usually are easily treated with food. However, in rare instances, usually in the elderly with renal or liver disease, severe and life-threatening hypoglycemia may develop.

3. **Glipizide (Glucotrol, Glucotrol XL):** Initial dose 5 mg qd. Increase slowly over weeks to 20 mg bid, according to blood glucose response. **Glucatrol XL:** A timed-release glipizide preparation; may be taken as a single daily dose of 5 or 10 mg (maximum 20 mg/day).

4. **Glyburide (DiaBeta, Glynase PresTab, Micronase):** Initial 2.5 mg qd. Increase slowly over weeks to 10 mg bid, according to blood glucose response. Taken once or twice daily; should not be used in patients with significant renal insufficiency.

5. All first- and second-generation sulfonylureas are available in generic form, except Glynase PresTab and Glucotrol XL.

6. When used in combination with insulin, sulfonylureas are usually given in the morning and NPH is given at dinner or at bedtime.

| Sulfonylureas: | Duration (hr) | Dose (mg/day) |
|---|---|---|
| Chlorpropamide (Diabinese) | 100 | 100-500 |
| Glyburide (DiaBeta, Micronase) | 24 | 1.25-20 |
| Glipizide (Glucotrol) | 15-24 | 2.5-40 |
| Glyburide micronized (Glynase PresTab) | 24 | 1.5-12 |
| Glipizide (Glucotrol XL) | 24-48 | 5-20 |

B. Contraindications to Oral Hypoglycemic Therapy: 1) type I diabetes, 2) pregnancy and lactation, and 3) severe concurrent diseases, such as sepsis or trauma, where insulin is needed. Allergies to sulfonylurea compounds are very rare.

C. **Metformin (Glucophage):**

1. Metformin belongs to the biguanide class of drugs, and it lowers blood glucose levels by decreasing peripheral and hepatic insulin resistance. It does not increase insulin production by beta cells; therefore, hypoglycemia is not a problem with metformin.

2. **Side Effects:**
   a. Common side effects include nausea, bloating, diarrhea, and abdominal cramping; the incidence of these side effects is 30%, and they usually disappear with time.
   b. Lactic acidosis is rare and has an incidence of 0.03 cases per 1,000 patient years.

3. **Contraindications to Metformin Therapy:**
   a. Renal dysfunction (creatinine level >1.5 mg/dL in men, >1.4 mg/dL in women)
   b. Liver dysfunction
   c. History of alcohol abuse or binge drinking
   d. Acute or chronic metabolic acidosis
   e. Conditions predisposing to renal insufficiency and/or hypoxia:
      (1) Cardiovascular collapse
      (2) Acute myocardial infarction or acute congestive heart failure
      (3) Severe infection
      (4) Use of iodinated contrast media
      (5) Major surgery

4. Start with 500 mg bid for a week, increase to 1,000 mg in the morning and 500 mg in the evening for a week, and then increase to 1,000 mg bid. Dosage of up to 850 mg tid a day may be needed [500-mg and 850-mg tablets].

5. Metformin can be used as monotherapy for type II diabetes and as combination therapy with the sulfonylureas or alpha-glucosidase inhibitors (acarbose). Combination therapy is especially successful in morbidly obese, insulin-resistant patients.

D. **Acarbose (Precose):**

1. Acarbose is an alpha-glucosidase inhibitor that delays the breakdown and absorption

of carbohydrate in the gut, resulting in decreased glucose levels.

2. Acarbose may be used as monotherapy or in combination with other oral hypoglycemic drugs or insulin.  On average, acarbose can lower Hb A1c values 1% when they are used as monotherapy or in combination with another agent.

3. Alpha-glucosidase inhibitors do not cause lactic acidosis or hypoglycemia.

4. Gastrointestinal side effects are mild and are dose-related and include cramping, gas, and diarrhea; occurring in up to 40% of patients; symptoms tend to disappear after initial dose.

5. Given three times a day with the first bite of the meal [25-mg, 50-mg, and 100.mg tablets].  Greater efficacy is seen with a higher dose, although some patients do well with a minimum dose.

**I.  Recommended Treatment Regimens for Type II Diabetes**

A.  **Monotherapy:**

1. The first choice oral hypoglycemic agent monotherapy for most patients is a sulfonylurea. They are effective and can be given once a day initially. Maximum effectiveness is reached when given twice a day. Side effects are limited.

2. Monotherapy with metformin may be of greater advantage in morbidly obese, insulin-resistant patients, and in patients who have clinical hypoglycemia or other side effects of sulfonylureas, and in patients who are hyperlipidemic. It may be less effective in thin patients with type II disease, who may be more insulin-deficient.

3. Acarbose can be used as monotherapy in any patient with type II diabetes. It is safe with no restrictions and may be of value as a first-line drug in elderly patients, those with mild to moderate elevation of HbA1c values, or those in whom metformin and sulfonylureas are contraindicated. It decreases HbA1c to a lesser degree than sulfonylureas and metformin, and it must be given three times a day.

4. Patients who do not respond to sulfonylurea monotherapy usually will not respond when switched to metformin monotherapy.  Failure of maximum monotherapy with either drug should lead directly to consideration of combination therapy.

5. Patients who fail to respond to acarbose monotherapy should usually be switched to monotherapy with one of the sulfonylureas or with metformin because acarbose is not be as effective as drugs from the other two classes.

B.  **Combination Therapy:**

1. Combination therapy may be accomplished with a sulfonylurea and metformin, or with acarbose and either a sulfonylurea or metformin.

2. For severe hyperglycemia and an Hb A1c value over 10%, the addition of an oral hypoglycemic agent from another class probably will not reduce the level to less than 8%. Traditional combination therapy with insulin and either a sulfonylurea or metformin or acarbose may be optimal for these patients.

C.  **Insulin therapy:** If glucose goals are not met with the foregoing regimens, a full insulin schedule should be initiated as a combined injection of NPH and regular insulin at least twice a day.

**II.  Therapeutic Monitoring**

A.  The objective of therapy is to maintain blood glucose at levels as near-normal as possible.

B.  Most stable type II diabetics treated with oral hypoglycemic agents may be adequately monitored with quarterly glycohemoglobin testing and office glucose checks.

C.  Insulin-treated type II diabetics should perform daily home blood glucose testing. Stable patients may be adequately monitored by one test per day performed at rotating times.

D.  **Goals for Glycemic Control In Non-Insulin Dependent (type II) Diabetes:**

|  | Normal | Goal value | Critical values |
|---|---|---|---|
| Fasting or preprandial plasma glucose (mg/dL) | <115 | <120 | <80 or >140 |
| Postprandial plasma glucose (mg/dL) | <140 | <180 | >180 |
| Glycosylated hemoglobin (%) | 4-6 | <7 | >8 |

E. **Additional Testing:**
   1. Urinalysis annually
   2. Timed urine collection specimen (24 h or overnight) for microalbuminuria annually in patients who have had diabetes for 5 yr or more. If albumin/creatinine ratio is abnormal, measure serum creatinine or urea nitrogen and assessment of glomerular filtration.
   3. Lipid profile should be checked after diabetes is diagnosed and glucose control established annually.
F. **Drugs That Antagonize Sulfonylurea Action and Cause Hyperglycemia:** Chronic alcohol use, rifampin, beta-Blockers, diuretics (thiazides, furosemide), estrogens, glucocorticoids, indomethacin, isoniazid, nicotinic acid, phenytoin, levothyroxine (Synthroid).

VIII. **Complications of Type II Diabetes**
   A. **Heart Disease, Stroke, and Peripheral Vascular Disease:**
      1. These disorders occur earlier and with greater frequency in diabetics. Angina is less likely to be symptomatic because of autonomic nervous system insufficiency.
      2. Treadmill stress tests should be considered in patients with risk factors for coronary artery disease.
      3. Hyperlipidemia should be treated more aggressively in diabetics. Niacin raises blood glucose and may therefore worsen diabetic control. Gemfibrozil (Lopid) is an excellent choice because it lowers triglycerides and raises HDL cholesterol.
   B. **Hypertension:**
      1. Hypertension should be treated more aggressively in diabetics.
      2. The angiotensin-converting enzyme inhibitors and the calcium channel blockers are the agents of first choice because they do not adversely affect glycemic or lipid profiles, they do not blunt the symptoms of hypoglycemia, and they may have a protective effect on diabetic nephropathy.
      3. **Second-line Agents:** Alpha blockers, such as terazosin (Hytrin), prazosin (Minipress), or doxazosin (Cardura), do not adversely affect glucose or lipids.
      4. Thiazide diuretics should be avoided in diabetics because they can raise glucose levels, adversely affect the lipid profile, and contribute to dehydration and hypokalemia.
      5. Beta blockers should be avoided because they adversely affect glycemic control and lipid profile, and may mask the symptoms of hypoglycemia.
   C. **Retinopathy:**
      1. 50% of all patients with diabetes have some degree of retinopathy after 10 years of disease. More than 80% of all patients with diabetes will have retinopathy 15 years after diagnosis.
      2. A dilated pupillary exam by an ophthalmologist should be done at the baseline evaluation, and yearly after 5 years of diabetes. Any rapid deterioration of visual acuity should be referred for ophthalmologic evaluation.
      3. Proliferative retinopathy is indicated by the development of new blood vessels and fibrous tissue. Proliferative retinopathy and hemorrhages lead to a loss of vision and dictate urgent ophthalmologic consultation.
   D. **Nephropathy:**
      1. In patients older than 40, the incidence of diabetic renal disease is 5 to 10%.
      2. Significant renal disease is heralded by the onset of microalbumninuria, which in turn leads to proteinuria and eventually to an elevation of BUN and creatinine.
      3. At the level of microalbuminuria, a reversal of nephropathy may be possible with careful diabetic control, lowering of blood pressure, and the use of ACE inhibitors or calcium channel blockers (even in normotensive patients).
      4. **Microalbuminuria Screening**
         a. Periodic screening for microalbuminuria in patients with either type I or type II diabetes is recommended. Microalbuminuria is a sensitive index of early nephropathy.
         b. Assessment of microalbuminuria is accomplished by checking urine

albumin/creatinine ratio checked annually on all diabetic patients.

   c. If albumin is high--exceeding 30 mg/g on at least two occasions--the adequacy of blood sugar and hemoglobin A1c levels should be reevaluated.

   d. If glycemic control is the best that can be achieved and microalbuminuria persists, an angiotensin-converting enzyme inhibitor should be given, even if the patient's blood pressure is normal.

E. **Neuropathy:**

   1. Foot problems are common in diabetic patients, and they should be instructed to regularly inspect their feet, and a foot examination should be a part of every clinic visit. The physician should check for neuropathy, vasculopathy, ulcers, or infection.

   2. The patient should be warned never to walk in bare feet and not to wear poorly fitting shoes. Patients with a history of diabetic foot problems should be instructed to wear only soft-soled shoes with a wide and high toe box.

# Hypothyroidism

## I. Clinical Evaluation

A. The most common cause of hypothyroidism is autoimmune thyroiditis. Other causes include radioactive iodine, thyroidectomy, thioamide drugs, and iodine ingestion. Transient hypothyroidism can occur in patients with acute thyroiditis.

B. **Symptoms of Hypothyroidism:** Fatigue, intolerance to cold, lethargy, drowsiness, constipation, dry skin, memory impairment, menstrual disorders, muscle cramps, weakness, weight gain.

C. **Physical Examination:** Bradycardia, brittle hair, cool dry skin, gravelly voice, hypothermia, large tongue, puffy face and hands, delayed relaxation phase of reflexes.

## II. Differential Diagnosis of Hypothyroidism

| Cause: | Clues to Diagnosis: |
|---|---|
| Autoimmune thyroiditis (Hashimoto's disease) | Family or personal history of autoimmune thyroiditis or goiter |
| Idiopathic (possible end-stage autoimmune disease) | |
| Iatrogenic: Ablation, medication, surgery | History of thyroidectomy, irradiation with iodine 131, or thioamide drug therapy |
| Diet (high levels of iodine) | Kelp consumption |
| Subacute thyroiditis (viral) | History of painful thyroid gland or neck |
| Postpartum thyroiditis | Symptoms of hyperthyroidism followed by hypothyroidism 6 months postpartum |

## III. Thyroid Function Tests

A. **Sensitive TSH assays:** Immunoradiometric assays can detect abnormally low or high TSH levels.

B. A sensitive TSH assay is the test of choice for screening when hypothyroidism is suspected.

C. Assessment of free T4 concentrations with a free T4 index or free T4 assay can confirm the diagnosis and rule out hypothyroidism secondary to pituitary or hypothalamic failure, which causes low levels of TSH and low levels of T4.

## IV. Subclinical Hypothyroidism

A. The diagnosis of hypothyroidism is straightforward when the TSH level is clearly elevated (>20 mcU/mL) and the free T4 level is decreased. Subclinical hypothyroidism is defined as a mildly elevated TSH level (5.1-20 mcU/mL) with a normal or slightly low free T4 level and no clinical signs of hypothyroidism. Most prevalent in the elderly and in women.

B. Treatment with levothyroxine (Synthroid) is recommended for all patients with subclinical hypothyroidism.

## V. Euthyroid Sick Syndrome

A. Alterations in thyroid function tests occur in euthyroid patients who have chronic and acute, non-thyroidal illness and catabolic states. Thyroid function tests are abnormal in up to 70% of all hospitalized patients. Medications can alter results of thyroid function tests.

B. If the patient has not received dopamine, corticosteroids, or T4 replacement therapy, a normal TSH value eliminates the possibility of primary hypothyroidism. A very high TSH level (>20 mcU/mL) with a low T4 concentration indicates hypothyroidism, and thyroid replacement therapy is appropriate.

## VI. Drugs that Affect Thyroid Function Testing

A. **Amiodarone HCl (Cordarone):** Induces hypothyroidism and hyperthyroidism; interferes with T4 metabolism

B. **Corticosteroids:** Suppress TSH; block conversion of T4 to T3

C. **Iodinated Cough Medications:** Can induce hypothyroidism

D. **Dopamine HCl (Dopastat, Intropin):** Suppresses TSH

E. **Lithium:** Induces hypothyroidism by blocking release of T4 and T3

F. **Phenytoin (Dilantin):** Interferes with binding of T4 to plasma proteins; may decrease free T4 level

**Laboratory Values, Diagnosis, and Management of Hypothyroid Disorders:**

| TSH (mcU/mL): | free T4: | Diagnosis: | Management: |
|---|---|---|---|
| High (>20) | Low or borderline | Primary hypothyroidism | Treatment and monitoring of TSH level |
| Borderline-high (5.1-20) | Low or normal | Possible hypothyroidism | Treatment or follow-up |
| Normal (0.3-5) | Low | Euthyroid sick syndrome | Follow-up |
| Low (<0.3) | High | Hyperthyroidism | Treatment |
| Low (<0.3) | Low | Possible pituitary or hypothalamic dysfunction | Evaluation of pituitary and hypothalamus with TRH stimulation test |

VII. **Treatment of Hypothyroidism**

A. Treatment with levothyroxine (Synthroid, Levoxine) is recommended. Desiccated thyroid preparations (Armour Thyroid), synthetic T3, and mixtures of T3 and T4 should be avoided.

B. The starting dose of levothyroxine (Synthroid) is 100 mcg (0.1 mg) per day in young, healthy patients. In elderly patients and in those at risk of coronary artery disease, the initial daily dose should be 25 to 50 mcg; increase slowly every 4-6 weeks, as tolerated, until the optimal dose of 75 to 150 mcg is reached. Check for manifestations of thyrotoxicity before any dosage increase.

C. TSH should be checked after equilibrium is established, usually after 4-6 weeks of treatment, or the last dosage change.

D. Periodic monitoring should be done every 6-12 months for patients who do not have symptoms. Serum TSH assay is the only test needed; a normal result implies adequate treatment. A low or undetectable TSH level indicates overtreatment. A TSH >20 mcU/mL indicates undertreatment or noncompliance.

E. Risks of treatment of hypothyroidism include exacerbation of existing angina, arrhythmias, myocardial infarction. Treatment may result in osteoporosis if desiccated thyroid preparations (Armour Thyroid) are used or if overtreatment occurs.

# Obesity

## I. Management of Obesity

### A. Restricted Diets:

1. A nutritionally adequate Low Calorie Diet (LCD) of 1200-1500 kcal/day or 12-15 kcal/kg/day, and weight loss of 0.5 kg/week is recommended for most patients.
2. Very-low-calorie diets (VLCD) of 800 kcal/day (6-10 kcal/kg body weight) must be conducted under close supervision; these diets are restricted to severely overweight persons.

### B. Altering the proportion of the calories from fat, carbohydrate, and protein can have a limited effect on weight loss; however, the effects are small in comparison with the direct effect of caloric restriction. There is no conclusive evidence to show that a diet high in fiber produces satiety or weight loss.

### C. Meal Frequency: Patients should consume more frequent, smaller meals.

### D. Nutrition Education: Education by a dietitian should be provided with emphasis on dietary restriction, and modifications of current eating habits. Encourage appropriate eating habits, nutritional intake, and a life-long adoption of a proper eating style.

### E. Exercise: Exercise is an important part of weight reduction programs as a way to increase energy expenditure; exercise diminishes the tendency for rapid post-program weight gain. 20-30 minute sessions to a minimum intensity of 60% of the maximum heart rate (200-age) at least 3 times a week is recommended. Aerobic exercise such as walking or swimming is preferable.

### F. Behavior Modification:

1. Behavior modification techniques include self-monitoring, stimulus control, cognitive restructuring, teaching the consequences of eating behavior, stress management, and improving self-esteem.
2. Behavior therapy involves 1) identifying eating or related life-style behaviors to be modified, 2) setting specific behavioral goals, 3) modifying determinants of the behavior to be changed, and 4) reinforcing the desired behavior. The goal of behavior treatment is to modify eating and physical activity habits, focusing on gradual changes.

## II. Drug Treatment of Obesity

### A. Appetite suppressant drugs are effective in suppressing appetite and inducing weight loss. When drug therapy is stopped, weight may be rapidly regained.

### B. Drug therapy combines two drugs--phentermine (Fastin, Adipex-P) and fenfluramine (Pondimin)--with exercise, dietary changes, and behavioral modification.

### C. Phentermine (Fastin):

1. Phentermine is an appetite suppressant, amphetamine derivative with significantly less sympathomimetic and stimulant activity than amphetamine. Given as an oral sustained release resin complex, peak plasma concentrations occur within 8 hours, therapeutic concentrations persist for at least 20 hours, with a t ½ of 20 to 24 hours.
2. Phentermine, given as a single 30 mg dose qAM, significantly reduces hunger ratings and food intake. Available as 30 mg capsules or tablets. DEA schedule IV.
3. Phentermine is more effective than placebo in promoting weight loss in patients with uncomplicated obesity and in obese diabetics.
4. Patients may regain lost weight when taken off the drugs, and some obese patients may need to be kept on diet medications for the rest of their lives.
5. Side effects are mainly minor and rarely require stopping treatment. Mild insomnia, nervousness, irritability, dry mouth, and headache are common. Depression, diarrhea, disorientation may occur. Side effects may be reduced by decreasing the dose.
6. Phentermine has been given successfully to patients with moderate hypertension and to diabetics.

D. **Fenfluramine (Pondimin)**
1. Fenfluramine (Pondimin) acts by partially inhibiting reuptake of serotonin and release of serotonin from nerve endings.
2. Its anorectic action appears to be mediated through activating serotoninergic rather than catecholaminergic pathways in the brain. Fenfluramine induces people to eat more slowly and to feel full earlier.
3. It has no stimulant activity, and it may have slight depressant effects. In addition to its central action, there is evidence that fenfluramine has a peripheral effect on muscle glucose uptake.
4. Fenfluramine has a t ½ of approximately 20 hours, and steady-state plasma concentrations are reached within 4 to 5 days.
5. Fenfluramine reduces hunger ratings in a dose-related manner following administration of single doses of 20, 40, and 80 mg. Food intake is significantly suppressed by single doses of 40, 60 and 80 mg.
6. Initial dosage is 20 mg PO tid; max 120 mg/d.
7. **Adverse Effects:** Gastrointestinal disturbances (nausea or diarrhea), drowsiness and lethargy are often experienced during the initial stages of treatment.
8. Abrupt withdrawal of fenfluramine can lead to severe depression; the dose should always be reduced gradually.
9. The incidence of adverse effects can be minimized by increasing the dose gradually over several weeks to the maximum tolerated dose.

III. **Controversial Weight Loss Therapies**
A. **Human Chorionic Gonadotrophin:** There is no evidence of any specific effect on weight loss.
B. **Gastric bubble or balloon** is no more effective than the low calorie diet. Weight lost is usually regained after removal.
C. **Liposuction:** Not a treatment for generalized obesity; used for the removal of localized areas of fat.

# Rheumatology and Hematology

## Low Back Pain and Osteoarthritis

**Initial Classification of Acute Low Back Symptoms**
A. **Potentially Serious Spinal Conditions:** Tumor, infection, spinal fracture, or a major neurologic compromise, such as cauda equina syndrome.
B. **Sciatica:** Back-related, lower limb symptoms suggesting lumbosacral nerve root compromise.
C. **Nonspecific Back Symptoms:** Occurring primarily in the back and suggesting neither nerve root compromise nor a serious underlying condition.
D. In the absence of signs of dangerous conditions, special studies are not required since 90% of patients will recover spontaneously within 4 weeks.
E. **Nonmechanical Causes of Low Back Pain:**
   1. **Rheumatologic Disease:** Polymyalgia rheumatica, fibrositis, ankylosing spondylitis, Reiter's syndrome, psoriatic arthritis, enteropathic arthritis.
   2. **Infection:** Vertebral osteomyelitis, diskitis, epidural abscess
   3. **Tumor:** Osteoma, multiple myeloma, skeletal metastases.
   4. **Endocrinologic and Metabolic Disorders:** Osteoporosis with fracture, osteomalacia.
   5. **Referred Pain:** Abdominal aortic aneurysm, kidney stone, pyelonephritis.
F. **Markers for Potentially Serious Conditions:**

| Fracture | Tumor or Infection | Cauda Equina Syndrome |
|---|---|---|
| Major trauma, such as a vehicle accident or fall from height. New onset or worsening of back pain after minor trauma or strenuous lifting in an older or potentially osteoporotic patient. | Age >50 or <20. History of cancer, fever, chills, weight loss. Pain worsens at rest or when supine; severe nighttime pain. Risk Factors for Spinal Infection: Recent bacterial infection, UTI, IV drug abuse, diabetics, immune suppression. | Saddle anesthesia. Bladder dysfunction (urinary retention, frequency, overflow incontinence). Severe or progressive neurologic deficit in the lower extremity. Laxity of the anal sphincter. Perianal/perineal sensory loss. Major motor weakness. |

**Clinical Evaluation of Low Back Pain**
A. Assess present symptoms, limitations, duration of symptoms, and history of previous episodes of pain or injury. Symptoms may include constant or intermittent pain, numbness, weakness, and stiffness located primarily in back, leg, or both.
B. Ascertain results of any previous testing or treatment.
C. Pain drawings and pain-rating scales may help further document the patient's perceptions and progress. Sciatica commonly follows a specific dermatome.
D. Sudden onset of pain is most likely to arise from a disk, while pain with a slow onset or with frequent, milder recurrences, is more likely to be ligamentous in origin.
E. Certain body positions or movements may exacerbate or relieve pain. Determine the time of day when pain appears. Herniated disk pain causes great difficulty sitting or bending, while pain of ligamentous origin causes inability to remain in any position for a long time without moving to relieve the pain.
F. Obtain an occupational and recreational history; assess degree of disability and modifications of activity. Determine how much weight the patient can lift.

G. Spinal stenosis is associated with vague bilateral leg pain that occurs with walking or standing.

## III. Physical Examination

A. **Observation and Regional Back Examination:**
   1. Severe guarding of lumbar motion in all planes may indicate spinal infection, tumor or fracture.
   2. Vertebral point tenderness to palpation may suggest fracture or infection.
   3. Assess range of motion of the back (disk problems tend to limit range of motion asymmetrically). Ask patient to bend forward, backward, and from side to side noting pain.
   4. Palpate the back to identify tender areas or trigger point areas over the interspinous, posterior sacroiliac, and iliolumbar ligaments. Disk problems often cause very little tenderness, while chronic ligament strains cause specific tender points.

B. **Neurologic Screening:**
   1. **Testing for Muscle Strength:**
      a. Ask patient to toe walk (calf muscles, S1 nerve root), heel walk (ankle and toe dorsiflexor muscles, L5 and some L4 nerve roots), squat and rise (quadriceps, L4 nerve root).
      b. Test the dorsiflexor muscles of the ankle or great toe (L5 or some L4 nerve root) hamstrings and ankle evertors (L5-S1), and toe flexors (S1).
   2. **Circumferential Measurements:** Muscle atrophy can be detected by measurements of the calf and thigh circumference. Differences of less than 2 cm may be normal.

C. **Reflexes:** Ankle jerk reflex tests the S1 nerve root; knee jerk reflex tests the L4 nerve root.

D. **Sensory Examination:** Test light touch or pressure in the medial (L4), dorsal (L5), and lateral (S1) aspects of the foot.

E. **Clinical Testing for Sciatic Tension:**
   1. Straight leg raising (SLR) test can detect tension on the L5 and/or S1 nerve root related to disc herniation.
   2. Sitting knee extension tests sciatic tension in the same way as SLR. Patients with significant nerve root irritation will have pain or will lean backward to reduce tension on the nerve.

F. Anal sphincter tone and sphincter reflex (scratching perianal area and watching for constriction) should be tested. Intact perianal innervation indicates intact bladder innervation. Failure to detect impairment of bladder innervation may result in bladder distention and permanent hypotonicity.

## IV. Initial Treatment of Low Back Pain

A. **Nonsteroidal Anti-inflammatory Drug Therapy:**
   1. The classification of NSAIDs by chemical class has little clinical significance for treating acute pain. Categorization of NSAIDs by half-life is more useful. When short-term analgesia is the primary goal, the key consideration is rapid onset. Athletic injuries and soft-tissue trauma are common conditions which require a rapid-onset NSAID.
   2. In patients with chronic mild to moderate pain, intermediate- and long-acting NSAIDs may improve compliance because of once- or twice-daily dosing. They are not recommended as first-line therapy in the elderly or those with compromised renal or hepatic function because of a greater risk of toxic accumulation. Long-acting NSAIDs are not useful for more severe pain.
   3. The newer NSAID drugs nabumetone and etodolac have not been reported to produce as many GI adverse effects. NSAIDs should be taken with food to reduce GI upset.
   4. A loading dose (usually twice the standard dose) is recommended for agents with a slower onset--naproxen, naproxen sodium, or diflunisal. Loading doses are unnecessary when using ibuprofen, ketoprofen, etodolac.

5. NSAIDs should be prescribed with caution in patients being treated with antihypertensives or anticoagulants.

## Dosages for NSAIDs with half-life <4 h

| Drug and Maximum Dosage | Dosage |
|---|---|
| Ibuprofen (Motrin) 3,200 mg/d | 300 mg qid; or 400 mg, 600 mg, or 800 mg tid or qid; usually the agent of choice |
| Ketoprofen (Orudis) 300 mg/d | 25-75 mg tid-qid |
| Tolmetin (Tolectin) 2,000 mg/d | 400 mg tid to start; 600-1,800 mg/d in 3-4 divided doses |
| Ketorolac (Toradol) 40 mg/d | 30-60 mg IM, followed by 15-30 mg IM q6h; max 120 mg/day; or 10 mg PO q6h prn [10 mg]. |

## Suggested Dosages for NSAIDs with Half-Life >5 h

### Half-Life 5-15 h

| | |
|---|---|
| Diflunisal (Dolobid) 1,500 mg/d | 1000 mg, followed by 500 mg q 8-12h |
| Etodolac (Lodine) 1,200 mg/d | 200-400 mg q6-8h |
| Diflunisal (Dolobid), 1,000 mg | 400 mg tid or bid; 300 mg qid, tid, or bid |
| Ketoprofen, extended release (Oruvail) 300 mg/d | 200 mg once a day |
| Naproxen sodium (Anaprox, Aleve) 1,375 mg/d | 550 mg, followed by 275 mg bid-tid |
| Naproxen (Naprosyn) 1,250 mg/d | 500 mg, followed by 250-500 q6-8h. [250, 375, 500 mg]; slower onset than naproxen sodium. |
| Sulindac (Clinoril) 400 mg/d | 150 mg bid |

### Half-Life >15 h

| | |
|---|---|
| Nabumetone (Relafen) 2,000 mg/d | Starting dose, 1,000 mg taken as a single dose, then 500-750 mg qd-bid. [500, 750 mg]. |
| Piroxicam (Feldene) 20 mg/d | 20 mg/d in a single dose [10,20 mg] |

B. **Management of NSAID Therapy:**
1. Patients receiving NSAIDs over a long period of time should be monitored for occult blood loss. After obtaining a baseline hematocrit, repeat every 6-12 months. Chemistry profile including electrolytes and urinalysis are recommended if an NSAID is to be used chronically.
2. Hepatic toxicity from NSAID therapy occurs less frequently than renal toxicity. Liver function tests should be done at 6-12-month intervals.
3. If the desired effect is not achieved after two weeks, consider an increase in dosage. If the therapy is still unsatisfactory, switch to another NSAID with a similar half-life.
4. If full dosages of an NSAID fail to provide adequate relief, consider adding acetaminophen 650-1,000 mg q4h concurrently; the effect of both drugs may be synergistic. Acetaminophen spares the gastric mucosa, but has the potential for hepatic toxicity.
5. An NSAID may be used in conjunction with propoxyphene HCL (Darvon) or another narcotic analgesic with the NSAID taken regularly and the narcotic agent taken prn.

C. **Lessening the Risk of Gastric Ulceration:**
1. **H2-Blockers:**
   Ranitidine (Zantac) 150 mg hs. The patient can add another 150-mg dose in the morning if symptoms persist.
   Cimetidine (Tagamet) is given 400 mg hs

Famotidine (Pepcid) is 20 mg hs
Nizatidine (Axid) can be prescribed at 150 mg hs

2. Misoprostol (Cytotec) is the prophylactic agent of choice to prevent NSAID-induced gastric ulcers in high-risk patients. Can cause colic and diarrhea. Contraindicated in pregnancy, irritable bowel syndrome. The dosage of misoprostol should usually be adjusted from a test dosage of 100 mcg 2-4 times daily taken with food. Recommended dosage is 100-200 mcg qid.

D. **Muscle Relaxants:** Muscle relaxants seem no more effective than NSAIDs for low back symptoms, and using them in combination with NSAIDs has no demonstrated benefit. Side effects including drowsiness. Should only be prescribed for less than one week.
   -Cyclobenzaprine (Flexeril) 10 mg PO tid [10 mg];
   -Methocarbamol (Robaxin) 500-750 mg PO bid-tid [500, 750 mg].
   -Carisoprodol (Soma) 350 mg PO tid-qid [350 mg]

E. **Antidepressants:**
   1. Patients with chronic pain frequently benefit from low-dose amitriptyline (Elavil) or another tricyclic in addition to their pain medication.
   2. Imipramine (Tofranil) may also offer pain relief 50-150 mg PO qhs [10, 25, 50 mg], fluoxetine (Prozac) may also be useful; 20 mg PO qAM.

## V. Physical Methods

A. **Activity Alteration:**
   1. Most patients will not require bed rest. Prolonged bed rest (more than 4 days) has potentially debilitating effects, and its efficacy is unproven. Two to four days of bed rest are reserved for patients with the most severe limitations (due primarily to leg pain).
   2. Patients can minimize the stress of lifting by keeping any lifted object close to the body at the level of the navel. Twisting, bending, and reaching while lifting also increase stress on the back. Patients should avoid prolonged sitting. A soft support placed at the small of the back and armrests to support some body weight may make sitting more comfortable.
   3. After acute inflammation has subsided, extension and flexion exercises should be used to increase strength and flexibility in the back. Aerobic exercise such as walking, swimming, and light jogging may be recommended to help avoid debilitation from inactivity.

B. Traction applied to the spine is not effective for treating acute low back symptoms. Massage, diathermy, ultrasound, biofeedback, transcutaneous electrical nerve stimulation (TENS), low back corsets and back belts have no proven efficacy.

C. Needle acupuncture and injection of steroids or lidocaine, in the epidural space have no proven benefit.

D. Shoe lifts are not effective in treating acute low back symptoms when the difference in lower limb length is less than 2 cm.

E. Soft shoe insoles are an option for patients who must stand for prolonged periods.

## VI. Special Diagnostic Studies

A. Routine testing and imaging studies are not recommended during the first month of back symptoms except when there is a suspicion of a dangerous condition. If a patient's limitations, due to low back symptoms, do not improve in 4 weeks, reassessment and further diagnostic studies may be indicated.

B. **Laboratory Tests:** Erythrocyte sedimentation rate, complete blood count, and urinalysis (UA) can be useful to screen for suspected infection, tumor, or rheumatologic conditions.

C. **Imaging:** MRI or CT-scan should be considered if there are definitive nerve findings on physical examination and when surgery is being considered.

D. **Lumbosacral radiographs** are usually not helpful.

E. **Bone Scan:** Rarely useful, but can detect suspected spinal tumors, infection, or occult fractures.

F. **Electromyography (EMG):** May be useful to identify focal neurologic dysfunction in patients with leg symptoms lasting longer than 3-4 weeks.

G. **Sensory Evoked Potentials (SEPs):** May be indicated if spinal stenosis or spinal cord myelopathy is suspected.

VII. **Surgical Considerations**
  A. **Criteria for Nerve Root Decompression:**
   1. Sciatica is both severe and disabling.
   2. Symptoms of sciatica persist without improvement for longer than 4 weeks or with extreme progression.
   3. There is strong physiologic evidence of dysfunction of a specific nerve root with intervertebral disc herniation confirmed by an imaging study.   .
  B. Surgery is an elective procedure unless progressive motor deficits, cauda equina syndrome or other emergency is present.
  C. Consider urgent orthopedic referral if severe, unremitting leg pain is unresponsive to physical therapy, or if significant acute neurologic deficits, especially in the distribution of S1 and S2, because of the risk of bladder hypotonicity.

# Gout

## I. Etiology of Gout

A. Hyperuricemia and deposition of uric acid crystals in connective tissue can result from any disturbance that increases the synthesis of uric acid or decreases the excretion of uric acid.

B. **Causes of Hyperuricemia:** Overproduction of uric acid occurs in some genetic conditions (enzyme disorders of purine metabolism), however, the great majority of patients with gout have decreased renal excretion of uric acid. Other causes include hematologic malignancy, alcohol abuse, and use of diuretics that decrease urate excretion.

## II. Epidemiology

A. Gout occurs mainly in middle-aged men. The peak onset is between ages 30 and 49 in men, and after menopause in women.

B. Hyperuricemia is the primary risk factor for gout, as designated by a serum uric acid concentration $\geq 7$ mg/dL in men, or $\geq 6$ mg/dL or greater in women. Increased serum urate levels do not invariably lead to crystal deposition.

## III. Stages of Gout

A. **Acute Gouty Arthritis:**

1. An acute arthritis affecting a single joint is the typical presentation. About half of all initial attacks involve podagra--inflammation of the great toe.
2. **Other Common Sites:** Ankle, heel, instep, and knee. The arms and hands are less frequently affected.
3. Usually begins abruptly in a single joint, often during the night, and is characterized by a very painful, swollen, warm, red, and tender joint. 80% to 90% of initial gouty attacks are monarticular and may be accompanied by low-grade fever, elevated ESR and increased WBC count.
4. Attacks of gout subside in 3-10 days, even without treatment.

B. **Intercritical Period:** Following resolution of the inflammation, the patient enters a symptom-free interval between acute gout attacks. Most patients experience another attack within months or years.

C. **Chronic Tophaceous Gout:**

1. Tophi (deposits of urate crystals) involving the joints may cause a destructive arthropathy if patients are not treated.
2. Developing over years (about 10 years), tophi occur most commonly in the olecranon bursa, Achilles tendon, extensor forearm surfaces, and in the ear helix.
3. May cause deforming arthritis, and renal disease is a potential problem in late phases; crystals deposit in the renal interstitium, and uric acid stones form in collecting ducts.

## IV. Diagnosis of Acute Gouty Arthritis

A. **Joint Aspiration:** Identification of uric acid crystals is the best way to establish the diagnosis of gout. An infectious cause should be ruled out; however, infection may rarely coexist with gout.

B. Prepare a wet mount, and examine the fluid under a compensated, polarizing microscope. Gout is diagnosed by finding uric acid crystals that are needle-shaped and negatively birefringent; they appear yellow when the long axis is parallel to the axis of the first ordered compensator. Identification of crystals within polymorphonuclear leukocytes is diagnostic for gout.

C. If polarized microscopy is not available, look for needle-shaped crystals under a regular light microscope, but such identification is not specific for gout. Light microscopy of Gram stain, and culture of the aspirate may be used to exclude an infectious cause.

D. Radiologic studies are not clinically helpful in the diagnosis of gout.

E. Serum uric acid concentration may not be elevated during acute gout; the level is normal in 25% of acute attacks. Conversely, an elevated serum uric acid level alone cannot serve as a sole criterion for the diagnosis of gout.

F. **When Fluid Cannot Be Aspirated from the Affected Joint, a Presumptive Diagnosis of Gout Is Supported by the Following Factors:**
   1. Prior history of acute monarticular arthritis (especially of the big toe) followed by a symptom-free period.
   2. Hyperuricemia.
   3. Rapid resolution of symptoms after colchicine therapy.
G. **Tophi** should be carefully searched for in patients with acute monarthritis. Tophi are classically found in the helix of the ear. Other locations include the ulnar aspect of the forearm, olecranal and prepatellar bursae, Achilles tendons, and hands.
H. Acute gout may follow excessive alcohol, or repetitive joint trauma, or may follow the introduction of medication to lower uric acid levels. Patients with acute monarthritis in the postoperative period also often have gout.

## Therapy For Acute Gouty Arthritis

A. **NSAIDs** are the drugs of choice in acute gout and they are highly effective.
B. Indomethacin is the drug of choice because of its short half-life and ease of administration; 50 mg PO tid with meals; other rapid acting NSAID's such as ibuprofen may also be used.
C. Administer the maximum dosage of the NSAID until symptoms are relieved (approximately 4 to 5 days), then taper over 2 weeks and discontinue.
D. Hypouricemic drugs (allopurinol) are contraindicated during an acute attack because they may exacerbate the attack. However, do not discontinue hypouricemic agents unless they were recently started and may have caused the attack.
E. If NSAIDs are contraindicated (active peptic ulcer disease, recent GI bleeding, renal insufficiency, hypersensitivity, concomitant anticoagulant medication) or if they are ineffective, glucocorticoids may be used for acute gout.
   1. Oral prednisone may be used if only one joint is involved, 40 mg/d PO for 3-5 days; then gradually taper by 5 mg/d over the next 10-14 days, and discontinue; or give an intraarticular injection of triamcinolone (10-40 mg depending on size of joint). Never inject glucocorticoids into an infected joint.
   2. Corticotropin, 40 to 80 IU IM in a single injection, is beneficial for acute gout when two or more joints are involved.
F. **Colchicine:**
   1. Although colchicine is highly effective, it is not recommended for acute gout because of its side effects (nausea, vomiting, diarrhea, abdominal discomfort in 80%) and because of its high toxicity relative to that of NSAIDs or glucocorticoids. Not useful in attacks lasting longer than 5 days.
   2. Colchicine 0.5 mg PO every hour until relief or side effects occur. Maximum total dose 5-6 mg; reduce dose in elderly or renal or hepatic disease.

## Therapy For Chronic Gout

A. **Diet:** Alcohol intake should be reduced, and patients should limit foods that are extremely high in purine, such as organ meats, anchovies, and shellfish.
B. **Colchicine** is recommended for prophylaxis in patients who have recurrent attacks of gouty arthritis. A low dosage (0.6 mg, once or twice daily) is usually well tolerated; 0.6 mg/d if renal insufficiency.
C. **Hypouricemic Therapy** should be started when colchicine alone has failed to prevent a second episode of acute gout.
   1. **Probenecid:**
      a. Probenecid increases renal excretion of uric acid and may be used when there is evidence of decreased uric acid excretion (as measured in a 24-hour collection).
      b. Administer colchicine (0.6 mg/d) for at least 14 days before starting the uricosuric agent to avoid exacerbating acute gouty arthritis.
      c. Start probenecid at 250 mg bid. Increase the dosage to 500 mg bid after 1 week, then increase by 500-mg increments every 4 weeks while monitoring the serum uric acid level, which should be maintained below 6.5 mg/dL. Max dose 1 g bid; average maintenance dosage is 500 mg bid.

    d. Patients should drink ample fluid daily to decrease the likelihood of stone formation. Probenecid is contraindicated if decreased renal function or nephrolithiasis. Common side effects are GI upset and rash.

2. **Allopurinol:**

    a. Allopurinol decreases serum uric acid by reducing production. It is extremely effective, but should be used only for the following patients:

    Over age 60 (among whom there is a high incidence of renal insufficiency)
    Increased uric acid production (>800 mg in 24 hour urine collection)
    Renal insufficiency (creatinine clearance <50 mL/min)
    History of kidney stones
    Gouty nephropathy
    Severe tophaceous deposits
    Tumor lysis syndrome
    Intolerance or to uricosuric agents
    Resistance to uricosuric agents

    b. Initiation of allopurinol may exacerbate an acute attack of gout by altering uric acid metabolism. Therefore, colchicine (0.6 mg/d) should be administered for at least 14 days preceding initiation of allopurinol.

    c. Start allopurinol at 100 mg/d; increase by 100-mg increments per week until uric acid levels are <6.5 mg/dL. Max 800 mg/d. The usual maintenance dosage is 300 mg/d; reduce dosage if renal insufficiency.

    d. The most common side effects are a benign erythematous rash and GI intolerance. Exfoliative dermatitis and toxic epidermal necrolysis have been reported. Other less common side effects include bone marrow suppression, hepatitis, jaundice and vasculitis.

## VII. Asymptomatic Hyperuricemia

A. Hyperuricemia (serum urate >7 mg/dL in men, >6 mg/dL in women) without evidence of gout or renal disease should be managed with dietary modifications (weight loss, restriction of organ meat, decreased alcohol) rather than pharmacologic therapy.

B. Hypouricemic agents should be used only if actual gouty arthritis has occurred.

C. Allopurinol may be used if profuse overproduction and overexcretion of urate occurs.

## VIII. Calcium Pyrophosphate Dihydrate Crystal Disease

A. Calcium pyrophosphate dihydrate crystal disease may resemble gout. The diagnosis is confirmed by synovial fluid analysis. CPPD crystals are more pleomorphic than uric acid crystals, commonly rod or rhomboid-like in shape, and, unlike uric acid, are fairly birefringent and show positive elongation under compensated polarized light.

B. Synovial fluid white blood cell counts are usually less than 50,000/mm$^3$ in CPPD disease. Rule out joint infection if signs of septic arthritis.

C. **Treatment of CPPD Joint Deposition Disease:**

1. NSAID's such as indomethacin are the first choice for acute treatment.
2. Effusion aspiration, alone or with intra-articular corticosteroid injection, often provides relief.
3. **If Attacks Are Frequent:** NSAID's or colchicine can be used for prophylaxis in a dose similar to that used for gout.

# Rheumatoid Arthritis

### Pathophysiology
A. Rheumatoid arthritis (RA) is a chronic systemic inflammatory disease with a prevalence of 1%. It affects the synovial lined joints and can also affect the pulmonary, cardiac, nervous, integumentary, and reticuloendothelial systems.
B. RA is 2-4 times more common in women than men, and the incidence increases with advancing age.
C. 75% of patients with RA have circulating rheumatoid factor (RF).

### Clinical Evaluation of Rheumatoid Arthritis
A. Malaise and fatigue are common symptoms of RA and a symmetric pattern of joint inflammation commonly affects the wrists, metacarpalphalangeal and proximal interphalangeal joints of the hands, elbows, shoulders, cervical spine, hips, knees, ankles, and metatarsalphalangeal joints of the feet. RA usually spares the distal interphalangeal joints.
B. Pain and stiffness of the involved joints is the dominant symptom; a phenomenon known as "gelling" often occurs in which the joints are more stiff after a period of rest, such as in the morning. Swelling, warmth, and tenderness with motion or palpation of the involved joints often occurs.
C. Frequent joint effusions and palpable synovial hypertrophy are found. Subcutaneous rheumatoid nodules may occur at pressure points, such as on the olecranon.
D. With longstanding disease, multiple joint deformities may often occur requiring joint replacement surgery. Osteoporosis may develop, particularly if steroids have been used.

### Laboratory Findings
A. Mild anemia of chronic disease, elevated sedimentation rate, and a positive rheumatoid factor are characteristic. Synovial fluid white cell counts of 5,000-20,000/mcL with 50% neutrophils occur.
B. X-ray Findings: Erosions of bone are common; periarticular osteopenia is seen first in the hands and feet. Erosion of the lateral aspect of the head of the fifth metatarsal, and joint space narrowing due to loss of articular cartilage are common.

### Complications of Rheumatoid Arthritis
A. Vasculitic lesions manifest as infarcts of the digital pulp, postcapillary venulitis, or leukocytoclastic vasculitis. Vasculitis affects the peripheral nerves, resulting in mononeuritis multiplex and foot or wrist drop.
B. Pericarditis and, rarely, pericardial tamponade may occur. Exudative pleural effusions are typified by low glucose levels.
C. Pulmonary nodules may occur in the subpleural area or intraparenchymally. Interstitial fibrosis and pneumonitis sometimes occur.
D. Dry eyes, episcleritis, or scleritis may occur.
E. High-titer RF levels are associated with more severe disease.

### Treatment of Rheumatoid Arthritis
A. Regular physical/occupational therapy should be instituted very early in the disease process.
B. Medications can be divided into those that can provide symptomatic relief and those that may modify disease.
C. First Line Symptomatic Therapy: Nonsteroidal anti-inflammatory drugs (NSAID's) and glucocorticoids.
D. Second Line Therapy: Hydroxychloroquine.
E. Third Line Therapy:
   1. Parenteral gold compounds or methotrexate. Methotrexate has the advantages of rapid onset of action within weeks, and convenient once-weekly oral dosing.
   2. Azathioprine should be added if there has been failure to respond to gold or methotrexate, or both.

3. If severe, progressive, refractory disease, add cyclophosphamide or cyclosporine.

F. **Surgical Therapy:** Tenosynovectomy, tendon repair, and joint replacement may be required in severe disease.

G. **Nonsteroidal Anti-inflammatory Drugs (NSAID's):**
   1. Classification of these drugs by their chemical structure predicts neither clinical response nor toxicity in an individual patient. The selection of a particular NSAID is largely empiric. An adequate clinical trial of at least two weeks and maximum dose is necessary; combination therapy should not be used because of increased toxicity.
   2. **Laboratory Monitoring:** Complete blood count and serum chemistry profile should be obtained every 6 months for patients on chronic NSAID therapy.
   3. **Carboxylic Acid Derivatives:**
      -Meclofenamate sodium (Meclomen) 200-400 mg/d divided tid or qid
      -Mefenamic acid (Ponstel) 250 mg PO qid [250 mg].
   4. **Salicylates:**
      -Salicylate combination (Trilisate) 1 tab PO q4-8h [500, 750, 1000 mg].
      -Salsalate (Disalcid) 3000 mg/d in divided doses bid-tid [500, 750 mg].
      -Magnesium Salicylate (Magan) 650 mg PO q4h or 1000 mg tid [325, 500, 545, 600 mg].
      -Diflunisal (Dolobid) 1,000 mg loading dose, then 500 mg PO bid [250, 500 mg].
   5. **Acetic Acids:**
      -Diclofenac (Voltaren) 50 mg PO bid-tid [25, 50, 75 mg].
      -Nabumetone (Relafen) initial dose 1000 mg PO qd with or without food; 1000 mg PO qd-bid [500, 750 mg].
      -Sulindac (Clinoril) 150-200 mg PO bid [150, 200 mg].
      -Tolmetin (Tolectin) 600-1800 mg/d divided tid
   6. **Propionic Acids:**
      -Fenoprofen calcium (Nalfon) 1200-3200 mg/d divided tid-qid
      -Flurbiprofen (Ansaid) 50-100 mg PO bid-qid [50, 100 mg].
      -Ibuprofen (Motrin) 300-800 mg PO qid [200, 300, 400, 600, 800 mg].
      -Ketoprofen (Orudis) 50-75 mg PO tid [25, 50, 75 mg].
      -Naproxen (Naprosyn) 250-500 mg PO bid-tid [250, 375, 500 mg].
      -Naproxen Sodium (Anaprox) 275-550 mg PO tid-qid [275, 550 mg].
      -Oxaprozin (Daypro) 1200-1800 mg/d PO qd
   7. **Pyranocarboxylic Acid and Enolic Acid Derivatives:**
      -Etodolac (Lodine) 200-400 mg PO tid-qid [200 mg].
      -Piroxicam (Feldene) 10-20 mg PO qd [10, 20 mg].
   8. **Pyrrolopyrrole:**
      -Ketorolac (Toradol) loading dose 30-60 mg IM, followed by 15-30 mg IM q6h; max 120 mg/day [15, 30 mg/mL]; or 10 mg PO q6h prn, max 40 mg PO qd [10 mg].

H. **Systemic Corticosteroid Treatment of Rheumatoid Arthritis:**
   1. Intraarticular injection of a long-acting corticosteroid may provide palliative, temporary relief. Triamcinolone hexacetonide [Aristospan], 40 mg, max 2-3 injections a year.
   2. Low-dose prednisone (2.5-10 mg/day) or a short course of high dose pulse methylprednisolone (Solu-Medrol) 1,000 mg/day IV for 2 or 3 days may be used for severe cases of rheumatoid arthritis.
   3. Use corticosteroids only if unable to achieve symptom control with NSAID's. Dramatic symptomatic improvement may result; does not modify the disease process and long-term toxic effects are common.

I. **Disease-Modifying Anti-Rheumatic Drugs for Rheumatoid Arthritis**
   1. **Hydroxychloroquine:**
      a. Improvement occurs in about 50%; well tolerated; used in conjunction with NSAID's in mild to moderate disease. Nausea may occur occasionally.
      b. Ocular toxicity is uncommon and reversible; ophthalmologic examination is required every 6 months for the first year then annually.

   c. 400 mg/day in divided doses.
2. **Methotrexate:**
   a. Low-dose methotrexate therapy is often the initial disease-modifying treatment; it has a rapid onset of action, good efficacy, and is well tolerated. Nausea, vomiting, and stomatitis may occur. Hepatic fibrosis may develop in 30% after extended periods.
   b. Measure complete blood count, liver function tests, prothrombin time, and albumin every 4-6 weeks. Liver biopsy may be indicated after 2 years of therapy.
   c. Abrupt onset of pulmonary interstitial fibrosis is less common than hepatotoxicity, but potentially fatal unless the drug is discontinued.
   d. **Dosage:** 7.5 mg/wk, as single IM dose weekly, or 2.5 mg at 12-hr intervals (up to 22.5 mg/wk). Concomitant use of folic acid may reduce mucocutaneous side effects.
   e. Usually combined with a nonsteroidal anti-inflammatory drug. Low doses of prednisone may be used with MTX during the initial 6-8 weeks it takes for MTX to achieve efficacy.
3. **Gold Compounds:**
   a. Maximum response may not occur for as long as 3 months.
   b. **Adverse reactions:** Rash, pruritus, oral ulcers, weakness, dizziness, nausea, vomiting, flushing. A CBC and urinalysis should be checked regularly.
   c. **Dosage:** 10 mg/wk IM, increasing to 50 mg/wk IM to cumulative dose of 1 g; or oral (Auranofin), 3 mg PO bid.
4. **Azathioprine:**
   a. Commonly used when gold or methotrexate therapy has failed.
   b. Bone marrow suppression may occur; check complete blood cell count monthly.
   c. **Dosage:** 1 mg/kg (50-100 mg) daily as single dose; may increase after 6-8 wk.

# Deep Venous Thrombosis

## I. Pathophysiology

A. If venous thrombi of the lower extremely are not treated, 50% may embolize to the lung. The source of symptomatic pulmonary emboli is usually thrombosis in the larger veins above the knee rather than thrombosis in the veins of the calf.

B. Deep venous thrombosis can be found in at least 80% of pulmonary emboli.

## II. Risk Factors for Deep Venous Thrombosis

A. **Venous Stasis:** Prolonged immobilization, stroke, myocardial infarction, heart failure, obesity, varicose veins, anesthesia, age > 65 years old.

B. **Endothelial Injury:** Surgery, trauma, central venous access catheters, pacemaker wires, previous thromboembolic event (especially if precipitating factors are not eliminated).

C. **Hypercoagulable State:** Malignant disease, high estrogen level (pregnancy, oral contraceptives).

D. **Hematologic Disorders:** Polycythemia, leukocytosis, thrombocytosis, antithrombin III deficiency, protein C deficiency, protein S deficiency, antiphospholipid syndrome, inflammatory bowel disease.

## III. Signs and Symptoms of Deep Venous Thrombosis

A. Signs and symptoms of DVT are absent in about 50%, and they range from subtle to obvious.

B. May be asymptomatic or the patient may complain of pain, swelling, "heaviness," aching, or the sudden appearance of varicose veins. Recognized risk factors may be absent.

C. DVT may be characterized by an edematous limb with a erythrocyanotic appearance, dilated superficial veins, elevated skin temperature, tenderness in the thigh or calf. Absence of clinical signs does not preclude the diagnosis.

D. A swollen, tender leg with a palpable venous "cord" in the popliteal fossa strongly suggests popliteal DVT. The lack of a palpable cord does not rule out DVT. Marked discrepancy in limb circumference supports the diagnosis of DVT, but most patients do not have measurable swelling.

E. The clinical diagnosis of DVT is correct only 50% of the time; therefore, diagnostic testing is mandatory.

## IV. Diagnostic Testing

A. **Impedance Plethysmography** depends on the detection of impaired venous emptying of the leg. High false negative rate, and over 30% of cases may be missed. Plethysmography must be used in conjunction with duplex scanning.

B. **Duplex Scanning:**
1. **Doppler Studies:** Uses Doppler shifts to detect blood flow in the veins.
2. **Ultrasound Imaging:** Two-dimensional ultrasonography produces an image of the deep veins.
3. When Doppler measurement of blood flow is added to ultrasound imaging, the combination is referred to as a duplex scan.

C. When results of impedance plethysmography and duplex scanning are positive, these techniques are adequately specific. Results that do not support the clinical impression should be investigated with venography.

D. **Contrast Venography:**
1. When impedance plethysmography and ultrasound techniques fail to demonstrate a thrombus, venography is the diagnostic "gold standard" for patients at high clinical risk. The test is negative if contrast medium is seen throughout the deep venous system.
2. Venography can cause iatrogenic venous thrombosis in 4%, and allergic contrast reactions occur in 3% of patients.

E. **MRI** is a relatively new approach to the detection of DVT. MRI may have an accuracy comparable to that of contrast venography, and it may soon replace contrast venography as the "gold standard" of venous imaging.

# V. Treatment of Deep Vein Thrombosis

## A. Heparin Anticoagulation:

1. Continuous intravenous heparin is the standard of therapy for deep venous thrombosis at any site.
2. Anticoagulant therapy should be initiated as soon as venous thrombosis is clinically recognized as likely while awaiting the completion of a diagnostic workup.
3. The amount of heparin needed for effective anticoagulation is higher than was once taught; a 5,000-U bolus and a drip of 1,000 U/hr usually does not produce a therapeutic aPTT within the first 48 hours.
4. **Initial Bolus:** 10,000 U of heparin by intravenous push
5. **Initial Maintenance Drip:**
   Mix 20,000 U of heparin in 500 cc of D5W or normal saline (40 U/cc)
   Start drip beginning at 32 cc/hr (1,280 U/hr)
6. Check aPTT 6 hr after giving initial bolus. **Therapeutic Range:** Activated PTT 1.5-2.0 times control.
7. **Maintenance Dose Adjustment:**

| aPTT | Hold drip | Adjust drip | Check aPTT |
|---|---|---|---|
| <50 sec | 0 min | Increase 3 cc/hr | 6 hr later |
| 50-59 sec | 0 min | Increase 3 cc/hr | 6 hr later |
| 60-85 sec | 0 min | No change | Next morning |
| 86-95 sec | 0 min | Decrease 2 cc/hr | Next morning |
| 96-120 sec | 30 min | Decrease 2 cc/hr | 6 hr later |
| >120 sec | 60 min | Decrease 4 cc/hr | 6 hr later |

8. Heparin must be continued until the anticoagulant effects of warfarin have become established (usually 3 to 5 days after initiation). Subcutaneous low-molecular weight heparin may replace intravenous heparin in the next few years but is not generally available at present.
9. Monitor platelet count during heparin therapy; thrombocytopenia develops in up to 5%. Heparin rarely induces hyperkalemia, which resolves spontaneously upon discontinuation. Ambulation can begin once the activated PTT is in the therapeutic range.

## B. Oral Anticoagulants:

1. Oral anticoagulants should be started only after effective anticoagulation with heparin has been established because they increase coagulability and thrombogenesis during the first few days of administration. There is a high incidence of progressive thrombosis and embolization when oral warfarin is started without adequate prior heparinization.
2. **Warfarin (Coumadin)**, initial dose 10 mg; subsequent doses should be based on a daily PT values and its rate of change.
3. After heparin therapy has overlapped with warfarin therapy for 3-5 days and the PT is 1.3-1.5 times control (or International Normalized Ratio 2.0-3.0), heparin can be safely discontinued. Outpatients receiving oral anticoagulants should have their PT checked weekly.
4. **Length of Warfarin Therapy:** Oral anticoagulation should be maintained for 3 months after a first episode of DVT or pulmonary embolism. Indications to prolong therapy to 6-12 months include persistent risk factors, extensive or complicated thrombosis, or recurrent thrombotic episodes.

## C. Thrombolytic Therapy:

1. Thrombolytics clear the thrombus more rapidly, and preserve venous valvular function.
2. **Indications for Thrombolytics in DVT:**
   a. Patients with extensive DVT.
   b. Those with severe venous outflow obstruction (phlegmasia cerulea dolens).
3. **Contraindications to Thrombolytics:**
   a. **Absolute Contraindications:** Active bleeding, recent stroke, central nervous

system tumor.
   b. **Relative Contraindications:** Surgical procedure within preceding 10 days; recent gastrointestinal bleeding; uncontrolled hypertension; recent trauma (cardiopulmonary resuscitation), pregnancy, endocarditis, renal or hepatic failure, left-sided heart thrombus.
4. The thrombus should usually be demonstrated by venography before thrombolytics are used.
5. The agent should be delivered as close to the thrombus as possible. Catheter-induced thrombosis in the axillary or subclavian vein or superior vena cava can best be lysed by direct infusion through the involved catheter.
6. Monitor complete blood count, PT or international normalized ratio (INR), activated PTT, and fibrinogen levels twice daily.
7. **Streptokinase:** Duration required for complete clot lysis is substantially longer with streptokinase than with tissue plasminogen activator (tPA); much less expensive than tPA. **Dosage:** bolus of 250,000 U IV followed by 100,000 U/hr
8. **Tissue Plasminogen Activator:** tPA is "clot-selective", and may promote clot lysis more rapidly than other agents. **Dosage:** 100 mg over a 2-3 hour period.

D. **Thrombectomy** for DVT may be indicated for phlegmasia cerulea dolens (severe DVT) after thrombolytic therapy has failed.

E. **Vena Caval Interruption Methods:**
   1. Pulmonary embolism can be prevented by percutaneous filter interruption of the inferior vena cava. Filters have a patency rate of 95% and are effective in preventing 95% of emboli.
   2. **Indications for Vena Cava Filter:** Pulmonary embolism despite adequate anticoagulation, contraindications to anticoagulants, prevention of recurrent pulmonary embolism in high-risk patients.

## VI. Superficial Non-Septic Phlebitis
1. Patients with isolated thrombosis in a calf vein or with purely superficial phlebitis should remain ambulatory and wear compression stockings.
2. Patients with superficial non-septic phlebitis, in whom ultrasound imaging has excluded deep-system thrombosis, may be treated with nonsteroidal anti-inflammatory drugs.

## VII. Prevention of Deep Vein Thrombosis
A. Prophylaxis should be given to patients at risk (most hospitalized patients).
B. Low dose of heparin (5,000 U subcutaneously every 12 hours) or pneumatic compression stockings are effective in reducing the occurrence of thrombosis.

# Pulmonary Embolism

## I. Pathophysiology
A. Pulmonary embolism is usually caused by an embolism from a thrombosis in the larger veins above the knee.
B. A deep venous thrombosis can be found in at least 80% of cases of pulmonary emboli.

## II. Risk Factors For Pulmonary Embolism
A. **Venous Stasis:** Prolonged immobilization, stroke, myocardial infarction, heart failure, obesity, varicose veins, anesthesia, age > 65 years old.
B. **Endothelial Injury:** Surgery, trauma, central venous access catheters, pacemaker wires, previous thromboembolic event.
C. **Hypercoagulable State:** Malignant disease, high estrogen level (pregnancy, oral contraceptives).
D. **Hematologic Disorders:** Polycythemia, leukocytosis, thrombocytosis, antithrombin III deficiency, protein C deficiency, protein S deficiency, antiphospholipid syndrome, inflammatory bowel disease.

## IV. Diagnosis of Pulmonary Embolism
A. **Signs and Symptoms of Pulmonary Embolism:** Pleuritic chest pain, shortness of breath, tachycardia, hypoxemia, hypotension, hemoptysis, cough, syncope.
B. Classic triad of dyspnea, chest pain, and hemoptysis is seen in 20% of patients; the majority of patients have only a few subtle or ambiguous symptoms. Most pulmonary emboli are clinically inapparent or completely asymptomatic.
C. A deep venous thrombosis may be indicated by an edematous limb with an erythrocyanotic appearance, dilated superficial veins, and elevated skin temperature.
D. The best diagnostic approach to pulmonary embolism is search for an alternative diagnosis that can be more readily proved. If this is accomplished, the workup for pulmonary embolism can be brought to a close. However, if no other satisfactory explanation can be found in a patient with findings suggestive of pulmonary embolism, the workup must be pursued to completion.

## V. Frequency of Symptoms and Signs in Pulmonary Embolism

| Symptoms | Frequency (%) | Signs | Frequency (%) |
|---|---|---|---|
| Dyspnea | 84 | Tachypnea (>16/min) | 92 |
| Pleuritic chest pain | 74 | Rales | 58 |
| Apprehension | 59 | Accentuated S2 | 53 |
| Cough | 53 | Tachycardia (>100/min) | 44 |
| Hemoptysis | 30 | Fever (>37.8°C, 100°F) | 43 |
| Sweating | 27 | Diaphoresis | 36 |
| Non-pleuritic chest pain | 14 | S3 or S4 gallop | 34 |
| Syncope | 13 | Thrombophlebitis | 32 |
| | | Lower extremity edema | 24 |
| | | Cardiac murmur | 23 |
| | | Cyanosis | 19 |

## VI. Diagnostic Evaluation
A. **Chest Films** are nonspecific and insensitive for pulmonary embolism. The chest film may be normal, or it may show an elevated hemidiaphragm, focal infiltrates, large or small pleural effusions, or atelectasis.
B. **Electrocardiogram** abnormalities are also nonspecific. The tracing is often normal; the most commonly seen abnormality is sinus tachycardia. Occasionally, acute right ventricular strain causes tall and peaked P waves in lead II, right axis deviation, right bundle branch block, a classic S1-Q3-T pattern, or atrial fibrillation.
C. **Blood Gas Studies:**
1. There is no level of arterial oxygen that can rule out pulmonary embolism. Most

patients with pulmonary embolism have a normal arterial oxygen. Impaired gas exchange is best assessed by using the alveolar-to-arterial (A-a) oxygen gradient.

   2. On room air at sea level, the gradient may be calculated with the following formula:

$$\text{A-a oxygen gradient} = 147 - [\,1.2\,(PCO_2) + \text{measured } pAO_2\,]$$

   3. A normal gradient should be no higher than 10 plus one tenth of the patient's age.

   4. A normal A-a oxygen gradient is seen in 5-15% of patients with pulmonary emboli but is inconsistent with massive pulmonary embolism and hypotension. An elevated gradient is quite nonspecific and may be produced by almost any pulmonary disease.

D. **Ventilation-perfusion Scan:** Virtually all patients suspected of having pulmonary emboli need a V/Q scan. Unfortunately, the V/Q scan is most often nondiagnostic; patterns other than "normal" and "high-probability" are nondiagnostic. Further workup is necessary when the V/Q scan is nondiagnostic.

E. **Venous Imaging:**

   1. If the V/Q scan is nondiagnostic, a workup for deep venous thrombosis (DVT) should be pursued using duplex ultrasound and impedance plethysmography, or contrast venography. The positive identification of DVT in a patient with signs and symptoms suggesting pulmonary embolism virtually proves the diagnosis of pulmonary embolism.

   2. Inability to demonstrate a source of DVT does not significantly lower the likelihood of pulmonary embolism because clinically asymptomatic DVT may be difficult to find.

   3. Patients with a nondiagnostic V/Q scan and no demonstrable site of DVT should proceed to pulmonary angiography.

F. **Angiography:**

   1. Contrast pulmonary arteriography is the "gold standard" for the diagnosis of pulmonary embolism with unmatched sensitivity and specificity.

   2. False-negative results may occur in 2% to 10% of patients. False-positive results are extremely rare.

VII. **Management of Acute Pulmonary Embolism for Patients in Stable Condition**

A. Intravenous access and oxygen should be provided for all patients.

B. **Heparin Anticoagulation:**

   1. In the absence of specific contraindications, heparin therapy should be started as soon as the diagnosis of pulmonary embolism is seriously considered. It is rarely appropriate to delay heparin therapy while awaiting a firm diagnosis. Full anticoagulating doses of heparin can be given immediately after major surgery.

   2. For an average-sized adult, the initial bolus of heparin should be 10,000 to 20,000 U and the initial drip rate should be at least 1,280 U/hr (20,000 U in 500 cc D5W at 32 cc/hour). Heparin dosing for pulmonary embolism is the same as that for deep venous thrombosis.

   3. Check activated partial thromboplastin time (PTT) 4-6 hours after therapy is initiated or after the dosage is adjusted. Therapeutic Range: PTT 1.5-2.0 times control.

   4. **Maintenance Dose Adjustment:**

| aPTT | Hold drip | Adjust drip | Check aPTT |
|------|-----------|-------------|------------|
| <50 sec | 0 min | Increase 3 cc/hr | 6 hr later |
| 50-59 sec | 0 min | Increase 3 cc/hr | 6 hr later |
| 60-85 sec | 0 min | No change | Next morning |
| 86-95 sec | 0 min | Decrease 2 cc/hr | Next morning |
| 96-120 sec | 30 min | Decrease 2 cc/hr | 6 hr later |
| >120 sec | 60 min | Decrease 4 cc/hr | 6 hr later |

   5. Heparin should be continued for a 5-day course.

   6. Monitor platelet count during heparin therapy; thrombocytopenia develops in up to 5%. Heparin rarely induces hyperkalemia, which resolves spontaneously upon

discontinuation.

7. After full anticoagulation has been established with heparin (often within 6 hours), oral warfarin (Coumadin) may be initiated. It is not safe to start warfarin without prior heparinization, because the drug causes a hypercoagulable state during the early stages of its use. Ambulation can begin once the PTT is in the therapeutic range.

C. **Warfarin (Coumadin) Therapy:**
1. Initial dose of warfarin is 10 mg; subsequent doses should be based on a daily INR (on PT) value and its rate of change.
2. Administration of heparin and warfarin should overlap for a minimum of 3-5 days. Once heparin therapy has overlapped with warfarin therapy for 3-5 days and the International Normalized Ratio is 2.0-3.0 (or the PT is 1.3-1.5 times control), heparin can be safely discontinued.
3. **Length of Warfarin Therapy:** If risk factors (prolonged inactivity) have been corrected, a 3-6 month course of warfarin is sufficient. Persistent risk factors, extensive or complicated thrombosis, or recurrent thrombotic episodes may be indications to prolong therapy to 6-12 months. Outpatients receiving oral anticoagulants should have their PT checked weekly.

VIII. **Management of Acute Pulmonary Embolism for Patients in Unstable Condition**
A. Patients with pulmonary embolism who have severe hypoxemia or any degree of hypotension are considered to be in unstable condition.
B. **Heparin and oxygen** should be started immediately.
C. **Fluid and Pharmacologic Management:**
1. In most cases of acute cor pulmonale, gentle pharmacologic preload reduction unloads the congested pulmonary circuit and reduces right ventricular pressures.
2. Hydralazine, isoproterenol, or norepinephrine may be required.
3. Pulmonary artery pressure monitoring is essential.
D. **Thrombolysis and Embolectomy:**
1. When a patient with proven pulmonary embolism is in unstable condition, immediate clot removal by thrombolytic therapy or by emergency surgical embolectomy is the accepted standard of care. The benefits of intervention far outweigh any relative contraindications.
2. Full dose heparin should always be started along with the infusion of any thrombolytic agent.
3. Thrombolytic therapy usually is indicated only when the diagnosis of pulmonary embolism has been proved beyond a reasonable doubt. However, it may be impossible to prove the diagnosis rapidly enough to save the life of a patient in unstable condition, and thrombolysis should be attempted as a last-ditch effort in an otherwise moribund patient with a diagnosis of suspected massive pulmonary embolism.
4. The fastest-acting thrombolytic agent available, tissue plasminogen activator (Activase), should be used.
5. **Contraindications to Thrombolytics:**
   a. **Absolute Contraindications:** Active bleeding, recent stroke, central nervous system tumor.
   b. **Relative Contraindications:** Surgical procedure within preceding 10 days; recent gastrointestinal bleeding; uncontrolled hypertension; recent trauma (cardiopulmonary resuscitation); pregnancy. Advanced age, menstruation, and controlled hypertension are not contraindications to thrombolysis or heparin.
6. The catheter used for pulmonary arteriography should pulled back into the inferior vena cava for infusion of thrombolytics since there is no advantage to leaving the catheter in the pulmonary artery unless the distal tip can be embedded into the thrombus.
7. Monitor complete blood count, PT or international normalized ratio (INR), activated PTT, and fibrinogen levels twice daily.
8. **Alteplase, (tPA, Activase)** total dose of 100 mg is given over period of 90 min, as follows:

- 15 mg initial bolus
- 50-mg infusion over first 30 min
- 35-mg infusion over next hour

The dose should always be adjusted for patients who weigh less than 70 kg (154 lb). If the patient weighs 10% less than 70 kg, each component of the dose is reduced by 10%.

9. **Streptokinase:** The duration required for complete clot lysis is substantially longer with streptokinase than with tissue plasminogen activator. Bolus of 250,000 U IV followed by 100,000 U/hr.

## IX. Emergency Thoracotomy

A. Emergency surgical removal of embolized thrombus is reserved for instances when there is an absolute contraindication to thrombolysis or when the patient's condition has failed to improve after thrombolysis.

B. Cardiac arrest from pulmonary embolism is an indication for immediate thoracotomy.

C. **Femorofemoral cardiopulmonary bypass** has been used in cases of cardiopulmonary collapse due to pulmonary embolism while the patient is awaiting thrombolysis or embolectomy.

# *Gynecology*

## Cervical Cytology Screening

I. **Screening for Cervical Cancer**
   A. All women age who are 18 or older, or who have been sexually active should have an annual cervical smear and pelvic examination. After 3 or more consecutive normal annual examinations, the smear may be performed less frequently (every 2-3 years) if there are no risk factors for cervical cancer.
   B. Annual smears should be performed if there are risk factors for lesions of the cervix, including human papilloma virus or HIV infection, smokers, or multiple sexual partners.
   C. After removal of the uterus for benign disease, periodic cytologic evaluation of the vagina is recommended every 1-3 years.

II. **Technique of Cytologic Sampling**
   A. Sampling error is a major cause of false-negative smears. The scraping of the portio should include the entire transformation zone, and a cellular sample from the endocervical canal should be obtained with an endocervical brush. The entire portio should be visible when the smear is obtained.
   B. Collect sample prior to the bimanual examination to avoid contamination with lubricant.
   C. Pap smear should be done before tests for gonococcus and chlamydia.
   D. When large amounts of vaginal discharge are present, remove discharge before obtaining the smear being careful not to disturb the epithelium. Small amounts of blood will not interfere with evaluation, large amounts, as occurs during menses, will interfere with cytologic sampling. Vaginitis should be treated and cured before sampling.
   E. Obtain portio sample before the endocervical sample because bleeding from the endocervix may occur after brush use. When obtaining the endocervical sample, gently rotate brush in the endocervical canal. The endocervical and ectocervical samples are placed on a single slide.
   F. Uniformly apply the sample to the slide, without clumping, and rapidly fix. If spray fixatives are used, hold spray at least 10 inches away to prevent destruction of cells.

**The Bethesda System for Reporting Cervical/Vaginal Cytologic Diagnoses**

I.  **Descriptive Diagnoses**
    A.  **Benign Cellular Changes:**
        1.  **Infection:**
            Trichomonas vaginalis
            Fungal organisms consistent with *Candida* spp
            Predominance of coccobacilli consistent with shift in vaginal flora
            Bacteria morphologically consistent with Actinomyces spp
            Cellular changes associated with herpes simplex virus
        2.  **Reactive Cellular Changes Associated with:**
            Inflammation
            Atrophy with inflammation ("atrophic vaginitis")
            Intrauterine contraceptive device (IUD)
            Other: Radiation
    B.  **Epithelial Cell Abnormalities:**
        1.  **Atypical Squamous Cells of Undetermined Significance (ASCUS):** Qualify
            (reactive or premalignant)
        2.  **Low-grade Squamous Intraepithelial Lesion Encompassing:**
            HPV
            Mild dysplasia/CIN 1
        3.  **High-grade Squamous Intraepithelial Lesion Encompassing:**
            Moderate and severe dysplasia
            CIS/CIN 2 and CIN 3
        4.  **Squamous Cell Carcinoma**
    C.  **Glandular Cell Abnormalities:**
        Endometrial cells, cytologically benign, in a postmenopausal woman
        Atypical glandular cells of undetermined significance: Qualify (reactive or
        premalignant)
        Endocervical adenocarcinoma
        Endometrial adenocarcinoma
        Extrauterine adenocarcinoma
        Adenocarcinoma, not otherwise specified

III.  **Management of Abnormal Pap Smear Results**
    A.  **Satisfactory, but Limited by Few (or absent) Endocervical Cells:**
        1.  Endocervical cells are absent in up to 10% of Pap smears premenopause; up to
            50% postmenopausally.
        2.  Lower endocervical cell detection in pregnancy and in oral contraceptive users
        3.  Management: If benign diagnosis is given, either repeat annually or only recall
            women with previously abnormal Pap smears.
    B.  **Unsatisfactory for Evaluation:**
        1.  Repeat Pap smear midcycle in 6-12 weeks.
        2.  If atrophic smear, treat with estrogen for 6-8 weeks, then repeat Pap smear.
    C.  **Benign Cellular Changes:**
        1.  **Infection-Candida:**
            a.  Most cases represent asymptomatic colonization.
            b.  Offer treatment for symptomatic cases.
            c.  Repeat Pap at usual interval or 6-8 weeks after treatment.

2. **Infection-Trichomonas:**
   a. Determine whether recently treated. If not, offer treatment (may transmit sexually).
   b. Repeat Pap at usual interval or 6-8 weeks after treatment.
3. **Infection-Predominance of Coccobacilli consistent with Shift in Vaginal Flora:**
   a. Implies possible bacterial vaginosis, but finding is non-specific.
   b. Diagnosis should be confirmed by examination findings of homogeneous vaginal discharge, positive amine test, and clue cells on microscopic saline suspension.
4. **Infection-Actinomyces:**
   a. Seen more frequently in IUD users; usually due to colonization, not infection.
   b. Examine patient to exclude pelvic actinomycosis (presents like PID). Repeat Pap smear 1-2 months after first smear. If still positive, then remove IUD and recheck Pap smear in 1-2 months. If negative, then insert a new IUD. If still positive, then treat with penicillin for at least 30 days.
5. **Infection-Herpes Simplex Virus:**
   a. Pap smear has poor sensitivity but good specificity for HSV; a positive smear usually is caused by asymptomatic infection.
   b. HSV culture is usually negative by the time Pap smear result is available; therefore, it is not cost-effective to perform culture in the absence of a visible lesion.
   c. Inform patient of pregnancy risks and possibility of transmission.
   d. No treatment is necessary. Repeat Pap as for a benign result.
6. **Reactive-Non-Specific Inflammation:**
   a. May be metaplasia, chlamydial or gonococcal endocervicitis, or viral infection.
   b. Examine patient, culture for gonorrhea and test for chlamydia. Treat empirically if mucopurulent cervicitis is seen or await test results and treat if positive.
   c. Repeat Pap smear in 6-8 weeks if treated; repeat at usual interval if not treated.
7. **Atrophy with Inflammation:**
   a. Common in post-menopausal women or those with estrogen-deficiency states.
   b. If associated with atypical squamous cells of undetermined significance (ASCUS) or low-grade squamous intraepithelial lesion (LG-SIL), treat with vaginal estrogen for 4-6 weeks, then repeat smear.

D. **Squamous Cell Abnormalities:**
   1. **Atypical Squamous Cells of Undetermined Significance (ASCUS):**
      a. Indicates cells with nuclear atypia, but not due to HPV.
      b. The most common strategy is to repeat Pap smear at intervals of 3-6 months. If two consecutive smears are negative, then repeat yearly Pap smears. If repeat Pap smear shows ASCUS or more advanced stage changes, then colposcopy and biopsy are indicated.
      c. Many clinicians manage ASCUS by colposcopy and biopsy initially.
   2. **Low Grade Squamous Intraepithelial Lesion (LG-SIL):** LG-SIL includes human papilloma virus, koilocytosis atypia, mild dysplasia/CIN I. 60% of LGSIL lesions regress spontaneously; 15% progress to HG-SIL.
      a. **Management options for LG-SIL:**
         (1) **Colposcope with a single LG-SIL result:** If the Biopsy is normal, the patient should be reevaluated with Pap smear every 4-6 months for 2 years. Will occasional detect HG-SIL early
         (2) **Follow with Pap smears every 4-6 month for 2 years; if any two Paps show LG-SIL or ASCUS, refer for colposcopy:** Risk loss to follow-up. Risk delay of diagnosis of HG-SIL.
         (3) **High-Grade Squamous Intraepithelial Lesion (HG-SIL; moderate/severe dysplasia; CIN 2, CIN 3, carcinoma in situ):** Must be evaluated by colposcopy and directed biopsy.

E. **Glandular Cell Abnormalities:**
   1. **Endometrial Cells:**
      a. Insignificant in premenopausal woman with normal menstrual pattern.

      b. Must be evaluated with endometrial sampling in woman with abnormal bleeding
  2. **Atypical Glandular Cells of Undetermined Significance (AGCUS):**
      a. Could represent infection, HPV infection, adenocarcinoma in situ, or adenocarcinoma. Most common strategy is to repeat Pap smear at interval of 3-6 months.
      b. AGCUS/premalignant changes must be evaluated by endocervical curettage with colposcopic evaluation.
      c. Preinvasive or invasive adenocarcinoma is suspected from these studies diagnostic conization is indicated. Abnormal endometrial cells on cytology should be investigated by endometrial biopsy, fractional dilation and curettage or hysteroscopy to exclude endometrial adenocarcinoma.
  3. **Endocervical Adenocarcinoma, Endometrial Adenocarcinoma, Extrauterine Adenocarcinoma, Adenocarcinoma, not otherwise specified:** These diagnoses require thorough evaluation that may include endocervical curettage, cone biopsy, and/or endometrial biopsy.

## IV. Technique of Colposcopically Directed Biopsy

A. Liberally apply a solution of acetic acid 3-5% to cervix, and inspect cervix for abnormal areas (white epithelium, punctation, mosaic cells, atypical vessels). Obtain punch biopsies of any abnormal areas under colposcopic visualization.

B. Hemostatic agents such as Monsel solution or silver nitrate may be applied to stop bleeding. Record location of each biopsy.

C. **Endocervical Curettage:** ECC is usually done routinely during colposcopy, except during pregnancy.

## V. Treatment of Squamous Intraepithelial Lesions after Confirmation by Colposcopically directed Biopsy

A. **Typical (papillary) Condyloma Acuminata:** Use either cryotherapy, LEEP, or laser.

B. **Low Grade SIL (flat condyloma or CIN I):**
  1. **Aggressive Approach:** If the entire lesion is visualized and the limits of the transformation zone are seen, the lesion can be ablated or excised. Since 15% of these lesions progress to high grade squamous intraepithelial lesion (HSIL), ablation or excision is a reasonable treatment.
  2. **Conservative Approach:** Since the risk of progression is at most 20% and the lesion is not dangerous until it does progress, these lesions may be followed with repeat Pap smear in 4-6 months until evidence of progression to HG-SIL or persistence of low grade SIL. If the untreated lesion does not resolve after a year, reevaluation by colposcopy, biopsy, and ablation or excision are indicated.

C. **High Grade SIL (or treated LG-SIL):**
  1. **Following colposcopically directed biopsy, and exclusion of invasive disease,** perform ablative therapy to destroy the entire transformation zone.
  2. Ablation is appropriate if the entire lesion and transformation zone are seen and endocervical curretage is negative. After the lesion has been removed, Pap smears should be scheduled at 3-month intervals for 1 year.

## VI. Management Based on Biopsy Findings

A. **Benign Cellular Changes (infection, reactive inflammation):** Treat infection. Repeat smear every 4-6 months; after 2 negatives, repeat yearly.

B. **Squamous intraepithelial lesions (SIL) low-high grade, Dysplasia (mild/mod/severe), Carcinoma in situ, Condyloma:**
  1. Cryotherapy Double freeze technique: Freeze with lubricated, liquid nitrogen probe for 3 minutes, followed by 4-5 minute pause, repeat freeze for 3 min (or use LEEP, Cautery, laser).
  2. The entire lesion should be covered and a 5 mm margin of freeze should be visual iced. Then repeat Pap smear every 4-6 months for 1-2 years.

C.  **Inadequate colposcopy (non-visualization of transition zone or all of lesion) or positive ECC, or any question of malignancy, or significant Biopsy/Pap discrepancy:** Excisional conization (or LEEP, laser).

D.  **Microinvasive Carcinoma on Biopsy:** Excisional conization.

E.  **Invasive Carcinoma:** Consider referral for surgery and/or radiotherapy.

# Sexually Transmitted Diseases

I. **Gonorrhea**
   A. **Recommended Treatment of Uncomplicated Infections in Adolescents and Adults:**
      1. Ceftriaxone (Rocephin) 250 mg IM; active against incubating syphilis.
      2. Cefixime (Suprax) 400 mg po; active against incubating syphilis.
      3. Ciprofloxacin (Cipro) 500 mg po; contraindicated in pregnancy, lactation, and <17 years of age; not active against syphilis.
      4. Ofloxacin (Floxin)400 mg po; contraindicated in pregnancy, lactation, and <17 years of age.
      5. plus Doxycycline 100 mg po bid x 7 days for coexisting C. trachomatis infection; may abort incubating syphilis; contraindicated in pregnancy.
   B. **Alternative Regimens:**
      1. Spectinomycin 2 g IM; for patients who cannot tolerate cephalosporins or quinolones; safe in pregnancy and in adolescents; not effective for pharyngeal GC; resistant strains have been reported.
      2. Ceftizoxime 500 mg IM, Cefotaxime 500 mg IM, Cefotetan 1 g IM, Cefoxitin 2 g IM, Cefuroxime axetil 1 g po, Cefpodoxime 200 mg po.
      3. Enoxacin 400 mg po, Lomefloxacin 400 mg po, or Norfloxacin 800 mg po
      4. plus Doxycycline 100 mg po bid x 7d.
   C. **Indications for Immediate Empiric Treatment:**
      1. Mucopurulent cervicitis
      2. Pelvic inflammatory disease
      3. Contacts to GC or to presumptive GC infection
      4. Treatment of partners should be completed
   D. **Diagnostic Labs:**
      1. Culture is recommended for public health purposes.
      2. Test of cure is not necessary.
      3. Consider serologic testing for syphilis and HIV.

II. **Chlamydia Trachomatis**
   A. **Recommended Treatment of Uncomplicated Infections in Adolescents and Adults:**
      1. Doxycycline 100 mg po bid x 7d; contraindicated in pregnancy and nursing mothers
      2. Azithromycin (Zithromax) 1 g po ($27.37)
   B. **Alternative Regimens:**
      1. Ofloxacin (Floxin) 300 mg po bid x 7 d
      2. Erythromycin base 500 mg po qid x 7 d; not as efficacious as doxycycline; useful in pregnancy
      3. Test of care should be considered if alternative regimens are used.
   C. **Diagnostic Labs:**
      1. Culture and nonculture techniques for chlamydia are available.
      2. Test of cure is not recommended if a recommended regimen is used.
      3. Consider serologic testing for syphilis and HIV.

III. **Mucopurulent Cervicitis**
   A. Treatment for gonorrhea and chlamydia is recommended.
   B. Partner referral and treatment is recommended.

IV. **Pelvic Inflammatory Disease**
   A. The diagnosis of pelvic inflammatory disease should be considered in any woman of reproductive age who has pelvic pain. The pain is often dull and constant usually bilateral, and less than 2 weeks in duration. Sexual history may include multiple partners and exposure to sexually transmitted disease.
   B. Pain may be associated with an abnormal vaginal discharge, abnormal uterine bleeding, dysuria, dyspareunia, nausea, vomiting, fever. More likely to begin during the first half of the menstrual cycle after menses.

C. Other symptoms include postcoital bleeding, spotting, and gastrointestinal symptoms.

D. PID is characterized by fever, diffuse lower abdominal pain; adnexal tenderness and cervical motion tenderness; vaginal discharge.

E. **Differential Diagnosis:** Appendicitis, ectopic pregnancy, other intra-abdominal pathology.

F. Many episodes of PID go unrecognized; physicians should maintain a low threshold for diagnosis and immediate treatment. Early treatment reduces subsequent tubal infertility and ectopic pregnancy rates. Consider serologic testing for syphilis and HIV.

G. Complete blood cell count with differential, pregnancy test, electrolytes. Gonorrhea and chlamydia cultures.

H. Laparoscopy is the "gold standard" of PID; recommended when the diagnosis is unclear. Laparoscopy also detects ovarian cysts, ectopic pregnancy, appendicitis, or endometriosis.

I. Pelvic ultrasound may show tubo-ovarian abscess.

J. **Diagnostic Criteria:**
   1. No single historical, physical or laboratory finding is both sensitive and specific.
   2. Lower abdominal tenderness
   3. Adnexal tenderness
   4. Cervical motion tenderness
   5. **Additional Criteria:**
      a. Temperature > 38.3 C
      b. Abnormal cervical or vaginal discharge
      c. Elevated ESR
      d. Elevated C-reactive protein
      e. Elevated WBC count
      f. Cervical infection with GC or chlamydia trachomatis
      g. Laparoscope findings consistent with PID

K. **Indications for hospitalization of women with PID:**
   1. The diagnosis is uncertain and surgical emergencies such as appendicitis and ectopic pregnancy cannot be excluded
   2. Pelvic abscess is suspected
   3. Pregnancy
   4. Adolescent patient
   5. HIV infection
   6. Severe illness or nausea and vomiting preclude outpatient management
   7. The patient is unable to follow or tolerate an outpatient regimen
   8. Failure to respond clinically to outpatient therapy
   9. Clinical follow-up within 72 hours of starting antibiotic treatment cannot be arranged

L. **Outpatient Regimens:**
   1. Ceftriaxone (Rocephin) 250 mg IM or Cefoxitin (Mefoxin) 2 g IM plus Probenecid 1 g po plus Doxycycline 100 mg po bid x 14 d, or
   2. Ofloxacin (Floxin) 400 mg po bid x 14 d, plus Clindamycin 450 mg po qid x 15 d or Metronidazole 500 mg po bid x 15 d

M. **Inpatient Regimens:**
   1. Cefoxitin (Mefoxin) 2 g IV q6h or cefotetan (Cefotan) 2 g IV q12h plus doxycycline 100 mg IV po q12h
   2. Clindamycin 900 mg IV q8h plus gentamicin 2 mg/kg IV, followed by 1.5 mg/kg IV q8h, then complete 14 d of clindamycin 450 mg PO qid or doxycycline 100 mg PO bid

N. **Partner Referral:** Sexual contacts should be treated for GC and Chlamydia, independent of clinical and laboratory findings.

## V. Nongonococcal Urethritis

### A. Diagnosis:
1. Symptoms include dysuria, discharge
2. Testing to determine specific diagnosis is recommended
   a. Gram stain of intraurethral swab specimen or visible discharge; more than 5 WBC per oil immersion field is diagnostic.
   b. Leukocyte esterase test (LET) of 1+ or greater on first 15 mL of voided urine may be found.

### B. Treatment of Uncomplicated Infections in Adolescents and Adults:
1. **Recommended Regimens:**
   a. Doxycycline 100 mg po bid x 7 d
   b. Azithromycin (Zithromax) 1 g po
2. **Alternative Regimens:** Erythromycin base 500 mg po qid x 7 d or erythromycin base 250 mg po qid x 14 d
3. Sexual contacts should be treated.

# Vaginal Infections

## Clinical Evaluation

A. Determine type and extent of symptoms, including internal or external itching, swelling, odor, pelvic pain.

B. Change in sexual partners or sexual activity; recent changes in contraception method; medications (antibiotics, contraceptives); history of prior genital infections in patient or partner.

C. Use of nonprescription products, douching, new soaps, or deodorant sprays. Possibility of pregnancy.

D. **Physical Examination:**
   1. Examine for erythema, swelling, or lesions on perineum, vulva, vagina, or cervix.
   2. Note the color, texture, and odor of vaginal or cervical discharge.
   3. **Saline Wet Mount:**
      a. Use one swab to obtain a sample from the pool of vaginal secretions in the posterior fornix, obtaining a "clump" of discharge if possible. Place the smear on a slide, add one drop of normal saline, and apply coverslip.
      b. Coccoid bacteria and clue cells (bacteria-coated, stippled, epithelial cells) are characteristic of bacterial vaginosis. Trichomoniasis is confirmed by identification of trichomonads--motile oval flagellates. White blood cells are usually visible as well.
   4. **Potassium Hydroxide (KOH) Preparation:**
      a. Place a second sample on another slide. Add one drop of 10% potassium hydroxide (KOH) and a coverslip. A pungent, fishy odor upon addition of KOH--a positive whiff test--strongly indicates bacterial vaginosis.
      b. The KOH prep may reveal yeast in the form of thread-like hyphae and budding yeast.
   5. **Cultures** are time-consuming and not routinely indicated, but they can verify candidiasis or trichomoniasis when a wet mount proves inconclusive.

E. **Screening for STDs:** Testing for gonorrhea and chlamydial infection should be considered for women with a new sexual partner, or purulent cervical discharge, cervical motion tenderness, symptoms of pelvic inflammatory disease, or if cervical friability and/or bleeding are noted after endocervical brushing.

## Differential Diagnosis

A. The most common cause of vaginitis is bacterial vaginosis, followed by Candida albicans with trichomoniasis on the decline.

B. The clinician must be alert to common non-vaginal etiologies, including contact dermatitis from spermicidal creams, latex in condoms, or douching. In addition, any STD can produce vaginal discharge.

## Bacterial Vaginosis

A. Bacterial vaginosis develops when a shift in the normal vaginal ecosystem results in replacement of the usually predominant lactobacilli with mixed bacterial flora. Bacterial vaginosis is the most common type of infectious vaginitis.

B. There is usually little or no inflammation of the vulva or vaginal epithelium. There is little itching, and no pain, and the symptoms tend to have an indolent course characterized by chronic vaginal discharge and some postcoital odor.

C. Vaginal discharge and a "fishy" odor may be more frequently noticeable after intercourse; may be asymptomatic.

D. **Diagnostic Findings:**
   1. Clue cells (saline slide shows epithelial cells covered with bacteria).
   2. Positive whiff test (fishy odor with KOH)
   3. Homogeneous, white, adherent discharge
   4. Culture for this organism should be avoided because of poor specificity.

E. **Recommended Treatment Regimen:**
   1. Bacterial vaginosis can be eliminated with oral or topical prescription therapies.

2. Metronidazole (Flagyl) 250 mg PO tid for 7 days. A single oral dose has a lower cure rate and a higher relapse rate compared with the longer regimen.

3. **Side Effects:** Nausea, heartburn, metallic taste. Emetic effect with alcohol (Antabuse effect); peripheral neuropathy, seizures rarely; contraindicated in the first trimester of pregnancy because of a small teratogenic potential.

4. **Topical Therapies:**
   a. Clindamycin vaginal cream, 2% (Cleocin) and metronidazole (MetroGel-Vaginal) provide a >90% cure rate and a low risk of adverse reactions.
   b. Clindamycin cream (Cleocin) one applicatorful (5 g) at bedtime for 7 nights. Cream mineral oil base may weaken latex condoms and contraceptive diaphragms.
   c. Metronidazole gel (MetroGel), one applicatorful bid, morning and evening, for 5 days.

5. Routine treatment of sexual partners is not recommended.

F. **Persistent Cases:** Reevaluate and exclude other infections, including trichomonas.
   1. Clindamycin, 300 mg orally bid for 7 days.
   2. Treatment of sexual partners should be considered in persistent or recurrent cases.

IV. **Candida Vulvovaginitis**
   A. Second most common diagnosis associated with vaginal symptoms. Found in 25% of asymptomatic women. True fungal infections account for less than 33% of all vaginal infections.
   B. **Possible Risk Factors:** Use of oral contraceptives, antibiotics, diabetes, intestinal colonization by Candida, tight clothing, sexual transmission, immunologic defects.
   C. **Symptoms and Signs:** Marked itching; thick, white, odorless discharge; vulvar or vaginal erythema. Thrush appears as white plaques loosely attached to the oral or vaginal mucous membranes.
   D. **Potassium Hydroxide Preparation:** Hyphae or budding yeast forms. Rapid tests for Candida antigens are more sensitive than KOH preparation.
   E. Cultures should be obtained only if treatment failure or recurrence of symptoms. Candida on Pap smear is specific but not sensitive.
   F. **Treatment of Candida Vulvovaginitis:**
      1. For severe symptoms and chronic infections use a 7-day course of treatment. In extensive vulvar involvement, use cream instead of a suppository preparation.

      Terconazole (Terazol 7), 0.4% cream, one applicatorful (5 g) intravaginally for 7 nights; or (Terazol 3) 0.8% cream, one applicatorful (5 g) intravaginally for 3 nights; or 80 mg suppository, 1 suppository for 3 nights; terconazole is superior to treatment with miconazole or clotrimazole.

      Butoconazole (Femstat) 2% cream, one applicatorful (5 g) intravaginally for 3 nights. Can be used for 6 d, if needed.

      Clotrimazole (Gyne-Lotrimin) 1% cream, one applicatorful (5 g) intravaginally for 7 nights; or 100 mg vaginal tablet for 7 nights (OTC); 100 mg vaginal tablet, two tablets for 3 nights; or 500 mg vaginal tablet, one tablet single application.

      Miconazole (Monistat 7) 2% cream, one applicatorful (5 g) intravaginally for 7 nights (OTC); or 200 mg vaginal suppository, one suppository for 3 nights; or 100 mg vaginal suppository, one suppository for 7 nights (OTC).

      Tioconazole, 6.5% (Vagistat), one applicatorful (5 gm) intravaginally one time.

      Nystatin vaginal tablets, (Mycostatin), one tablet PO at bedtime for 14d.

      Creams and suppositories are oil-based and may weaken latex condoms and diaphragms.

   G. **Oral Regimens for Resistant or Recurrent Candida Cases:**
      Fluconazole (Diflucan), 150 mg PO one time [150 mg]
      Ketoconazole (Nizoral), 200 mg PO bid for 5 nights
      Itraconazole (Sporanox), 200 mg PO one time

   H. **Resistant or Recurrent Cases:**
      1. Reexamination and possibly culture.
      2. Repeat topical therapy for a 14-21-day course. Oral regimens have enhanced patient compliance and the potential for eradicating rectal reservoirs.

3. Treatment of sexual partners and condom usage should be considered.
4. Patients with recalcitrant disease should be evaluated for diabetes and HIV because these patients may have a higher incidence of vaginal candidiasis.

I. **Prophylactic Regimens for Frequent Infections:**
Fluconazole (Diflucan), 100-150 mg PO once each week for six months [100,150 mg]
Clotrimazole (Gyne-Lotrimin), one 500-mg vaginal tablet each week for six months
Ketoconazole (Nizoral), 100 mg PO qd for six months.

J. **Personal Practices:** Advise loose-fitting cotton undergarments and use of sanitary napkins rather than tampons. Advise against douching.

## Trichomonas Vaginitis

A. Flagellated anaerobic protozoan; a sexually transmitted disease.
B. Typically elicits an acute inflammatory response of the vaginal epithelium. Produces severe vaginal and vulvar itching or irritation, dysuria, dyspareunia, or an abnormal vaginal odor.
C. Fiery red vaginal mucosa, and a profuse, yellow-green, bubbly, vaginal discharge. Asymptomatic in 50% of women and 90% of men.
D. A strawberry cervix (scattered red macules) is uncommonly seen.
E. **Diagnosis:** Motile trichomonads on normal saline preparation; >10 white blood cells per high-power field. Diagnosis of Trichomonas by Pap smear is unreliable and should be confirmed by saline mount prep. Culture documentation by modified Diamond is usually not required.
F. **Treatment of Trichomonas Vaginitis:**
1. Metronidazole (Flagyl), 2 g PO in a single dose for both the patient and sexual partner, or 500 mg PO bid for 7 days, or 250 mg tid for 7 days. Metronidazole should be taken with food to avoid GI distress.
2. Topical therapy is not recommended because the organism may persist in extravaginal sites such as the urethra and Skene's glands after local therapy.
3. Evaluate for coexisting sexually transmitted diseases.
4. **Persistent Cases:** Consider noncompliance, reinfection, metronidazole resistance, inaccurate diagnosis, or infection with multiple sexually transmitted diseases.
5. If persistence of trichomonas, retreatment of the patient and partner is indicated using standard dosages. Higher dosages may be used, metronidazole 2 g PO qd for three days or 500 g PO bid for 14 days with intravaginal metronidazole gel (MetroGel-Vaginal), 5 g intravaginally bid for 5 days.

## Other Diagnoses Causing Vaginal Symptoms

A. One-third of patients with vaginal symptoms will not have laboratory evidence of bacterial vaginosis, Candida, or Trichomonas.
B. Other causes of the vaginal symptoms include multiple infections, cervicitis, allergic reactions, or vulvodynia.
C. **Atrophic Vaginitis** should be considered in postmenopausal patients with burning and dyspareunia. The mucosa appears pale and thin with flat folds; wet-mount findings will be negative. Treatment is oral hormone replacement therapy.
D. **Allergy** is a very unusual cause of vaginal symptoms. Symptoms can result from Candida allergy or semen protein allergy. Systemic antihistamines may be helpful.

## Management of Recurrent Vaginitis

A. Treatment failure needs to be distinguished from reinfection or a new infection.
B. The initial diagnosis and treatment may have been incorrect, or the patient may not have completed the course of treatment.
C. More than one organism may have been responsible for the first infection, and treatment eradicated only the most prominent culprit.
D. With trichomoniasis, the patient may have been reinfected by an untreated partner. With candidiasis, the patient may have been reinfected by organisms from the GI tract.
E. A noninfectious condition such as allergy, chemical irritation, cystitis, or urethritis may be responsible for the symptoms.

# Evaluation of Breast Masses

## I. Clinical Evaluation of Breast Masses

A. A detailed history and physical examination should determine the presence of associate pain (especially if cyclical), nipple discharge, duration of mass; change in size. Color any nipple discharges.

B. Determine patient age and menopausal status. The incidence of breast cancer rise rapidly in the fifth decade. Breast cysts are common before menopause and vary in siz with menses.

C. Determine results of and time since the last clinical breast examination and the la mammogram; and breast self-examination practices; previous breast masses ar biopsies.

D. **Risk Factors for Breast Cancer:**
1. Female sex
2. Age over 50 years old
3. Previous breast cancer
4. Family history, particularly in first degree, maternal, or premenopausal relatives.
5. 80% of women with breast cancer have no risk factors other than being women an over 50 years old.

E. **Physical Examination:**
1. First examine the patient in the supine position with her arms up and behind her hea This flattens the breast tissue and compresses it for examination.
2. Then have the patient sit up with arms first at her side and then behind her head. Thi facilitates examination of the breast contours and allows visualization of nippl inversion or tethering.
3. Examine for dimpling, asymmetry, lumps, thickened areas, changes in shape contour; palpate both breasts and the axillae. Compress nipples to identify ar discharge. Make a drawing of any irregularities and masses.
4. The characteristics of a lump have limited diagnostic value. Very discrete, smoot nodules are more likely to be benign; tenderness is usually associated with benignit If the physical characteristics of the mass suggest benignity, it is reasonable monitor a nodule during one menstrual cycle.
5. Assess mass for singular or multiple components, mobility, tenderness, and cystic c solid qualities.

## II. Differential Diagnosis by Age of the Patient

A. **<30 Years Old:** The common causes are fibroadenoma, papillomatosis, absces (especially if lactating), or fat necrosis.

B. **30-50 Years Old:** Consider fibrocystic mastopathy, cancer, fat necrosis, or cystosarcom phylloides.

C. **If Older than 50:** Cancer is the primary diagnosis, followed by fibrocystic mastopathy, fa necrosis, and cyst.

## III. Evaluation of Breast Masses

A. If physical characteristics support the diagnosis of a cyst, needle aspiration should b done.
1. Swab the area of the breast with Betadine, and inject 1% lidocaine into the overlyin skin, using a 27-30 gauge needle.
2. Insert a 22 gauge needle into the mass and evacuate the cyst.
3. Non-bloody fluid should not be sent for cytology. If grossly bloody, the fluid should b analyzed by cytology, and biopsy considered. A compression dressing is placed ove the breast, and the patient reexamined in 3-4 weeks.

B. If the lesion is solid or if no fluid is obtained, use the same 22 gauge needle to aspirat tissue (fine needle aspiration cytology).

C. **Fine-Needle Aspiration:**
1. Sensitivity 65-98%. False-positive results are rare, but false-negative rates may b as high as 22%. If fine-needle aspiration is negative, biopsy is required.

2. Use a 10- or 20-mL syringe with a 22 gauge needle. When the needle enters the mass, apply suction by retracting the plunger and advance the needle. Direct the needle to different areas of the mass, maintaining suction on the syringe.
3. Slowly release suction before the needle is withdrawn from the mass. Place the contents of the needle onto glass slides or put the cells in a fixative solution for pathologic examination.

D. Recurrence of cyst, residual mass after aspiration, or presence of bloody aspirate requires further evaluation by ultrasound and/or biopsy.

IV. **Nonpalpable (occult) Breast Lesions Detected by Mammogram**
   A. **Evaluate with Breast Ultrasound:**
      1. **If Solid:** Use mammographic localization, followed by open, needle-localization biopsy.
      2. **If Cystic:** Cyst aspiration may be considered as above or follow the mass with breast self exam, ultrasound, clinical exam, and mammography. If the lesion becomes solid, evaluate with biopsy or aspiration cytology. If remains cystic, continue follow-up examinations.

V. **Important Diagnostic Caveats**
   A. A normal mammogram is meaningless in the presence of a mass, and a mammogram can not rule out cancer.
   B. Assure a follow-up examination for all patients, even if there is absolute certainty that the mass is insignificant or benign.
   C. A breast mass in a pregnant patient warrants the same timely evaluation as in a non-pregnant patient.
   D. Routine use of mammography in women less than 35 years old is usually unrewarding and potentially misleading and dangerous, even in the presence of a dominant mass. Dense, hormonally active breast tissue in this group makes interpretation difficult and can not reliably define malignancy.

# Amenorrhea

## I. Pathophysiology of Amenorrhea

A. Amenorrhea may be caused by either failure of the hypothalamic-pituitary-gonadal axis, or by absence of end organs, or by obstruction of the outflow tract. The underlying etiology of amenorrhea should always be determined.

B. Menses usually occur at intervals of 28 ± 3 days in two-thirds of women, with a normal range of 18-40 days.

C. The duration of amenorrhea that is considered pathologic is arbitrary, and any woman who has concerns should be evaluated.

D. Amenorrhea is defined as the absence of menstruation for 3 or more months in a women with past menses (secondary amenorrhea) or the absence of menarche by the age of 16 years in girls who have never menstruated (primary amenorrhea).

## II. Differential Diagnosis of Amenorrhea

A. **Pregnancy:** The possibility of pregnancy should be excluded.

B. **Anatomic causes** include abnormal differentiation of the genital tract, intrauterine adhesions (synechiae).

C. **Ovarian failure** includes disorders in which the ovaries are devoid of germ cells, and disorders in which the germ cells do not respond to follicle-stimulating hormone.

D. **Endocrine Imbalances** include hypothalamic or pituitary dysfunction, adrenal and thyroid disorders, inappropriate steroid feedback such as polycystic ovarian syndrome (PCO).

## III. Clinical Evaluation of Amenorrhea

A. Establish the timing of pubertal milestones, life style changes, dietary and exercise habits; medications or drugs; environmental and psychologic stress.

B. Previous pelvic surgery; evidence of increased androgen (acne, hirsutism, temporal balding, deepening of the voice, increased muscle mass, and decreased breast size).

C. Evidence of decreased estrogen includes hot flushes, night sweats, and dyspareunia.

## IV. Physical Examination

A. **Body Dimensions and Habitus:** Assess the distribution and extent of androgen-stimulated body hair; extent of breast development; breast secretions. Examine external and internal genitalia.

B. Breast development indicates exposure to estrogens, whereas the presence of pubic and axillary hair indicates exposure to androgens.

## V. Differential Diagnosis

A. **Hypothalamic Chronic Anovulation** may be caused by emotional and physical stress, dieting, excessive exercise. Significant weight loss associated with amenorrhea may be due to anorexia nervosa or bulimia.

B. **Androgen Insensitivity Syndrome (Testicular feminization syndrome):** Suggested by significant breast development in the absence of a normal amount of pubic and axillary hair; blind ending or absent vagina; confirmed by karyotype or by the measurement of testosterone concentrations which are in the adult male range.

C. **Imperforate Hymen, Vaginal and Uterine Aplasia, or Vaginal Septa:** A bulging perineum and a pelvic mass are commonly present.

D. **Intrauterine Synechiae or Adhesions (Asherman syndrome):** Should be considered if oligomenorrhea or amenorrhea develop following curettage, or bacterial or tuberculous endometritis; confirmed by hysterosalpingography or hysteroscopy.

E. **Ovarian Failure:** Should be considered if menopausal symptoms occur, especially hot flushes or dyspareunia.

F. **Increased Androgen Activity or Hypoprolactinemia:** Suggestive symptoms include presence of excess body hair or galactorrhea, and signs of adrenal or thyroid dysfunction.

G. **Kallmann Syndrome (isolated gonadotropin deficiency or familial hypogonadotropic hypogonadism):** Indicated by primary amenorrhea, absent sexual development, anosmia or hyposmia, color blindness, cleft lip and cleft palate. Secondary sex characteristics fail to develop or progress after puberty. Endocrine testing establishes diagnosis.

### H. Polycystic Ovarian Syndrome (PCO), or Chronic Hyperandrogenic Anovulation:

1. Heterogeneous disorder with clinical and biochemical variability.
2. Anovulation may occur because of inappropriate feedback signals to the hypothalamic-pituitary unit, and may be characterized by luteinizing hormone-dependent excess androgen production.
3. Generally presents with amenorrhea, hirsutism, and obesity from puberty, but may also present with irregular and profuse uterine bleeding; may not always be associated with hirsutism or obesity.

## VI. Diagnostic Approach to Amenorrhea

### A. Progestin Challenge Test:

1. Progestin is administered as a clinical aid to diagnosis and to evaluate estrogen levels. This test determines whether the outflow tract is intact.
2. **Administer:**Medroxyprogesterone acetate (Provera) 10 mg orally daily for 7 days or progesterone in oil 100 mg IM.
3. Any genital bleeding within 10 days of completion of progesterone regimen indicates a positive test. Such a positive result indicates that an outflow tract (uterus) is intact. A positive result suggests (but does not prove) chronic anovulation, rather than hypothalamic-pituitary insufficiency or ovarian failure.
4. If the test is negative (suggesting low levels of estrogen), then the regimen is repeated with estrogen and a progestin together.
   Conjugated estrogen, 1.25 mg PO daily for 21 days, together with
   Medroxyprogesterone acetate (Provera) 10 mg PO for the last 5 days of estrogen therapy.
5. This regimen should induce bleeding if the endometrium is normal. If bleeding occurs, the problem is localized to the hypothalamic-pituitary axis or ovaries, and anatomic causes are excluded.
6. If bleeding occurs after estrogen-progesterone challenge, measure basal concentrations of LH, FSH to evaluate ovarian failure.

### B. Prolactin, thyroid-stimulating hormone (TSH) should be measured to rule out hyperprolactinemia and hypothyroidism.

### C. Hypothyroidism: Elevated levels of TSH indicate primary hypothyroidism.

### D. Hyperprolactinemia:

1. If the basal prolactin level is elevated (>20 ng/ml) on initial testing, review the patient's medications. Repeat the test with the patient in a relaxed, fasting state because prolactin levels may be increased by stress, exercise, anxiety, sleep, and food ingestion.
2. If thyroid function is normal and prolactin levels are elevated, then MRI evaluation of the sella turcica is indicated to rule out a pituitary adenoma.

### E. Ovarian Failure:

1. Increased FSH levels (>40 mIU/ml) indicate ovarian failure.
2. Perform a karyotype in women under age 30 to identify those with gonadal dysgenesis or mosaicism in whom a Y chromosome is present.

### F. Polycystic Ovarian Syndrome:

1. If basal prolactin, TSH, and FSH levels are within the normal ranges or even low, then free testosterone levels should be determined.
2. Increased levels of free testosterone and dehydroepiandrosterone sulfate (DHEA-S) imply PCO; however, circulating androgen levels are sometimes normal in PCO. Increased circulating levels of LH (>20 mIU/ml) or an LH/FSH ratio >2.5 may also aid in diagnosing PCO.

### G. Androgen Secreting Neoplasms:

1. In women with evidence of hirsutism or virilization, both total testosterone and DHEA-S levels should be determined.
2. Total testosterone levels >200 ng/ml or DHEA-S levels >7.0 ng/dl should lead to an

investigation for an androgen-secreting neoplasm.

H. **Cushing's Syndrome:**
1. An estimate of cortisol secretion is indicated in women with amenorrhea who present with stigmata of Cushing syndrome (truncal obesity, striae).
2. Basal level of 17-hydroxyprogesterone or 24-hour urinary excretion of pregnanetriol is warranted if 21-hydroxylase deficiency is suspected. Some degree of sexual ambiguity may be present.

## VII. Treatment of Amenorrhea

A. Management of amenorrhea should be instituted only after the etiology has been determined.

B. **Hypothalamic Chronic Anovulation:**
1. Characterized by a positive progesterone challenge test. There is a history of weight loss, increased psychosocial stress, or excess exercise. Normal or low body weight and normal secondary sex characteristics are usually present. TSH is normal; prolactin is normal or low.
2. A change in lifestyle may be effective in inducing ovulation (reduce stress, adequate nutrition).
3. If pregnancy is desired, ovulation may be induced with clomiphene (Clomid).
4. Hypoestrogenic patients who do not desire pregnancy should be treated with estrogen and progesterone to prevent osteoporosis or endometrial hyperplasia. Treatment is similar to that prescribed for menopausal women. Sexually active individuals may use low-dose oral contraceptive agents.

C. **Abnormalities of the Outflow Tract:** Outflow tract obstruction associated with a normal uterus should be corrected by hysteroscopic lysis to prevent tubal damage and adhesions caused by intra-abdominal menstrual blood.

D. **Hypergonadotropic Amenorrhea (Premature Ovarian Failure):**
1. Women with hypergonadotropic amenorrhea should receive a karyotype; the presence of a Y chromosome requires excision of gonadal tissue to eliminate the 25% risk of malignancy.
2. Associated autoimmune (often endocrine) disorders should be treated.
3. Hormone replacement therapy is indicated. Contraception should be used by sexually active women who do not desire pregnancy because pregnancy may still occur in up to 10%.

E. **Hyperprolactinemic Chronic Anovulation:** Bromocriptine is recommended for individuals with microadenomas (<10 mm in diameter) and for those with no radiographic evidence of a pituitary lesion. Initial therapy for macroadenomas consists of bromocriptine for at least 6 months. Surgery may be considered later.

F. **Polycystic Ovarian Syndrome:** Treatment aims to resolve infertility, control hirsutism, and to prevent endometrial hyperplasia from unopposed estrogen secretion.

# bnormal Uterine Bleeding

### Physiology of Normal Menstruation
A. In response to gonadotropin-releasing hormone from the hypothalamus, the pituitary gland synthesizes follicle-stimulating hormone (FSH) and luteinizing hormone (LH) which cause the ovaries to produce estrogen and progesterone.
B. During the follicular phase of a normal ovulatory cycle, estrogen stimulation causes an increase in endometrial thickness. After ovulation, progesterone production increases, and the luteal phase begins. Progesterone causes endometrial maturation and secretory changes. If fertilization does not occur, estrogen and progesterone levels decline and menstruation occurs.
C. The normal menstrual interval is 21-35 days. Normal duration of menstrual flow is 2-6 days. Average blood loss per cycle is 20-60 mL.
D. **Criteria for Abnormal Bleeding:** Bleeding that occurs at intervals of less than 21 days, or more than 36 days, lasting longer than 7 days, or blood loss greater than 80 mL.

### Clinical Evaluation of Abnormal Uterine Bleeding
A. Obtain a menstrual and reproductive history including last menstrual period, regularity, duration and frequency, number of pads per day, postcoital or intermenstrual bleeding.
B. Evaluate for the presence of stress, exercise, weight changes, systemic diseases; particularly thyroid, renal, hepatic diseases, or coagulopathies. Assess the possibility of pregnancy and birth control.
C. Determine whether the patient is having ovulatory or anovulatory cycles. Ovulatory cycles are characterized by menstrual flows occurring at regular intervals preceded by molimina changes (breast tenderness or fullness, cramping, edema).
D. Further confirmation of ovulatory status may be obtained by basal body temperature graphs or a serum progesterone level greater than 5 ng/mL during the luteal phase.
E. If cycles are anovulatory, the patient has dysfunctional uterine bleeding. If bleeding occurs during ovulatory cycles, further evaluation is necessary to rule out uterine pathology, see "Evaluation of Abnormal Ovulatory Bleeding" below.

### Dysfunctional Uterine Bleeding
A. Defined as abnormal uterine bleeding with no organic or anatomic cause.
B. DUB is synonymous with anovulatory bleeding, and is a diagnosis of exclusion. Nonuterine causes must be excluded: Foreign bodies, trauma, inflammatory or neoplastic conditions of the vulva or vagina.
C. Most young, non-pregnant women with abnormal uterine bleeding are found to have dysfunctional uterine bleeding.
D. DUB occurs most often at the extremes of the reproductive years. Anovulatory cycles are common during the year following menarche and during perimenopause.
E. **Bleeding Patterns Associated with Chronic Anovulation:** Metrorrhagia, menometrorrhagia, polymenorrhea, oligomenorrhea, and amenorrhea. With chronic anovulation, extended episodes of copious bleeding are common and these are separated by long intervals with no bleeding.

### Management of Dysfunctional Uterine Bleeding
A. Rule out pregnancy with a blood beta HCG test or urine pregnancy test. Hemoglobin/hematocrit.
B. Sample the endometrium in older women with intermenstrual bleeding.
C. **Oral Contraceptive Therapy:** Prescribe a 21-day package of oral contraceptives containing 35 mcg of estrogen. Take one pill tid for 7 days. During the 7 days of therapy, bleeding should subside and following treatment, heavy flow will occur. After 7 days off the hormones, begin another 21-day package of oral contraceptives, taking one pill a day for 21 days.
D. **Cyclic Progesterone Therapy:**
   1. This therapy is useful for patients who do not desire contraception.
   2. Medroxyprogesterone acetate (Provera) 10 mg on days 1-10 each calender month.

This therapy results in a more regular bleeding pattern and prevents endometr carcinoma, but does not inhibit ovulation.

E. **Suppression of Severe Bleeding:**
1. Stop bleeding by giving medroxyprogesterone acetate (Provera) three 10 mg ta daily x 10 days.
2. Then allow regular bleeding by using cyclic progesterone therap Medroxyprogesterone acetate 10 mg tab daily on days 1-10 each calender month

F. **Other Agents:** Ferrous sulfate 325 mg PO tid-qid and docusate (Colace) 100 mg PO b

G. Long-term unopposed estrogen stimulation in anovulatory patients can result endometrial hyperplasia, which can progress to adenocarcinoma. In perimenopaus patients who have been anovulatory for an extended interval, the endometrium should sampled by biopsy or dilation and curettage.

## V. Evaluation Abnormal Ovulatory Bleeding

A. **Causes of Abnormal Bleeding with Ovulatory Cycles:** Anatomic abnormalitie coagulopathies (thrombocytopenia, leukemia, Von Willebrand's disease), renal or hepa disease.

B. **Anatomic and Inflammatory Causes of Bleeding:** Cervical polyps, endometrial polyp leiomyomas, cervical cancer, cervicitis, and endometritis.

C. **Evaluation of Uterine Causes of Abnormal Bleeding:**
1. Check platelet count, bleeding time, prothrombin time, and partial thromboplastin tim renal and hepatic diseases should be ruled out.
2. Cervical polyps are usually visible within the cervical os, and should be removed an evaluated pathologically at the time of examination.
3. **Dilation and Curettage or Hysteroscopy:** In the evaluation of menorrhagi hysteroscopy with selected biopsy or curettage is superior to blind dilation ar curettage.

## VI. Treatment of Abnormal Ovulatory Bleeding

A. Women with ovulatory cycles who have menorrhagia and whose endometrial samplin evaluation is normal, can be treated with hormones or surgery.

B. **Hormonal Treatment:** Medroxyprogesterone 10 mg tid from day 5 to day 25 of menstru cycle. Side effects: weight gain, abdominal bloating, mood changes, anxiety, an depression.

C. **Surgery:** Reserved for patients whose bleeding is refractory to medical therapy and wh do not desire fertility. Options include hysterectomy or endometrial ablation.

# Menopause

## Physiology of the Menopausal Transition
A. The average age of menopause is 49 years, with a range of 41-55. Menopause before age 41 is considered premature. Menopause is often diagnosed by irregular menses accompanied by hot flashes and an elevated follicle-stimulating hormone (FSH) level.
B. In the period before menopause, irregular menses begin to occur -- shortening, then lengthening, then cessation of menses.

## Climacteric Syndromes
A. **Hot Flushes:**
   1. Most frequently occurring climacteric symptom; episodic occurrence of sudden skin flushing and perspiration.
   2. Hot flush frequency varies from less than one daily to 3 episodes per hour; duration is usually 3-4 minutes.
B. **Lower Urinary Tract Atrophy:**
   1. After menopause, atrophic changes occur in the urethra and periurethra. Loss of pelvic tone and prolapse of the urethrovesicular junction occurs.
   2. Dysuria, urgency, frequency, suprapubic discomfort, stress, and urge incontinence often occur.
C. **Genital Changes:**
   1. Loss of vaginal elasticity is associated with shortening of the vaginal canal and loss of rugae. Epithelial thinning, friability, and alkaline pH predispose to bacterial vaginoses. Cervical atrophy and retraction of the cervix occurs; the squamocolumnar junction migrates upward.
   2. Atrophic vaginitis, dyspareunia, vaginal bleeding may occur.
D. **Osteoporosis:**
   1. Menopause is often associated with decreased bone mass and increased susceptibility to fractures; estrogen supplementation decreases hip and vertebral fracture risk by 50%.
   2. Hormone therapy initiated long after menopause may stabilize bone mass in women who have delayed using hormonal therapy.
E. **Cardiovascular System:** Estrogen replacement offers protection from cardiovascular disease in menopausal women.

## Laboratory Tests
A. Laboratory tests are sometimes indicated to exclude or confirm other diagnoses that may cause amenorrhea (thyroid disease, hyperprolactinemia, pregnancy).
B. Diagnosis of menopause may be confirmed by an FSH serum level >25 mIU/mL.
C. A lipid profile, Pap smear, mammogram, and stool guaiac are often indicated for routine screening.
D. Bone density measurements are not usually needed. For woman who are undecided about hormone replacement therapy, a bone density test (dual-energy x-ray absorptiometry) can provide information about the presence of osteoporosis, allowing the patient to make a more informed decision.

## Overview of Menopause Treatment
A. Treatment can be aimed at the symptom reduction or at the prevention of osteoporosis and cardiovascular disease. Women who are still menstruating are eligible for hormone replacement therapy (HRT) if perimenopausal and troubled by symptoms of menopause.
B. Skin thickness and collagen content are increased by estrogen replacement. Estrogen replacement reduces the risk of Alzheimer's disease and improves the cognitive scores of women with Alzheimer's disease.
C. Estrogen replacement should be continued indefinitely, because stopping therapy results in rapid loss of bone. There is no upper age limit for starting estrogen replacement.
D. **Breast Cancer Risk:** Breast cancer risk is not significantly increased by hormone therapy.

E. **Hormone Replacement Regimens:**
   1. Estrogen can be administered daily (continuous regimen) or with an interruption therapy at the end of each month (cyclic regimen). Continuous administration recommended since cyclic therapy provides no specific benefit. Patients may disl cyclic therapy because of resumption of symptoms in the medication-free peri continuing menses, and the increased complexity. While bleeding may often occ during the first 3-6 months of continuous therapy, amenorrhea is achieved in 96 women by 6-12 months.
   2. Progestins should be added to postmenopausal hormone regimens to preve endometrial hyperplasia and to minimize risk of uterine cancer. Progesterone is indicated for women without a uterus.

## V. Contraindications to the Use of Non-Contraceptive Estrogens
A. **Absolute:**
   1. Previously diagnosed or suspected breast cancer
   2. Previously diagnosed or suspected endometrial cancer
   3. Active liver disease
   4. Active thromboembolic disease
B. **Relative:**
   1. Recently active endometriosis or history of severe endometriosis
   2. History of thromboembolic disease related to estrogen
   3. Obesity
C. Therapy is not contraindicated in women with fibroids, hypertension, diabetes mellitus cigarette smoking.

## VI. Hormone Replacement Therapy Regimens
A. **Estrogen and Progestogen Therapy For Patients With Uterus Present:**
   1. **Continuous Therapy:**
      a. **Estrogen:** Conjugated estrogens (Premarin) 0.625 mg PO daily **OR** Estrac (Estrace) 1 mg daily **OR** Estradiol transdermal patch (Estraderm) 0.5 mg twi weekly.
      b. **Progesterone:** Medroxyprogesterone acetate (Provera), 2.5 mg daily, in continuous fashion.
      c. Some spotting and bleeding is expected initially, but amenorrhea occurs approximately 40 percent of women within three months.
      d. In women who continue to experience spotting or bleeding three months after t start of continuous estrogen replacement therapy, the dosage medroxyprogesterone should be increased to 5 mg daily. If bleeding continu after six months of the 5-mg dosage of medroxyprogesterone, the dosage can increased to 10 mg per day.
      e. Follow-up endometrial biopsies are not routinely necessary. If irregular bleedi persists after the establishment of amenorrhea, further diagnostic work-up w endometrial biopsy or dilatation and curettage may be necessary.
   2. **Cyclical Therapy:**
      a. Conjugated estrogens (Premarin), 0.625 mg, on days 1 through 25, a medroxyprogesterone (Provera) acetate, 5 to 10 mg, on days 12 through 25.
      b. An easier cyclic schedule is estrogen every day of month, with progesterone adde for first 2 weeks.
B. **Hormone Replacement Side Effects:**
   1. Gastrointestinal symptoms due to estrogen (nausea) may respond to a switch transdermal estrogen, 0.5 mg patch twice weekly.
   2. Progestogens are associated with bloating, cramping, irritability. Decreasing the da progestogen dosage or taking it on alternate days may help alleviate these symptom

## VII. Estrogen-Only Therapy
   1. **Uterus Present:** Estrogen-only therapy is not recommended if a uterus is present d to an increased risk of endometrial hyperplasia and neoplasia. However, estrog

only therapy may be used if unacceptable progestogen side effects occur. Pretreatment endometrial biopsy and yearly follow-up biopsies are necessary.

2. **Uterus Removed:** Continuous daily estrogen-only therapy is recommended if a uterus is not present.

3. Estrogen doses are the same as those given above.

## VIII. Additional Menopausal Therapy

### A. Calcium and Vitamin D:

1. Recommendations on treatment with calcium and vitamin D are equivocal. Nevertheless, calcium and vitamin D supplementation should accompany estrogen therapy for women with poor dietary intake.

2. Women should have a calcium intake of 1,000 mg/day, including dietary intake. Calcium supplementation is unnecessary for women with adequate nutrition.

3. Vitamin D at 400 IU per day is recommended for patients with limited exposure to sunshine who do not drink Vitamin D fortified milk. Vitamin D has no benefit for other women.

### B. Exercise: Healthy woman should exercise at least three times a week for 30 minutes, although no additional benefit has been proven in ambulatory women.

# *Urology*

## Impotence in Male Patients

I. **Pathophysiology**
  A. Erectile dysfunction is the inability to achieve and maintain an erection adequate for satisfactory sexual functioning. A single failed episode is usually an isolated incident, and normal functioning resumes in the majority of cases. Alcohol consumption is a common cause.
  B. The prevalence of erectile dysfunction increases with age. Prevalence is 5% at age 40, increasing to 15-25% at age 65 and older.
  C. **Physiology of Erection:**
    1. Parasympathetic input initiates erection by dilation of the helicine arteries of the penis and entrapment of blood.
    2. Flaccidity occurs after constriction of the helicine arteries is induced by sympathetic innervation.
  D. Most of the medical disorders associated with erectile dysfunction affect the arterial system.
  E. Peripheral neuropathy may impair neuronal innervation of the penis or the sensory afferents.
  F. Androgens play a role in regulating sexual interest, and may also play a role in erectile function.
  G. Psychological processes such as depression, anxiety, and relationship problems can impair erectile functioning.
  H. Etiologic factors for erectile disorders may be categorized as neurogenic, vasculogenic, or psychogenic, but commonly all three are contributing factors.
  I. Peyronie's Disease: Formation of plaques or thickening of the tunica albuginea, causes curvature of the penis; most commonly occurring in men older than 40, and causes painful erections, inability to achieve full erection, and difficulty in vaginal penetration.
  J. **Risk Factors:**
    1. Diabetes mellitus, hypertension, vascular disease, hypercholesterolemia, neurogenic disorders, depression, alcohol ingestion; renal failure. Vasectomy has not been associated with an increased risk of erectile dysfunction.
    2. Pelvic trauma or surgery. Acute or chronic prostatitis, radical prostatectomy and external radiotherapy.
  K. **Prevention of Impotence:** Specific antihypertensive, antidepressant, and antipsychotic drugs can be chosen to lessen the risk of erectile failure.

II. **Evaluation of Erectile Dysfunction**
  A. Determine frequency of sexual difficulties and duration of problem; gradual or sudden onset. Quality, frequency, and duration of erections; presence of nocturnal or morning erections; ability to achieve sexual satisfaction, and ejaculation with masturbation.
  B. Home and work environment stress, use of tobacco, alcohol, and recreational drugs.
  C. **Psychosocial Factors:** Performance anxiety, the nature of sexual relationships, current sexual techniques.
  D. **Medical Conditions:** Diabetes or hypertension; surgical procedures.
  E. **Medications:**
    1. Note when the medication was begun, for what condition, and at what dosage.
    2. **Drugs Associated with Erectile Dysfunction:**
      a. **Addictive Substances:** Alcohol, marijuana, cocaine, heroin, methadone, tobacco
      b. **Antihypertensive Agents:** Beta-blockers, calcium channel blockers, diuretics, especially thiazides
      c. **Psychotropic Agents:** Antidepressants, benzodiazepines, lithium preparations, monoamine oxidase inhibitors, phenothiazines, tranquilizers

      d. **Other Medications:** Antihyperlipidemic agents, chemotherapeutic agents, histamine-receptor antagonists

## III. Physical Examination
A. Assess general state of health and emotional affect. Observe the gait for neurologic defects. Assess male secondary sex characteristics; femoral and lower extremity pulses.
B. **Signs of a Hormonal Abnormalities:** Abnormal hair distribution, gynecomastia, testicular atrophy.
C. Determine volume, consistency, and symmetry of the testicles; presence of hydrocele or varicocele. Examine the penis for size, sensation, shape; palpate for plaques suggestive of Peyronie's disease. Examine prostate.
D. **Neurologic Examination:** Perianal sensation, anal sphincter tone, and bulbocavernosus reflex.

## IV. Laboratory Tests
A. CBC, free testosterone, and serum prolactin. If the free testosterone level is abnormal, test luteinizing hormone (LH) and follicle-stimulating hormone (FSH). Creatinine, lipid profile, fasting blood sugar, thyroid function studies. Urinalysis.
B. **Assessment of Penile Vascular Function:**
   1. **Nocturnal Penile Tumescence Monitoring:**
      a. Healthy men will normally have 3-5 rigid erections each night, each lasting 15 minutes to an hour.
      b. **Snap Gauge Testing:** A ring device composed of three bands of increasing strength, which will break under increasing erectile force.
      c. **RigiScan Monitor:** Portable unit that is attached to the thigh and provides a precise record of erectile function.
   2. If normal sleep erections occur, it is unlikely that organic disorders are causing erectile dysfunction. A normal NPT indicates that psychogenic factors may be the cause.
   3. **Doppler Ultrasonography:** Aids in visualizing blood flow through the arteries that supply the penis, and identifies venous leakage disorders. Vasoactive agents may be injected intracorporeally.
   4. **Cavernosography and Cavernosometry:** Can be used to quantitate the severity of venous insufficiency.

## V. Therapeutic Measures
A. **Psychotherapy and/or Behavioral Therapy:** May be useful for patients with a psychogenic cause, and may be helpful in patients with an organic cause in addition to other treatments.
B. **Medical Therapy:**
   1. Treat reversible medical problems that may contribute to erectile dysfunction. If the problem developed shortly after initiating a new medication, consider discontinuation or substitution of another medication.
   2. **Hypogonadism:**
      a. Androgen replacement therapy may be effective in cases of proven low testosterone level.
      b. Testosterone enanthate 300 mg IM every 3-4 weeks. Sublingual or oral testosterone are unreliable.
      c. Transcutaneous testosterone patches may be an alternative; apply patch to scrotum; one patch per day [6 mg/d, 4 mg/day patches].
   3. **Yohimbine HCI (Yocon):** A derivative of tree bark that has alpha-adrenergic antagonist effects; there is little scientific evidence to suggest that it is any more effective than placebo; may be tried in cases of psychogenic impotence.
C. **Intracavernosal Injection Therapy:**
   1. Injection of vasodilator substances into the corpora of the penis is highly effective.
   2. Papaverine, phentolamine, and prostaglandin E are used in combination; occasionally causes priapism.

3. **Triple-drug Combination:**
   Papaverine, 19 mg/mL
   Phentolamine, 0.59 mg/mL
   Alprostadil (Prostaglandin E1) 5.9 mcg/mL
   Usual staring dose, 0.25 cc
4. **Single-drug Therapy:** Alprostadil 10 pg (If erection is inadequate, dosage can be increased up to 40 mcg).

D. The mixture is administered into either of the corpora cavernosa, avoiding neurovascular structures. To avoid hematoma, pressure should be applied to the puncture site for 2-3 minutes.

E. Priapism is the most serious immediate complication. Phenylephrine, is effective; intracavernosal injection of 2 mL of 0.1 mg/mL of solution.

F. Penile vasodilators may be problematic in patients who cannot tolerate transient hypotension, or anticoagulant therapy.

**acuum Constriction Devices:**

A. Vacuum constriction devices are effective and have a low incidence of side effects.

B. The flaccid penis is introduced into a vacuum cylinder, suction applied, and a constriction ring is placed at the base of the penis when the vacuum chamber is removed. After intercourse, the constriction ring is removed, and detumescence follows. Occasional minor ecchymoses and hematomas.

C. **Vascular Surgery:** Surgery of the penile vascular system may be effective in patients who have venous or arterial disease.

D. **Penile Prostheses:** Penile prostheses are available for patients who fail or refuse other forms of therapy; semirigid, malleable, and inflatable devices are available.

# Acute Epididymorchitis

I. **Clinical Evaluation of Testicular Pain**
   A. **History:** Epididymorchitis is indicated by a unilateral painful testicle and history of unprotected intercourse, new sexual partner, urinary tract infection, dysuria, discharge Symptoms may occur following acute lifting or straining.
   B. **Physical:** Epididymis and testicle are painful, swollen, tender; scrotum may be erythematosus and warm with associated spermatic cord thickening or penile discharge.
   C. **Differential Diagnosis of Painful Scrotal Swelling:**
      1. Epididymitis, testicular torsion, testicular tumor, hernia.
      2. Torsion is characterized by sudden onset, age<20, elevated testicle, previous scrotal pain. The epididymis will be located anteriorly on either side and there is absence of evidence of urethritis and UTI.
      3. Epididymitis is favored by fever, evidence of urethritis or cystitis, and increased scrotal warmth.

II. **Laboratory Evaluaition of Epididymorochitis**
   A. Epididymorchitis is indicated by leukocytosis (left shift); UA shows pyuria and bacteriuria.
   B. Midstream urine culture will reveal gram negative bacilli. Chlamydia and Neisseria cultures should be taken, although they are often unsuccessful. Epididymal aspirate may be indicated if there is poor treatment response or recurrent infection.

III. **Common Pathogens**
   A. **In Younger Men:** Usually associated with sexually transmitted organisms such as Chlamydia, gonorrhea.
   B. **Older Men:** Usually associated with concomitant urinary tract infection or prostatitis; E. coli, proteus, Klebsiella, Enterobacter, Pseudomonas.

IV. **Treatment of Epididymorchitis**
   A. Bed rest during acute phase; scrotal elevation with athletic supporter; ice pack, analgesics, and antipyretics. Avoid sexual and physical activity.
   B. **Empiric Antibiotics:**
      1. **Epididymitis is Presumed to be a Sexually Transmitted Disease in Young Sexually Active Males:**
         a. -Ceftriaxone 250 mg IM x 1 dose **AND** Doxycycline 100 mg PO bid x 10 days
         b. Treat sexual partners.
      2. **Epididymitis if Presumed Urinary Tract Infection:**
         a. Non-sexually transmitted organisms should be treated empirically with antibiotics. Urine cultures should guide therapy when available.
         b. TMP/SMX DS bid for 10 days or ofloxacin (Floxin) 300 mg PO bid for 10 days.
      3. **Alternative that will Cover Sexually Transmitted and Urinary Tract Infections:**
         a. Ofloxacin (Floxin) 300 mg po bid for 10 days **AND** Doxycycline 100 gm PO bid x 10 days.
         b. Treat sexual partners.
   C. **Acute Urethral Syndrome:**
      1. Ceftriaxone (Rocephin) 250 mg IM or 1 dose and doxycycline 100 mg PO bid x 7 days **OR**
      2. Ofloxacin (Floxin) 400 mg PO x 1 dose and doxycycline 100 mg PO bid x 7 days.

# Prostatitis and Other Disorders of the Prostate

### Classification of Prostatitis:
A. Acute bacterial prostatitis
B. Chronic bacterial prostatitis (with or without infected prostatic calculi)
C. Non-bacterial prostatitis
D. Prostatodynia

### I. Acute Bacterial Prostatitis
A. The least common type of prostatitis. Characterized by abrupt onset of fever and chills accompanied by symptoms of urinary tract infection or obstruction, low back or perineal pain, malaise, arthralgia, and myalgias. The patient appears acutely ill and is usually a younger man. Urinary retention may develop.
B. Prostate is enlarged, indurated, very tender and warm. Prostate massage is contraindicated because it is painful and may cause bacterial dissemination.
C. **Laboratory Evaluation:**
   1. **Mid-stream Urine (MSU):** Urine reveals WBC's. Culture reveals gram-negative organisms such as E coli or other Enterobacteriaceae.
   2. Nosocomial infections may be caused by Pseudomonas, enterococci, S. aureus.
   3. Imaging study may be needed in severely ill patients to rule out an abscess and need for surgery.
D. **Treatment:** Requires 14-28 days of antibiotic treatment. A fluoroquinolone, such as ofloxacin is the drug of choice.
   Ofloxacin (Floxin) 400 mg PO/IV q12h.
   Ciprofloxacin (Cipro) 500 mg PO bid.
   Norfloxacin (Noroxin) 400 mg PO bid.
   Trimethoprim/SMX (TMP-SMX, Septra) 160/800 mg (1 DS tab) PO bid.
   Doxycycline (Vibramycin) is the drug of choice for Chlamydia infection; 100 mg PO bid.

E. **Extremely Ill Septic Patients with High Fever:**
   1. Hospitalization for bed rest, hydration, analgesics, antipyretics, stool softeners.
   2. Ampicillin 1 gm IV q4-6h **AND** Gentamicin or tobramycin - loading dose of 100-120 mg IV (1.5-2 mg/kg); then 80 mg IV q8h (2-5 mg/kg/d) **OR**
   3. Ciprofloxacin (Cipro) 200 mg IV q12h.

### II. Chronic Bacterial Prostatitis
A. Characterized by recurrent urinary tract infections, typically in older patients. May be associated with perineal, low back or suprapubic pain, testicular, penile pain or discomfort, voiding dysfunction, post-ejaculatory pain, intermittent hematospermia. Chills and fever are not present. Often symptoms are subtle or absent.
B. **Exam:** Prostate is usually normal, occasionally enlarged and tender.
C. **Laboratory Evaluation:**
   1. Urinalysis and culture usually shows low grade bacteriuria (E. coli or other Gram negative Enterobacteriaceae, E. faecalis, S. aureus, coagulase negative staph).
   2. Express prostatic secretions onto a slide; place a coverslip, and examine under a microscope. More than 10-15 WBC's per high-power field is typical of prostatitis.
D. **Long-term Treatment (12-16 weeks):** Infection may be difficult to eradicate.
   1. A fluoroquinolone is the drug of choice.
   2. Ofloxacin (Floxin) 200-400 mg PO/IV Q12H.
   3. Ciprofloxacin (Cipro) 250-500 mg PO bid.
   4. Trimethoprim/sulfamethoxazole (TMP-SMZ, Septra) 160/800 mg (1 DS tab) PO bid.
   5. Doxycycline (Vibramycin) 100 mg PO bid.
   6. **Consider Suppression if Recurrent Symptomatic Infections:** Fluoroquinolone, TMP/SMX, erythromycin, or doxycycline.

## IV. Chronic Nonbacterial Prostatitis

A. The most common type of prostatitis is nonbacterial. Eight times more frequent tha[n] bacterial prostatitis. Characterized by perineal, suprapubic or low back pain; irritativ[e] or obstructive urinary symptoms; symptoms and exam are similar to chronic bacteri[al] prostatitis but with no recurrent UTI history.

B. Cultures are sterile and show no bacteria or uropathogens. Microscopic examinatic[n] reveals 10-15 WBC's per high-power field, indicating inflammation.

C. **Treatment (2-4 week trial of antibiotics):**
   1. Minocycline (Minocin), Doxycycline, or Erythromycin may relieve symptoms.
   2. Irritative symptoms may respond to nonsteroidal anti-inflammatory agents, musc[le] relaxants, anticholinergics, hot sitz baths, normal sexual activity, and regular mi[ld] exercise.
   3. Avoid spicy foods and excessive caffeine and alcohol.
   4. Serial prostatic massage may be helpful if congested prostate.
   5. Usually self-limited. In persistent cases rule out carcinoma of the prostate, urinar[y] bladder, and interstitial cystitis.

## V. Prostatodynia

A. Symptoms are similar to prostatitis, but no objective findings suggesting that symptom[s] arise in the prostate gland are present. Age range between 22-56 years.

B. Symptoms include a wide variety of pain or discomfort in the perineum, groin, testicle[s] the penis and urethra, or other prostatitis symptoms. Irritative or obstructive voidin[g] symptoms are predominant. No recurrent UTI history. Stress and emotional problem[s] are contributing factors.

C. Tender musculature may be found on rectal examination.

D. **Urine:** Normal (no WBC or bacteria), sterile for uropathogens. No inflammation in th[e] prostate gland and no urinary tract infection.

E. **Testing:** Formal urodynamic testing may detect uncoordinated voiding patterns. Cys[-] toscopic examination.

F. **Treatment:**
   1. Alpha-adrenergic blocking agents (terazosin 1-5 mg/day, and doxazosin 1-4 mg qc[ ] can be used to relax the bladder neck sphincter. Muscle-relaxing agents such a[s] diazepam (Valium 2-10 mg tid) may provide relief.
   2. Nonsteroidal anti-inflammatory agents, sitz baths, normal sexual activity, avoidanc[e] of stress, spicy foods, caffeine, and alcohol may be beneficial. Prostatic massag[e] is of no value.

# *Psychiatry*

## Depression

I. **Evaluation of Depression**
   A. Evaluation should identify characteristics of depressed mood, history of past episodes of depression.
   B. **Associated Symptoms:** Insomnia, weight loss, symptoms of anxiety, and vague somatic complaints. Inquire about hallucinations, paranoid thoughts, suicidal ideation and planning.
   C. **Substance Dependence or Abuse**: If alcohol or drug abuse is present, treatment should be provided.
   D. **Bipolar (manic-depressive) Disorder:** Characterized by alternating manic and depressive episodes. Before prescribing antidepressants, determine whether the patient has ever experienced a decreased need for sleep, racing thoughts, distractibility (symptoms of mania) because antidepressants may trigger manic episodes.
   E. **Core Depressive Symptoms:**
      **Sleep:** Insomnia or hypersomnia
      **Interest:** Loss of interest or pleasure in activities (anhedonia)
      **Guilt:** Feelings of excessive guilt, worthlessness, hopelessness
      **Energy:** Fatigue or loss of energy
      **Concentration:** Diminished ability to concentrate
      **Appetite:** Decreased or increased appetite, weight loss or gain
      **Psychomotor:** Psychomotor retardation or agitation
      **Suicidality:** Suicidal thoughts or ideation, suicide plan or attempt
   F. **Family History:** Depression or other mood disorders, suicide, drug or alcohol abuse.

II. **DSM-IV Diagnostic Criteria for Depression**
   A. At least five of the following symptoms must be present, including at least one of the first two for at least two weeks:
      1. Loss of interest or pleasure in usual activities
      2. Depressed mood
      3. Significant increase or decrease in weight or appetite
      4. Insomnia or hypersomnia
      5. Psychomotor agitation or retardation
      6. Fatigue or loss of energy
      7. Feelings of worthlessness or excessive or inappropriate guilt
      8. Diminished ability to think or concentrate; indecisiveness
      9. Recurrent thoughts of death or suicidal, with or without a specific plan.
   B. Symptoms must not be the result of an organic factor or a normal reaction to the death of a loved one. Delusions or hallucinations should not be present for 2 weeks in the absence of prominent mood symptoms.

III. **Medical Conditions Mimicking Depression**
   A. **Drug Intoxication:** Alcohol, barbiturates, cocaine, opiates.
   B. **Metabolic Disorders:** Diabetes, electrolyte imbalances (sodium, potassium, calcium); pernicious anemia, uremia.
   C. **Medications:** Amphetamines, antihypertensives, corticosteroids, oral contraceptives.
   D. **Neoplasms:** Brain tumors, occult lesions, pancreatic carcinoma.
   E. **Endocrinologic Disorders:** Adrenal disease, thyroid disease.
   F. **Neurologic:** Multiple sclerosis, normal-pressure hydrocephalus, Parkinson's disease, dementia, subdural hematoma.
   G. **Infections or Immunologic Disorders:** Hepatitis, HIV infection, mononucleosis, syphilis, tuberculosis, lupus erythematosus.

IV. **Laboratory Evaluation of Depression**
   A. CBC and blood chemistry series to look for anemia or hepatic or renal abnormalities.
   B. Thyroid-stimulating hormone level may be indicated to screen for hypothyroidism.
   C. If significant unexplained weight loss, obtain occult blood testing, mammography, or a Papanicolaou test to rule out malignancies in reproductive age females; pregnancy should be excluded.
   D. Obtain a baseline electrocardiogram if preexisting cardiac disease or elderly.

V. **Management of Depression**
   A. **Choosing an Antidepressant:**
      1. Consider the pattern of depression, patient's age, suicide potential, sleep habits, and any coexistent diseases or drug treatments.
      2. Determine if patient (or first-degree relative) has had a previous beneficial response to a given medication.
      3. Choose a sedating drug for patients with insomnia, or an SSRI over a tricyclic for a patient with anticholinergic sensitivity or orthostatic hypotension.
   B. All antidepressant drugs are equally effective, but have different side-effect profiles.
   C. Therapeutic response may not occur for 4-8 weeks at adequate dosage.
   D. Blood plasma levels should be measured to check compliance and therapeutic levels.
   E. **Anxiety:** If depression and anxiety are present, sedating antidepressants will help to control anxiety and depression.
   F. SSRIs, with their comparatively benign side-effect profile, allow once-daily dosing. SSRIs also present less danger from overdose because they lack the cardiovascular toxicity of the tricyclics.
   G. Electroconvulsive therapy is a safe and effective treatment; especially if high risk for suicide and insufficient time for a trial of medication.

| Drug | Recommended Dosage | Comments |
|---|---|---|
| **SECONDARY AMINE TRICYCLIC ANTIDEPRESSANTS** | | |
| **Class as a whole:** Side effects include anticholinergic effects (dry mouth, blurred vision, constipation) and alpha-blocking effects (sedation, orthostatic hypotension). Drug hangover is common but subsides within 7-10 d. May lower seizure threshold. Can induce cardiac rhythmic disturbances by slowing conduction. | | |
| Amoxapine (Asendin, generics) | Initial dosage 50 mg bid-tid, increase to 200-300 mg/d as tolerated. Max 600 mg/d. Elderly patients: reduce by 50% [25, 50, 100, 150 mg] | Risk of seizures in overdose. May be associated with tardive dyskinesia, neuroleptic malignant syndrome, galactorrhea. |
| Desipramine (Norpramin, generics) | 100-200 mg/d, gradually increasing to 300 mg/d as tolerated. Geriatric: 25-100 mg/d. [10, 25, 50, 75, 100, 150 mg] | No sedation; may have stimulant effect; best taken in morning to avoid insomnia. |
| Nortriptyline (Pamelor) | 25 mg tid-qid, max 150 mg/d. Elderly: 30-50 mg/d  [10, 25, 50, 75 mg] | Sedating |
| **TERTIARY AMINE TRICYCLICS** | | |
| **Class as a whole:** Anticholinergic effects and orthostatic hypotension may be more severe than with secondary amine tricyclics. | | |

| Amitriptyline (Elavil, generics) | 75 mg/d in divided doses, increasing to 150-200 mg/d. May be given in single bedtime dose. Elderly: 10 mg tid [10, 25, 50, 75, 100, 150 mg] | Sedative effect precedes antidepressant effect. High anticholinergic activity. |
|---|---|---|
| Clomipramine (Anafranil) | 25 mg/d, increasing gradually to 100 mg/d; max 250 mg/d; may be given once qhs [25, 50, 75 mg]. | Relatively high sedation, anticholinergic activity, and seizure risk. |
| Protriptyline (Vivactil) | 5-10 mg PO tid-qid; 15-60 mg/d [5, 10 mg] | Useful in atypical depression. |
| Doxepin (Sinequan, generics) | 50-75 mg/d, increasing up to 150-300 mg/d as needed [10, 25, 50, 75, 100, 150 mg] | Sedating. Also indicated for anxiety. Contraindicated in patients with glaucoma or urinary retention. |
| Imipramine (Tofranil, generics) | 75 mg/d in a single dose qhs, increasing to 150 mg/d; 300 mg/d. Elderly: 30-40 mg/d [10, 25, 50 mg] | High sedation and anticholinergic activity. Use caution in cardiovascular disease. |
| **TETRACYCLIC** | | |
| Maprotiline (Ludiomil, generics) | 75 mg/d initially, increasing gradually in 25-mg increments, max 225 mg/d. 75 mg/d [25, 50, 75 mg] | Sedating. Risk of seizures. May induce maculopapular rash in 3-10%. |
| **SELECTIVE SEROTONIN REUPTAKE INHIBITORS (SSRIs)** | | |
| Fluoxetine (Prozac) | 10-20 mg/d initially, taken in AM; max of 80 mg/d in 2 divided doses (morning and noon). Lower dosage for elderly patients or those with renal/hepatic impairment, or multiple medications [20 mg] | Longest half-life of any antidepressant (2-9 d). Discontinue 2 mo before a planned pregnancy. Common side effects: Anxiety, insomnia, agitation, nausea, anorgasmia, erectile dysfunction, headache, rash, anorexia, activation of mania. Also used for obsessive-compulsive disorder. |
| Paroxetine (Paxil) | 20 mg/d initially, given in AM; increase in 10-mg/d increments as needed to max of 50 mg/d. Elderly 10-40 mg/d [20, 30 mg] | Side effects: Headache, nausea, somnolence, dizziness, insomnia, abnormal ejaculation, anxiety, diarrhea, dry mouth. |
| Sertraline (Zoloft) | 50 mg/d, increasing as needed to max of 200 mg/d [50, 100 mg] | Side effects: Insomnia, agitation, dry mouth, headache, nausea, anorexia, sexual dysfunction. |
| Nefazodone (Serzone) | Start at 100 mg PO bid, increase to 150-300 mg PO bid as needed [100, 150, 200, 250 mg]. | Side effects: Headache, somnolence, dry mouth, blurred vision. Postural hypotension, impotence. |

| PHENYLETHYLAMINE | | |
|---|---|---|
| Venlafaxine (Effexor) | 75 mg/d in 2-3 divided doses with food; increase to 225 mg/d as needed. Taper when discontinuing [25, 37.5, 50, 75, 100 mg]. | Inhibits norepinephrine and serotonin; considered a "SSRI-plus". May be more effective than SSRIs. Side effects: hypertension, nausea, somnolence, insomnia, dizziness, abnormal ejaculation, headache, dry mouth, anxiety. |
| AMINOKETONE | | |
| Bupropion (Wellbutrin) | 100 mg bid; after at least 3 d, increase to 100 mg tid as needed [75, 100 mg] | Side effects: Agitation, dry mouth, insomnia, headache, nausea, vomiting, constipation, tremor. Good choice for patients with sexual side effects from other agents. |
| TRIAZOLOPYRIDINE | | |
| Trazodone (Desyrel, generics) | 150 mg/d, increasing by 50 mg/d every 3-4 d 400 mg/d in divided doses [50, 100, 150, 300 mg] | Rarely associated with priapism. Older, impotent men may benefit from the occasional propensity of trazodone to augment erectile function. Orthostatic hypotension in elderly. Sedating. |

H. **Tricyclic Agents:**
   1. Side effects (especially hangover) are worst during the first month of therapy, and usually become more tolerable afterward.
   2. Early in the course a patient may sleep better, but patients rarely describe affective improvement until at least 3-4 weeks.
   3. Prescribe only minimum quantities because of the overdose potential.

I. **Serotoninergic Agents:**
   1. Commonly used as first-line agents as well as secondary choices for patients whose depression does not respond to tricyclics. Although many patients take SSRIs with no adverse consequences, the most frequent side effects are insomnia, agitation, and sexual dysfunction. The SSRIs tend to be nonsedating, making them a good choice for patients who are lethargic or withdrawn.
   2. Sertraline or paroxetine are less energizing than fluoxetine, so these agents are better choices in depression combined with anxiety. Fluoxetine can have a stimulant effect on some patients, especially early in treatment. Sertraline and paroxetine are regarded as easier for some patients to tolerate.

J. **Antidepressant-Related Sexual Dysfunction:**
   1. Antidepressants cause sexual impairment in 20-30%, especially the selective serotonin reuptake inhibitors (SSRIs), though any antidepressant may be implicated.
   2. Impairments include erectile dysfunction or delayed ejaculation in men, inadequate lubrication or anorgasmia in women, and decreased libido in either sex.
   3. Bupropion (Wellbutrin) is a mildly stimulating antidepressant, and may be useful in patients who have had sexual impairment from other drugs. The short half-life of bupropion makes multiple daily doses necessary, complicating compliance.

K. **Monoamine Oxidase Inhibitors:**
   1. Contraindications discourage common use.
   2. Requires a tyramine-free diet. Risk of hypertensive crisis.
   3. **Drug Interactions** with epinephrine, meperidine (Demerol), and fluoxetine can be life-threatening.

L. **Follow-up Care for Patients with Depression:** Maintenance therapy is usually provided for up to one year followed by tapering of medication. For patients with repeated episodes of major depressive disorder, lifetime maintenance of drug therapy may be necessary.

# nxiety Disorders

### Generalized Anxiety Disorder
A. Generalized anxiety disorder (GAD) is the most common of the anxiety disorders.
B. It is defined as unrealistic or excessive anxiety and worry about two or more life circumstances for at least six months.
C. Chronic worry is a prominent feature of GAD as opposed to the intermittent terror that characterizes panic disorder.
D. Other features of GAD include insomnia, irritability, trembling, muscle aches, muscle twitches, clammy hands, dry mouth, and heightened startle reflex. Patients may also report palpitations, dizziness, difficulty breathing, urinary frequency, dysphagia, lightheadedness, abdominal pain, and diarrhea.
E. Patients may report that they "can't stop worrying," which may revolve around valid life concerns including money, job, marriage, health, and safety of children.
F. The presence of depression should be assessed because 30-50% of patients with anxiety disorders will also meet criteria for major depression.
G. Drugs and alcohol may contribute to anxiety disorders. Substance abuse is also a complication of anxiety disorders because patients often use alcohol to self-medicate anxiety.

### Panic Disorder
A. Patients with panic disorder report discrete periods of intense terror and doom that are almost intolerable.
B. Panic attacks are characterized by some or all of the following:
    1. Dizziness, unsteadiness, light-headedness, or faintness
    2. Chest pain or discomfort
    3. Chills or hot flushes
    4. Choking sensations
    5. Derealization or depersonalization
    6. Fear of dying
    7. Fear of losing control or "going crazy"
    8. Nausea or other abdominal distress
    9. Palpitations, pounding, or racing heart
    10. Sweating
    11. Trembling or shaking
    12. Paresthesias
    13. Smothering sensations or shortness of breath
C. The panic episode generally resolves within 10-30 minutes. This first panic attack generally is precipitated by a recent major life event. Agoraphobia may develop, with anticipatory anxiety and phobic avoidance.
D. Panic disorder is diagnosed only when panic attacks are unexpected and cannot be attributed to other conditions.
E. Panic attacks may occur in posttraumatic stress disorder and social phobia, and in some medical disorders, notably hyperthyroidism and pheochromocytoma.
F. Many patients have mixed anxiety and depression. Changes in appetite, weight, sleep, fatigability, irritability, concentration and sexual desire should be sought.

### Medical Disorders Causing Panic-like Symptoms
A. **Hyperthyroidism** may cause anxiety, tachycardia, palpitations, sweating, dyspnea.
B. **Hypoglycemia** can produce panic-like symptoms, but is uncommon in nondiabetics.
C. **Cardiac rhythm disturbances** and mitral valve prolapse may cause panic symptoms.
D. **Substance abuse or dependence** with withdrawal symptoms may resemble panic disorder.
E. **Pharmacologic Causes of Anxiety:**
    1. Analgesics (salicylate intoxication/NSAIDs)
    2. Sedatives (antihistamine intoxication/withdrawal)
    3. Sympathomimetics (phenylpropanolamine)

4. Psychotropics (akathisia), stimulants, selective serotonin reuptake inhibitors.
5. Large doses of caffeine may produce anxiety, insomnia.
6. Cocaine, amphetamines, theophylline, beta agonists, over-the-counter decongestants, steroids, and marijuana can precipitate panic attacks or anxiety.

IV. **Laboratory Evaluation of Anxiety Disorders**
   A. Chemistry profile (glucose, calcium and phosphate); electrocardiogram, TSH, and free T4.
   B. **Special Tests:** Urine drug screen, cortisol, urinary catecholamine levels.

V. **Treatment of Anxiety Disorders**
   A. Develop an empathetic---not sympathetic--response to the patient's story, and demonstrate an understanding by paraphrasing what the patient has told you.
   B. Treatment of anxiety disorders has two stages--stabilization and management. Stabilization usually includes drug therapy. In the management phase, patients learn to control their fears and their reactions to them.
   C. **Nondrug Approaches to Anxiety:**
      1. Discontinue caffeinated beverages and avoid excess alcohol.
      2. Exercise daily and get adequate sleep, with the use of medication if necessary.
      3. **Cognitive Psychotherapy:** Identify and correct the patient's perceptions of the harmful consequences of anxiety symptoms. Relaxation exercises and biofeedback are also useful.

VI. **Drug Therapy Anxiety Disorders**
   A. Tricyclic antidepressants SSRIs and are widely used to treat panic disorder and generalized anxiety disorder. Their onset of action is much slower than that of the benzodiazepines, but they have no addictive potential and may be more effective. An antidepressant is the agent of choice when elements of depression are present in addition to anxiety.
   B. Sedating antidepressants often have an early effect of promoting better sleep, although 2-3 weeks may pass before a patient experiences an antidepressant benefit. Better sleep usually brings some relief from symptoms, and the patient's functional level begins to improve almost immediately.
   C. Anxious patients benefit from the sedating effects of imipramine (Tofranil), amitriptyline (Elavil), and doxepin (Sinequan). The daily dosage should be at least 50-100 mg, and plasma levels should be 125 mg per mL, or greater.
   D. Desipramine (Norpramin) is useful if sedation is not desired. Desipramine has been found to be as effective as imipramine and has fewer anticholinergic and sedative effects. Most of the selective serotonin reuptake inhibitors (fluoxetine [Prozac]) will worsen panic symptoms before relieving them.
   E. **Benzodiazepines:**
      1. Tolerance to their sedative effects develops, but not to their antianxiety properties.
      2. Patients with depression and anxiety should not receive anxiolytics because benzodiazepines may worsen depression.
      3. A withdrawal syndrome occurs in 70 percent of patients which includes anxiety, dysphoria, sleep and perceptual disturbances, appetite suppression, and weight loss. Slow tapering of benzodiazepines is crucial.
      4. Benzodiazepines should be used for patients with panic disorder because of the need for more rapid relief.
      5. Alprazolam (Xanax), diazepam (Valium), lorazepam (Ativan), and clonazepam (Klonopin) are effective for panic disorder because of quick onset of action.
      6. Benzodiazepine can be used in conjunction with an antidepressant. Therapy starts with alprazolam and an SSRI or tricyclic antidepressant. The alprazolam is then tapered after 2-3 weeks, when the antidepressant has started to take effect.
      7. Clonazepam (Klonopin) has onset at about one hour and lasts about 8-12 hours, making it the better choice for a low-dose bid or tid regimen and around-the-clock symptom control for frequent or unpredictable panic.

8. Diazepam (Valium) remains a good choice in either situational or generalized anxiety.
9. Properly used, benzodiazepines can almost always relieve anxiety if given in adequate doses. Dependency becomes a problem with use daily for more than two or three weeks. If a patient cannot function without pharmacologic relief from stressful situations, some degree of dependency may be manageable.

| Drug | Dosage | Comments |
|---|---|---|
| **BENZODIAZEPINES** | | |
| Alprazolam (Xanax) | 0.25-0.5 mg tid; increase by 1 mg/d at 3-4 day intervals. 0.75-4 mg/d | Intermediate onset. Least sedating drug in class. Strong potential for physiologic dependence. |
| Chlordiazepoxide (Librium, generics) | 5 mg tid; 15-100 mg/d | Intermediate onset. Also indicated in acute alcohol withdrawal. |
| Clonazepam (Klonopin) | 0.5 mg tid; 1.5-20 mg/d | Intermediate onset. Has anti-panic effects. Long half-life; much less severe withdrawal. |
| Clorazepate (Tranxene, generics) | 7.5 mg bid; 15-60 mg/d | Fast onset. |
| Diazepam (Valium, generics) | 2 mg bid; 4-40 mg/d | Very fast onset. |
| Halazepam (Paxipam) | 20 mg tid; 60-160 mg/d | Intermediate to slow onset. |
| Lorazepam (Ativan, generics) | 1 mg bid; 2-6 mg/d | Intermediate onset. |
| Oxazepam (Serax, generics) | 10 mg tid; 30-120 mg/d | Intermediate to slow onset. |
| Prazepam (Centrax) | 10 mg bid; 20-60 mg/d | Slow onset. |
| **MISCELLANEOUS** | | |
| Buspirone (BuSpar) | 10 mg bid; max 40 mg/d; increase to 10 mg tid prn | Antidepressant; nonaddicting, nonsedating. For generalized anxiety and social phobia, not for prn usage; requires 2-3 wk to become effective. |
| Doxepin (Sinequan, generics) | 75-150 mg/d, max 300 mg/d | A tricyclic antidepressant with antianxiety effects. |
| Propranolol | 20 mg bid | Generalized anxiety disorder, social phobia |

| Atenolol (Tenormin) | 50 mg qd | Social phobia |
|---|---|---|

F. **Buspirone:**
  1. Buspirone is a nonbenzodiazepine anxiolytic. It is most effective for generaliz[ed] anxiety in patients who have never taken benzodiazepines. Buspirone takes long[er] to work than benzodiazepines--about two weeks and it may not improve sleep[.] is unlikely to cause dependence, and it has some antidepressant effects. Usua[lly] ineffective in panic disorder.
  2. Combined benzodiazepine-buspirone therapy may be used for anxiety, with subs[e]quent tapering of the benzodiazepine.

G. **Beta Blockers:**
  1. Propranolol HCL (Inderal) and other beta-blockers are very effective [in] performance anxiety or social phobia, but they can provoke depression.
  2. A beta blocker one hour before an anticipated stressful event can markedly redu[ce] performance anxiety.
  3. Dosage can be quite low (Inderal [propranolol] 10 mg qid), or it can be used as p[rn] only before anticipated stress.

## VII. Psychotherapeutic Techniques

| Therapy type | Description | Example |
|---|---|---|
| Supportive | Focuses on strengths, accepts limitations of unfavorable conditions, provides guidance. | Patient with low self-esteem [is] praised for strengths and encouraged to focus on them[.] |
| Cognitive | Cognitive therapy instructs in ways to separate realistic thoughts from unrealistic thoughts; deep breathing and relaxation exercises. | Patient records events in ord[er] that cause stress; moves up the list as sessions progress. |
| Behavioral Biofeedback | Monitoring of visceral or muscle functions with relaxation techniques. | Patient uses physiologic monitor as a focus for controlling anxiety. |
| In vivo exposure | Patient progressively experiences feared situation; relaxation techniques and slow breathing exercises. | Patient who is fearful in socia[l] groups experiences social encounters with first one, the[n] increasing numbers. |
| Systematic desensitization | Patients learn to relax in the presence of stimuli that produce anxiety. | Patient with fear of needles is[s] trained to relax while envisioning contact with need[le] and syringe. |

# nsomnia

### Causes of Insomnia

A. **Transient Insomnia** is the most common form of insomnia, and is due to factors such as stress, attempting to sleep in a new place, changes in time zones, and changing bedtimes due to shift work.

B. **Chronic Insomnia** is most commonly caused by dysthymia, depression, anxiety disorders and substance abuse.

C. **Medical Disorders** can cause insomnia resulting from pain, nausea, dyspnea, gastroesophageal reflux, sleep apnea, and myoclonus.

D. **Drugs Associated with Insomnia:** Antihypertensives, caffeine, diuretics, oral contraceptives, phenytoin, selective serotonin reuptake inhibitors, protriptyline (Vivactil), corticosteroids, stimulants, theophylline, thyroid hormone.

### Psychiatric Illnesses Associated with Insomnia

A. **Depression** is the most common psychiatric diagnosis associated with insomnia. Depression often develops in of patients with chronic insomnia.

B. **Chronic Anxiety:** 10% of chronic insomnia is secondary to chronic anxiety or panic disorder. Chronic use of long-acting benzodiazepines may be indicated for these patients.

### Behavioral Treatment of Insomnia

A. The patient should go to bed only when sleepy.

B. Use the bed for sleeping only. Reading, watching TV, or eating in bed should be discouraged.

C. If unable to sleep, get up and move to another room. Stay up until sleepy, then return to bed.

D. Set the alarm and get up at the same time every morning, regardless of how well you slept during the night. The patient should develop a consistent sleep-wake rhythm.

E. Naps and caffeinated beverages during the day should be eliminated.

### V.  Pharmacotherapy of Insomnia

A. Hypnotics should be given for only a limited time, usually less than two to four weeks.

B. Sedating antidepressants, such as doxepin (Sinequan), trazodone (Desyrel), or amitriptyline (Elavil), can also be used to treat insomnia, and are especially useful when the patient has underlying depression.

C. If benzodiazepines are used, patients with difficulty in falling asleep will benefit from short-acting agent like zolpidem. Patients who have early morning insomnia will benefit from a longer acting agent such as estazolam.

D. **Effects of Benzodiazepines on Sleep:** Slow wave sleep and rapid eye movement (REM) sleep are reduced; REM sleep latency is prolonged. REM sleep and slow wave sleep have important functions in learning, memory, and adaptation to stress.

E. **Long-acting Benzodiazepines:** Generally are not suitable for insomnia, but may be useful in treating insomnia that is associated with chronic anxiety.

F. **Zolpidem (Ambien):**
1. A nonbenzodiazepine, although it acts on the benzodiazepine receptor. It has a minimal effect on sleep stages and is reputed to promote a more natural sleep; zolpidem has a rapid onset of action; lacks withdrawal effects, no rebound insomnia and little or no tolerance.
2. No impairment of performance is evident during the day.

## Sedative-Hypnotic Benzodiazepines

| Drug | Dose | Half-life (hours) | Potency | Daytime drowsiness | Side Effects | Positive Effects |
|---|---|---|---|---|---|---|
| Flurazepam (Dalmane) | 15-30 mg [15, 30 mg] | 48-120 | +++ | 24% | Daytime drowsiness, confusion; sedative interactions. Intermediate- to long-acting. | Suppresses daytime anxiety; relative lack of withdrawal. |
| Triazolam (Halcion) | 0.125-0.5 mg [0.125, 0.25 mg] | 2-6 | +++ | 14% | Amnesia; confusion; rebound insomnia; Abrupt onset and offset of action. Side effects can be unpredictable. | Short duration results in less daytime sedation and in less accumulation in elderly patients. |
| Temazepam (Restoril) | 15-30 mg [7.5, 15, 30 mg] | 8-20 | + | 17% | Rebound insomnia. Has slowest onset (30-60 min) | Daytime alertness after use. Short- to intermediate-acting. |
| Estazolam (ProSom) | 1-2 mg | 8-24 | +++ | 20% | REM sleep suppression; withdrawal symptoms | Short- to intermediate-acting. Daytime sedation occurs. |
| Quazepam (Doral) | 15 mg | 48-120 | +++ | 12% | Same side effects as flurazepam | Lack of withdrawal effects; daytime alertness after use. Intermediate- to long-acting. |
| Zolpidem (Ambien) | 10 mg; begin with 5 mg in elderly | 3-8 | +++ | 5% | Potential for idiosyncratic side effects | Daytime alertness after use; lack of withdrawal; usually no suppression of REM. Very short-acting. |

# Smoking Cessation Therapy

## Clinical Evaluation of Nicotine Withdrawal

A. **Symptoms:** Anxiety, craving, insomnia, depression, difficulty concentrating; hunger, impatience, insomnia, irritability, and restlessness.

B. If the patient has failed to quit smoking because of these withdrawal symptoms, then pharmacotherapy is indicated.

## II. Pharmacologic Aids

A. **Transdermal Nicotine:**

1. **First-Line Therapy:** Transdermal nicotine more reliably decreases craving than nicotine gum or clonidine. Compliance is higher than with nicotine gum or clonidine.

2. **Side Effects:** Pruritus, erythema, and burning at application site.

3. **Nicotine Toxicity:** Smoking while using patch or using multiple patches may cause toxicity manifest by nausea, dizziness, hypotension, convulsions, angina, and respiratory failure.

4. **Dosages:**
   -Transderm Nicotine (Nicoderm, Habitrol) initial dose 21 mg/day for up to 6 weeks, then 14 mg/day for 2 weeks, then 7 mg/d for 2 weeks; max 8 weeks [7, 14, 21 mg/patch].
   -Transderm Nicotine (ProStep) initial dose 22 mg/day for 4-8 weeks then 11 mg/day x 2-4 weeks; max 12 weeks [11, 22 mg/patch].

B. **Nicotine Polacrilex (Nicorette):**

1. Must be chewed slowly over 30-45 minutes whenever urge to smoke occurs. 10-12 pieces/d; max 30 pieces per day [2 mg, 96 pieces/box].

2. May be appropriate for those smokers who have a strong desire for an oral nicotine method; has a bitter taste; longer durations of therapy (more than 3 months) appear to be helpful.

3. Nicotine polacrilex may be added to transdermal nicotine because the combination produces a greater suppression of withdrawal symptoms than does transdermal nicotine alone.

C. **Clonidine:** Has not shown significant efficacy, and is not approved for smoking cessation.

## III. Smoking Cessation Behavioral Therapy

A. **Set a Stop Date:** Share the date with supportive family and friends, and write the date in a written contract.

B. **Keep a smoking journal** of daily smoking habits for several days including time of day and the circumstances or situations associated with smoking.

C. **Identify Alternative Behaviors:** Chew sugarless gum to keep mouth busy; keep hands busy with other activities when experiencing the urge to smoke.

D. **Establish a Reward System:** Put all the money that previously would have been spent on cigarettes in a jar, and decide on a reward on which to spend the money. Mark smoke-free days on a calendar. Increase contact with friends who have quit.

E. **Behavioral therapy** in addition to nicotine therapy increases quit rates by a factor of 1.6-1.8. Behavioral therapy may be especially indicated in smokers with a history of psychiatric, alcohol and drug problems.

## V. Failed Attempts with Transdermal Nicotine

A. If dependent smokers fail to quit with transdermal nicotine therapy, determine the causes of the relapse and screen for psychiatric, alcohol and drug problems. Determine whether the patient experience relapse because of withdrawal (intense craving) or some nonwithdrawal event (receipt of bad news).

B. If the relapse was due to withdrawal, consider adding nicotine polacrilex to transdermal nicotine or consider using higher doses of transdermal nicotine (two patches, a 21-mg patch and a 14-mg patch).

C. If the relapse was due to a non-withdrawal event, then group behavioral therapy in addition to transdermal nicotine therapy is recommended.

# Alcohol and Drug Abuse

**I. Clinical Evaluation**

    A. Determine the amount and frequency of alcohol use and other drug use in the past month, week, and day. Ask about previous abuse of alcohol or other drugs.

    B. If the patient currently uses alcohol, determine how many days per week, on average, the patient drinks, how much alcohol is usually consumed and whether the patient ever consumes five or more drinks at a time.

    C. Effects of the alcohol or drug use on the patient's life: Problems with health, family, job or financial status or with the legal system.

    D. History of blackouts or motor vehicle crashes. Affect on family members or friends of the patient's drinking or drug use.

    E. **Drug Abuse History:**

        1. Have you felt that you ought to cut down on your drinking or drug use?

        2. Have people criticized your drinking or drug use?

        3. Have you ever had a drink or used drugs first thing in the morning (eye opener) to steady your nerves, get rid of a hangover or get the day started?

    F. **Psychologic/behavioral Manifestations of Drug Disorders:** Agitation, irritability, dysphoria, mood swings, hostility, violence, generalized anxiety, panic attacks, depression, psychosis.

    G. **Family Manifestations of Drug Disorders:** Family dysfunction, marital problems, behavioral problems, abuse and violence.

    H. **Social Manifestations of Drug Disorders:** Alienation and loss of friends, gravitation toward others with similar lifestyle.

    I. **Work/school Manifestations of Drug Disorders:** Decline in performance, frequent job changes, frequent absences (especially on Mondays), requests for work excuses.

    J. **Legal Manifestations of Drug Disorders:** Arrests for disturbing the peace or driving while intoxicated, stealing, drug dealing, prostitution.

    K. **Financial Manifestations of Drug Disorders:** Borrowing or owing money, selling of possessions.

**II. Physical Examination**

    A. Alcohol abuse may be signaled by labile or refractory hypertension, or by mild upper abdominal tenderness.

    B. Cocaine snorting may be identified by damaged nasal mucosa. Injection drug abuse may be evident by hypodermic marks.

    C. **Eye Examination:**

        1. Nystagmus is often seen in abusers of sedatives or hypnotics or cannabis.

        2. Mydriasis (dilated pupils) is often seen in persons under the influence of stimulants or hallucinogens or in withdrawal from opiates.

        3. Miosis (pin-point pupils) is a classic sign of opioid effect.

**III. Laboratory Testing:**

    A. Impaired liver function and hematologic disorders should be sought with LFT's and CBC.

    B. Spot checks of urine or breath may reveal the presence of undisclosed drugs or alcohol.

**IV. Treatment of Alcohol and Drug Abuse**

    A. **Outpatient Detoxification:**

        1. Many drug-dependent patients can safely undergo withdrawal as outpatients.

        2. To qualify for outpatient detoxification, the patient must clearly agree to abstain from using any mood-altering agent, and must also agree to participate in a treatment program. The patient also needs a sober and responsible family member or friend who will monitor the patient and assist with medications.

        3. Evaluate the patient daily until he has started a treatment rehabilitation program and the risk of withdrawal is minimal. This interval may range from three days for alcohol abuse to 10 days for methamphetamines, opioids and cocaine.

  B. **Inpatient Detoxification:**
1. Hospital treatment is more likely to be needed for withdrawal from sedative drugs, such as alcohol, barbiturates and benzodiazepines. Withdrawal from these drugs can be life-threatening. Hospital treatment is also indicated for patients who have very high tolerance, or who have developed seizures, delirium or psychosis during a previous withdrawal.
2. Medical indications for inpatient therapy include a history of recent head trauma, jaundice, liver failure, electrolyte imbalance, pneumonia, sepsis, dehydration, arrhythmias, angina, ischemic heart disease, hypertension, severe respiratory disease, and age greater than 65 years.
3. Hospitalization is usually not indicated for opiate detoxification, which is best accomplished through an outpatient methadone program.

## V. Pharmacotherapy of Alcohol and Drug Rehabilitation
  A. **Alcohol and Sedative Withdrawal:**
1. Detoxification may be necessary after prolonged use or when there are signs of abuse or addiction (extended periods of intoxication, multiple psychoactive prescriptions, unsuccessful attempts to discontinue).
2. Sedatives associated with withdrawal include alcohol, benzodiazepines, barbiturates, and chloral hydrate.
3. **Withdrawal Syndrome:**
   a. **Minor (stage 1) withdrawal:** Restlessness, anxiety, insomnia, agitation and tremor; tachycardia, low-grade fever, diaphoresis, and elevated blood pressure.
   b. **Major (stage 2) Withdrawal:** Includes signs associated with minor withdrawal plus visual or auditory hallucinations. Whole-body tremor, pulse exceeding 100 per minute, diastolic pressure >100 mm Hg, pronounced diaphoresis, and vomiting may also be present.
   c. **Delirium Tremens (stage 3):** Temperature exceeding 37.8°C (100°F); disorientation to time, place and person, global confusion; inability to recognize familiar objects or persons.
4. Alcohol withdrawal seizures may occur 12-48 hours after the last drink; seizures from barbiturates usually occur within 72 hours after the last use.
5. Withdrawal from long-acting benzodiazepines may not occur for up to a week or more.
6. **Detoxification of Patients Dependent on Alcohol and Sedatives:**
   a. Detoxification involves step-wise dose reduction or substitution of a cross-tolerant, longer-acting substance (such as diazepam) that has less risk of severe withdrawal symptoms.
   b. The cross-tolerated drug is given in gradually tapering doses. The treatment should relieve symptoms, and prevent stage 2 or 3 withdrawal and seizures.
   c. The triazolobenzodiazepines, triazolam [Halcion] and alprazolam [Xanax], may not be completely cross-tolerant with other sedatives. Patients dependent on alprazolam require a particularly gradual tapering from their initial dosage.

  B. **Stimulant Withdrawal:**
1. Stimulant Withdrawal Syndrome: Depression, hypersomnia, fatigue, headache, irritability, and poor concentration. Prolonged and intense drug craving, paranoia and acute psychosis may occur.
2. Usually no treatment other than support is needed for the initial phase of stimulant withdrawal.
3. Haloperidol (Haldol) and thioridazine (Mellaril) are the drugs of choice for treating symptoms of paranoid psychosis.
4. Antidepressants such as desipramine (Norpramin) or fluoxetine (Prozac) may be useful in treating depressive symptoms.
5. Panic attacks may be treated with an antidepressant or a benzodiazepine.

  C. **Opiate Withdrawal:**
1. **Grading of Opiate Withdrawal:**
   a. **Grade 0 Opiate Withdrawal:** Drug craving, anxiety, and intense drug-seeking behavior

b. **Grade 1 Opiate Withdrawal:** Yawning, sweating, lacrimation, and rhinorrhea
c. **Grade 2 Opiate Withdrawal:** Mydriasis (dilated pupils), goose-flesh, muscle twitching, and anorexia
d. **Grade 3 Opiate Withdrawal:** Insomnia, increased pulse, respiratory rate and blood pressure, abdominal cramps, vomiting, diarrhea, and weakness.

2. Methadone is the preferred drug in the treatment of opiate withdrawal. Methadone is a synthetic opioid agonist with a sufficiently long duration of action so that it may be given once a day. Usually patients receive the daily dose in a clinic.

3. If methadone is not available, some symptomatic relief may be obtained with clonidine (Catapres). Clonidine is a centrally acting alpha-adrenergic agonist that suppresses restlessness, lacrimation, rhinorrhea, and sweating. Many physicians prefer the use of clonidine patches. Treatment with clonidine may also include promethazine (Phenergan) or hydroxyzine (Atarax, Vistaril) for nausea and vomiting, loperamide (Imodium), for diarrhea, and methocarbamol (Robaxin) for muscle cramps and joint pain.

4. Levomethadyl (Orlaam) also produces stable opioid effects when ingested orally for the treatment of heroin addiction. Its long duration of action permits dosing three times a week.

5. Clinics licensed to treat narcotic addiction are the only facilities legally allowed to pre-scribe and dispense methadone or levomethadyl. Methadone can be administered to hospitalized patients.

D. **12-Step Programs:**

1. After detoxification, almost every addict should enroll in counseling plus attendance at a self-help group. Alcoholics Anonymous (AA), Narcotics Anonymous (NA), Cocaine Anonymous (CA) use the same 12-step model.

# Anorexia Nervosa and Bulimia Nervosa

I. **Anorexia Nervosa**
   A. Anorexia nervosa primarily affects young women, with onset generally between the ages of 12 and 25 years. Perfectionist lifestyle and performance-related stress predispose to anorexia nervosa.
   B. Prevalence is between 2-5% among adolescent and young adult women. Untreated, mortality can approach 20%.
   C. **Family History:** There is an increased incidence of affective disorders; one or both parents is usually obese; occurs most often in patients of upper-middle socioeconomic status.
   D. **Signs and Symptoms of Anorexia Nervosa:**
      1. Amenorrhea, emesis, aversion to meats; cold sensitivity, compulsive behavior; overactivity, hoarding of food, overexercise (often to exhaustion).
      2. Patients often have a distorted body image, and a need to maintain an ultra-thin silhouette; the patient sees herself as obese regardless of the degree of emaciation.
      3. "Paradoxic Satiety" -- the patients reports no hunger when fasting and may feel satiated when she does not eat.
      4. Secondary sexual characteristics are suppressed or even reversed; emaciated body habitus, hair loss, multiple upper respiratory infections and constipation are common.
   E. **Diagnostic Criteria for Anorexia Nervosa:**
      1. Refusal to maintain body weight over a minimal, normal weight for age and height. Weight loss leading to body weight 15% below expected; or failure to make expected weight gain during period of growth, leading to body weight 15% below expected.
      2. Intense fear of gaining weight or of becoming fat, even though underweight.
      3. Disturbance in body image; believes self to be "too fat" even when obviously underweight.
      4. Absence of at least three consecutive menstrual cycles in female patients.
   F. **Laboratory Findings in Anorexia:** Decreased serum albumin, globulin, calcium, potassium and sodium; anemia, leukopenia.

II. **Bulimia Nervosa**
   A. Patients may be given a diagnosis of both anorexia nervosa and bulimia nervosa if they are underweight and binge on a regular basis.
   B. Prevalence is 5% in adolescent females and 0.5% in adolescent males. Mortality is rare and is usually related to unintended aspiration of vomitus.
   C. **Signs and Symptoms of Bulimia:**
      1. Emesis, binge eating, diuretic abuse, high-fiber diet, laxative abuse, post-binge depression
      2. Dental etching on inner aspects of teeth; scarring of dorsum of one hand (acid injury during emesis), nail discoloration; abdominal distention, parotid gland enlargement, abdominal striae.
      3. Weight fluctuations of 10 or more pounds in a one-month period may occur.
   D. **Diagnostic Criteria for Bulimia Nervosa:**
      1. Recurrent binge eating episodes (rapid consumption of large amounts of food in a short period of time).
      2. Feeling of lack of control over eating behavior during eating binges.
      3. Regularly engages in either self-induced vomiting, use of laxatives or diuretics, strict dieting or fasting, or vigorous exercise in order to prevent weight gain.
      4. A minimum of 2 binge eating episodes a week for at least 3 months.
      5. Persistent preoccupation with body shape and weight.
   E. **Laboratory Findings in Bulimia:** Hypokalemia and metabolic alkalosis. Elevated serum cholecystokinin level may be present.
   F. **Differential Diagnosis:** Rule out other disorders that may mimic bulimia such as gastrointestinal carcinoma, migraine, mesenteric artery syndrome (obstruction of the duodenum by superior mesenteric artery after rapid weight loss).

III. **Medical Complications of Anorexia and Bulimia Nervosa**
   A. **Cardiovascular:**
      1. Accounts for the majority of clinical pathology seen in anorexia nervosa and bulimia nervosa.
      2. 60-80% present with postural hypotension; 90% have bradycardia. Occasionally atrial flutter or fibrillation, premature ventricular contractions, right bundle branch block are seen.
   B. **Electrolyte Imbalances:**
      1. Electrolyte imbalances occur in 60% of bulimic patients and 40% of anorectic patients. Critical hypokalemia is seen in 25% of all bulimic patients and in most end-stage anorectic patients.
      2. Chloride deficiency develops in about 20% of bulimic patients, and is associated with hypochloremic metabolic alkalosis. Metabolic acidosis occurs in anorexia as a result of starvation ketosis.
   C. **Endocrine:**
      1. Decreased fertility and amenorrhea are associated with low levels of luteinizing hormone (LH) and follicle stimulating hormone (FSH).
      2. Thyroid hormone levels are decreased in 10% of patients with anorexia.
      3. Hypocalcemia is associated with osteoporosis.
   D. **Gastrointestinal:**
      1. Decreased gastrointestinal activity, constipation and obstipation occur.
      2. Tearing, fissuring and scaring of the anus may be seen in bulimia due to the practice of inserting well-soaped fingers into the rectum to induce a bowel movement.
   E. **Other Complications:**
      1. Intense intolerance to cold temperatures.
      2. Increased susceptibility to viral and bacterial infections.
      3. Chronic herpes simplex blisters; chronic dull headaches.
   F. **Iatrogenic Complications:**
      1. Overfeeding abdominal distention.
      2. Excess fluid replacement for dehydration can precipitate cardiac insufficiency.
   G. **Medical Indications for Hospitalization:** Severe emaciation, hypokalemia, hyponatremia, abnormal electrocardiogram. Recurrent use of syrup of ipecac can be toxic to the muscular system, and may require admission. Severe depression usually requires hospitalization because of the risk of suicide. Failure of outpatient treatment, or recurrence of an eating disorder may require hospitalization.

IV. **Treatment of Eating Disorders**
   A. A nutritionist can assist with meal planning.
   B. **Psychotherapy:** Goal-directed, short-term cognitive or behavioral therapy, either individual or group, or long-term, insight-oriented psychotherapy can be effective. Family therapy is useful. Occupational therapy helps to develop productive activities that reduce obsession with body image.
   C. Nursing staff should provide a social structure, monitor weight, food consumption, activity, and provide a sympathetic outlet for the patient's conflicts.
   D. **Nutritional Rehabilitation and Weight Restoration:**
      1. Target weight can be selected based on premorbid weight and by using reference charts such as standard pediatric growth curves.
      2. Outpatients should be seen every 1-2 weeks to monitor weight gain. Check serum electrolyte levels twice weekly.
      3. Limiting the patient's participation in physical activities or exercise may be necessary.
      4. Weight gain of 1-2 lb weekly should be expected. Addition of liquid nutritional supplements is often useful.
   E. **Pharmacotherapy of Anorexia Nervosa:**
      1. Two-thirds of patients with anorexia or bulimia nervosa have a history of a major depressive episode.
      2. Amitriptyline (Elavil) may be effective in promoting weight gain. An electrocardiogram should be obtained. Initial dosage is 50 mg at bedtime, then increased by 50-mg

increments until 150 mg or 3.25 mg/kg/d is attained. Improvement is not usually observed until after 3-4 weeks.

3. Cyproheptadine (Periactin) is an anti-histamine with serotonin-blocking activity; may be effective for promoting weight gain. Mild antidepressant effect. Dosage: 16-32 mg per day.

4. Fluoxetine (Prozac) has been used successfully in the therapy of anorexia and bulimia; 10-20 mg PO qAM.

F. **Pharmacotherapy of Bulimia Nervosa:**

1. Antidepressant medications are useful in the treatment of bulimia nervosa, whether or not accompanied by major depression, because they reduce the symptoms of binging and purging.

2. Imipramine (Tofranil) or desipramine (Norpramin) are useful at low dosage (50 mg per day). Slowly increase dose by 50-mg increments every 3-4 days, until a daily dose of 150 mg; the serum drug concentration should be measured after 1 week.

# Preventive Care

**Routine Preventive Care Protocol in Adults:**

| Years of age | 18 | 25 | 30 | 35 | 40 | 45 | 50 | 55 | 60 | 65 | 70 | 75 > |
|---|---|---|---|---|---|---|---|---|---|---|---|---|
| Cholesterol | | | -----------------------------Every 5 years ------------- | | | | | | | | | |
| Hearing | | | | | | | | | | -- Periodically -- | | |
| Mammography | | | | | - q1-2 years (women) | | | | | | | |
| Pap smear | | ------------------- Every 1 to 3 years (women) ----------------------- | | | | | | | | | | |
| Sigmoidoscopy | | | | | | | ---------- Every 3 to 5 years ----- | | | | | |
| Stool occult blood | | | | | | | --------------- Yearly ---------------- | | | | | |
| Urinalysis | | | | | | | | | | ------Periodically ------ | | |
| Vision/glaucoma | | | | | | --------------- Every 2 years ------------------- | | | | | | |
| Breast Exam | | --------- Every 1 to 3 years (women) ----------------------------------------- | | | | | | | | | | |
| Examinations for cancer: for persons > 40 years: thyroid, mouth, skin, ovaries, testicles, lymph nodes, rectum; for men >50 years: prostate | | ------Every 3 years ------------- Yearly ------------------------------- | | | | | | | | | | |
| Tetanus-diphtheria | | ------------------------------ Every 10 years ------------------------------- | | | | | | | | | | |
| Pneumococcal | | | | | | | | -------------------------------------------------Every 6 years------------- | | | | |
| Influenza | | | | | | | | | | --- Yearly -------- | | |

Upper age limits should be individualized
Pneumococcal revaccination is recommended every six years.
Daily multivitamins with folic acid are recommended for women who might become pregnant.

**Preventive Care Not Routinely Recommended for Asymptomatic, Normal-Risk Persons:**
  Chest radiograph
  Electrocardiogram
  Exercise stress testing
  Multiple blood chemistry screens
  Sputum cytology testing
  Multivitamin prophylaxis

# Order Form

## Books from Current Clinical Strategies Publishing:

| | | |
|---|---|---|
| Current Clinical Strategies, Practice Parameters in Medicine, Primary Care, Family Practice, and Gynecology | #___ x | $18.75 |
| Current Clinical Strategies, PEDIATRIC Drug Reference | #___ x | $8.75 |
| Handbook of Anesthesiology, Mark Ezekiel, MD | #___ x | $8.75 |
| Manual of HIV/AIDS Therapy, Laurence Peiperl, MD | #___ x | $8.75 |
| Current Clinical Strategies, Medicine, Paul D. Chan, MD. New 1996 edition | #___ x | $8.75 |
| Current Clinical Strategies, Physician's Drug Resource (Adult dosages) | #___ x | $8.75 |
| Current Clinical Strategies, Surgery | #___ x | $8.75 |
| Current Clinical Strategies, Gynecology & Obstetrics, New 1995 edition | #___ x | $10.75 |
| Current Clinical Strategies, Pediatrics, New 1995 edition | #___ x | $8.75 |
| Family Medicine: Pediatrics, Medicine, Gynecology, Obstetrics, New Edition | #___ x | $26.25 |
| Diagnostic History and Physical Examination in Medicine | #___ x | $8.75 |
| Outpatient and Primary Care Medicine | #___ x | $8.75 |
| Critical Care Medicine, New Edition | #___ x | $12.75 |
| Psychiatry | #___ x | $8.75 |
| Handbook of Psychiatric Drug Therapy | #___ x | $8.75 |

**Our Books are available in Computer and Apple Newton Formats.** Call for more information.

| | |
|---|---|
| **Shipping and Handling, add $6.00 per Order** | $ _____ |
| **Total** | $ _____ |

Enclose the cover of your old edition, and take 20% off your order when you purchase the new edition.

**Please Complete Reverse Side**

**Order by Phone:** 714-348-8404. **FAX:** 714-348-8405. There will be an additional $3.00 COD charge for phone orders. An invoice will be sent with your order.

Order by Mail: Send order and check payable to:

Current Clinical Strategies Publishing
27071 Cabot Road, Suite 126
Laguna Hills, California 92653

Return Address (Print Clearly):

_____

_____

_____

_____

Phone Number: (_____)_____

Prices are in US dollars. Other countries, send equivalent amount in foreign check plus a $5.00 conversion charge. Prices and availability subject to change without notice.

Comments:

We appreciate your comments about our books.

Suggested additions or corrections:

_____

_____

_____

_____

_____

_____

_____

# Order Form

**Books from Current Clinical Strategies Publishing:**

| | | |
|---|---|---|
| Current Clinical Strategies, Practice Parameters in Medicine, Primary Care, Family Practice, and Gynecology | #____ x | $18.75 |
| Current Clinical Strategies, PEDIATRIC Drug Reference | #____ x | $8.75 |
| Handbook of Anesthesiology, Mark Ezekiel, MD | #____ x | $8.75 |
| Manual of HIV/AIDS Therapy, Laurence Peiperl, MD | #____ x | $8.75 |
| Current Clinical Strategies, Medicine, Paul D. Chan, MD. New 1996 edition | #____ x | $8.75 |
| Current Clinical Strategies, Physician's Drug Resource (Adult dosages) | #____ x | $8.75 |
| Current Clinical Strategies, Surgery | #____ x | $8.75 |
| Current Clinical Strategies, Gynecology & Obstetrics, New 1995 edition | #____ x | $10.75 |
| Current Clinical Strategies, Pediatrics, New 1995 edition | #____ x | $8.75 |
| Family Medicine: Pediatrics, Medicine, Gynecology, Obstetrics, New Edition | #____ x | $26.25 |
| Diagnostic History and Physical Examination in Medicine | #____ x | $8.75 |
| Outpatient and Primary Care Medicine | #____ x | $8.75 |
| Critical Care Medicine, New Edition | #____ x | $12.75 |
| Psychiatry | #____ x | $8.75 |
| Handbook of Psychiatric Drug Therapy | #____ x | $8.75 |

**Our Books are available in Computer and Apple Newton Formats.** Call for more information.

| | |
|---|---|
| **Shipping and Handling, add $6.00 per Order** | $ _____ |
| **Total** | $ _____ |

Enclose the cover of your old edition, and take 20% off your order when you purchase the new edition.

**Please Complete Reverse Side**

**Order by Phone:** 714-348-8404. **FAX:** 714-348-8405. There will be an additional $3.00 COD charge for phone orders. An invoice will be sent with your order.

Order by Mail: Send order and check payable to:

Current Clinical Strategies Publishing
27071 Cabot Road, Suite 126
Laguna Hills, California 92653

Return Address (Print Clearly):

_____

_____

_____

_____

Phone Number: (_____)_____

Prices are in US dollars. Other countries, send equivalent amount in foreign check plus a $5.00 conversion charge. Prices and availability subject to change without notice.

Comments:

We appreciate your comments about our books.

Suggested additions or corrections:

_____

_____

_____

_____

_____

_____

_____

# Order Form

## Books from Current Clinical Strategies Publishing:

| | | |
|---|---|---|
| Current Clinical Strategies, Practice Parameters in Medicine, Primary Care, Family Practice, and Gynecology | #____ x | $18.75 |
| Current Clinical Strategies, PEDIATRIC Drug Reference | #____ x | $8.75 |
| Handbook of Anesthesiology, Mark Ezekiel, MD | #____ x | $8.75 |
| Manual of HIV/AIDS Therapy, Laurence Peiperl, MD | #____ x | $8.75 |
| Current Clinical Strategies, Medicine, Paul D. Chan, MD. New 1996 edition | #____ x | $8.75 |
| Current Clinical Strategies, Physician's Drug Resource (Adult dosages) | #____ x | $8.75 |
| Current Clinical Strategies, Surgery | #____ x | $8.75 |
| Current Clinical Strategies, Gynecology & Obstetrics, New 1995 edition | #____ x | $10.75 |
| Current Clinical Strategies, Pediatrics, New 1995 edition | #____ x | $8.75 |
| Family Medicine: Pediatrics, Medicine, Gynecology, Obstetrics, New Edition | #____ x | $26.25 |
| Diagnostic History and Physical Examination in Medicine | #____ x | $8.75 |
| Outpatient and Primary Care Medicine | #____ x | $8.75 |
| Critical Care Medicine, New Edition | #____ x | $12.75 |
| Psychiatry | #____ x | $8.75 |
| Handbook of Psychiatric Drug Therapy | #____ x | $8.75 |

**Our Books are available in Computer and Apple Newton Formats.** Call for more information.

| | |
|---|---|
| **Shipping and Handling, add $6.00 per Order** | $ _____ |
| **Total** | $ _____ |

Enclose the cover of your old edition, and take 20% off your order when you purchase the new edition.

**Please Complete Reverse Side**

**Order by Phone:** 714-348-8404. **FAX:** 714-348-8405. There will be an additional $3.00 COD charge for phone orders. An invoice will be sent with your order.

Order by Mail:  Send order and check payable to:

Current Clinical Strategies Publishing
27071 Cabot Road, Suite 126
Laguna Hills, California 92653

Return Address (Print Clearly):

_____

_____

_____

_____

Phone Number:  (_____)_____

Prices are in US dollars. Other countries, send equivalent amount in foreign check plus a $5.00 conversion charge.  Prices and availability subject to change without notice.

Comments:

We appreciate your comments about our books.

Suggested additions or corrections: